Where to Wear

2001 Edition

The "Black Book" for New York Shopping

Fairchild Melhado & Clason
New York

This book would not have been possible without the help of Peter Melhado, our editor, whose thought and guidance are reflected on every page.

First Printing

Clason, Dina & Melhado, Jill Fairchild
Where to Wear, 2001 Edition
ISBN 1-930189-14-1

Copyright © 2000 Fairchild Melhado & Clason
Manhattan Maps © 2000 Eureka Cartography
Produced by Graphic Image, Inc.

All rights reserved.
Every effort has been made to ensure the accuracy of the information in this book. However, the publisher and authors make no claims to, and accept no liability for, any misrepresentations contained herein. No part of this book may be used or reproduced in any manner whatsoever without written permission except in the case of brief quotations embodied in critical articles and reviews.
For information, contact *Where to Wear* at:
666 Fifth Avenue
PMB 377
New York, NY 10103
TEL 212-969-0138
TOLL-FREE 1-877-714-SHOP (7467)
FAX 212-315-1534
E-MAIL wheretowear@aol.com

Printed and bound in Canada.

Table of Contents

Manhattan Overview Map	v
Introduction	vii
Where to Wear 2001	1
Best Picks	3
Shhh! (Best-Kept Secret)	3
Top-of-the-Line Men's Shirt Labels	3
Shop Talk	4
Best Dressing Rooms	4
Designers: Rising Stars	4
Where Designers Shop	5
Affordable Chic	5
Best Designer Sample Sales	5
Where Hollywood Shops	6
Penny Wise	6
Notable 2000 Closings	6
"Must-Haves"	7
Unique Interiors	7
Fashion Scoop	8
What's In	9
In-Store Restaurants	10
Restaurants	11
Size Conversion Chart	16
Coming Soon—Fall 2000/Spring 2001	17
Alphabetical Store Directory	23
Stores by Category	217
Stores by Neighborhood	241
Manhattan Walking Maps	242
Repairs and Services	279
Dry Cleaners	281
Mending and Alterations	282
Custom Design Tailors	283
Shoe Repairs	283
Leather Repairs (Handbags & Luggage)	284
Trimmings (Ribbons, Buttons, Feathers and Odd & Ends)	284
Thrift Shops	285
Health and Beauty	287

Barbers	289
Haircuts—Unisex	289
Haircuts—Children	290
Hair Salons	290
Hair Removal	292
Beauty Treatments	293
Manicure	294
Day Spas—Women	295
Day Spas—Men	297
Fitness Studios	297
Pilates/Mat Classes	299
Yoga	300
Massage Therapists	300
Tanning Salons	301
Bridal Consultants	301
Make-up Artists	301
Personal Shoppers	302
Glossary of Terms	303
Website Shopping Directory	307
Note from the Authors	315

Introduction

Dear Reader,

Welcome to the second edition of *Where To Wear*, Manhattan's premier shopping guide for apparel and accessories for men, women, and children. *Where To Wear 2001* is bigger and better than ever with an additional 200 store listings, a website shopping directory, a guide to in-store restaurants and other convenient lunch spots, a glossary of fashion terms, as well as detailed maps to point you in the right direction. In short, it's packed with all the information you'll need to look and feel great.

So who needs *W2W*? Everyone who either loves or hates to shop (and those in between, too.) Shop 'til you drop types will discover dozens of rare finds—new, off-the-beaten-path stores carrying unusual and exciting items. Death before shopping types will still have to shop occasionally (sorry), but now they can save some time and energy armed with their fact-filled, easy-to-use copy of *Where To Wear*, the most comprehensive (but concise) guide to apparel and accessory shopping in New York City. Well, actually, Manhattan. Surely there is exquisite raiment fit for a queen in the outer boroughs, but we simply ran out of room. *Where To Wear* has entries for over 1,000 stores, and we've been to every one to discover what's fabulous, functional, frumpy, fearless, and frightful in the city's stores this season. Stores are listed alphabetically, and with each entry you'll find a detailed description of what the store and its merchandise are all about, its target customer and a brief fashion overview. In every case, we've tried to provide the reader with both information and opinion. Fashion is a subjective thing, so you'll also get our opinions about style, color, cut, fabric and overall fashion sense.

Occasionally we have something sweet (or not so sweet) to say about the staff's helpfulness or attitude. Also included are the address, phone number, and store hours. *Where To Wear*'s index groups these shops by category and location with a quick address finder, so you'll have all the possible destinations at your fingertips. In addition, *Where To Wear* features a list of New York services, from beauty treatments, fitness studios, and spas to couture dry cleaners and shoe repair shops. The beginning of the guide includes several fun, new lists, such as "Shhh! (Best-Kept Secrets)," "Unique Interiors," "Designers: Rising Stars" and "Best Designer Sample Sales." These lists are based on our personal opinions and will no doubt change with the constant openings and closings of New York's retail shops.

Throughout the book, we've noted stores and services that merit special consideration with a ★.

You'll also find fashion maxims and anecdotes. Do you know who said "Thank god we're living in a country where the sky's the limit, the stores are open late and you can shop in bed thanks to television"? See page 17.

So let's get going. Dedicated and reluctant shoppers alike should keep *Where To Wear* in their handbag, briefcase, or backpack (if you happen to need one, see page 226). *Where To Wear* is your passport to convenient, smart, fun shopping! And who knows, you might even make next year's best-dressed list.

—Dina Clason and Jill Fairchild Melhado

Dina Clason graduated from Tufts University. She was a retail executive at Tiffany & Co. and Barneys New York for 11 years. Prior to that she owned Il Papiro in Washington, D.C.

Jill Fairchild Melhado, daughter of fashion world legend and "W" magazine founder John Fairchild, worked as an intern at Glamour *magazine,* GQ *and* Vogue*. Ms. Fairchild has worked for Ailes Communications, a television production company, and in the late 80's she founded and ran her own accessory company.*

Where to Wear 2001

Best Picks
Shhh! (Best-Kept Secret)
Top-of-the-line Men's Shirt Labels
Shop Talk
Best Dressing Rooms
Designers: Rising Stars
Where Designers Shop
Affordable Chic
Best Designer Sample Sales
Where Hollywood Shops
Penny Wise
Notable 2000 Closings
"Must-Haves"
Unique Interiors
Fashion Scoop
What's In
In-Store Restaurants
Restaurants
Size Conversion Chart

"New clothes are a bad investment." —*Winona Ryder*

"We used to build civilizations.
Now we build shopping malls." —*Bill Bryson*

"Bargain: something you can't use at a price you can't resist."
—*Franklin P. Jones*

Where to Wear 2001

Best Picks

Anya Hindmarch
Bergdorf Goodman
Bond 07
Brooks Brothers
Calypso St. Barths
Canyon Beachwear
Carolina Herrera
Coach
DieselStyleLab
Entre Nous
Eugenia Kim
Faconnable
Gamine
The Gap
Hennes & Mauritz
Jamin Puech
Jimmy Choo
Kirna Zabête
Keni Valenti
La Petite Coquette
Language
Liz Lange Maternity
Longchamp
Manolo Blahnik
Mark Schwartz
Martier
Michael Kors
Nancy Geist
Nanette Lepore
Nicole Miller
Paul Stuart
Plein Sud
Resurrection Vintage
Sacco
Shoofly
Sigerson Morrison
Takashimaya
Tracy Feith
Via Spiga
Wolford

Shhh! (Best-Kept Secret)

Bu and the Duck
Deco Jewels
Do Kham
Fisch for the Hip
Hello Sari
Himaya
Vilebrequin
Jay Kos
Jimin Lee/Translatio
Jutta Neumann
Keni Valenti
Lilliput/SoHo Kids
Liza Bruce
Lucy Barnes
Makie
Michelle Roth & Co.
Mom's Night Out/One
Night Out
Soco
Studio 109
Thread

Top-of-the-Line Men's Shirt Labels

Charvet
Ermenegildo Zegna
Faconnable
Fray
Jay Kos
Lorenzini
Ralph Lauren Purple Label
Robert Talbott
Seize sur Vingt
Thomas Pink
Turnbull & Asser

Where to Wear 2001

Shop Talk

Barry Kieselstein-Cord: Will open on Madison Avenue.

Bijan: Gone from Fifth Avenue location and rumored to be relocating to a three-story townhouse between 60th and 65th Streets.

Bliss Spa: Expands business by opening up Bliss Nail Salons across Manhattan.

Chanel: Signs retail space in Soho at 139 Spring Street scheduled to open in the next year.

Donna Karan: Spring 2001 is opening day for the Donna Karan Collection store.

Fiorucci: Will open 25,000-sq. ft. flagship store in Noho.

H & M: Union Square discounter Bradlees to become new H & M store.

Helmut Lang: Set to open a freestanding perfumery in Soho that will have an Old-World European apothecary feel.

Jean Paul Gaultier: Rumored to be opening his own boutiques funded by Hermes.

Marc Jacobs: Opening new store called "Marc" to showcase his secondary line.

Max Mara: To build 6,000-sq. ft. store at 450 West Broadway in Soho.

Prada: To occupy the former Soho Guggenheim Museum space.

Tahari: Sets sight on 510 Fifth Avenue to house the majority of its operations, as well as a retail space on the ground floor.

Best Dressing Rooms

Bergdorf Goodman	Plein Sud
Henri Bendel's	Ralph Lauren
Jeffrey New York	Tocca
Nicole Farhi	

Designers: Rising Stars

Alice Roi	Nicolas Ghesquiere
Barbara Berghino	Pamela Dennis
Bruce	Rebecca Taylor
Jeremy Scott	Roberto Menichetti
Leigh Bantivoglio	Tracy Feith
Miguel Adrover	Veronique Branquinho
Miguelina	

Where Designers Shop

Alexander Lind: Chuckies and Scoop
Anna Sui: Resurrection Vintage
Carolina Herrera: Brooks Brothers and Vanessa Noel
Diane von Furstenberg: Manolo Blahnik
Manolo Blahnik: Banana Republic and Brooks Brothers
Matt Nye: Barneys New York and Bergdorf Goodman Men
Michael Kors: Banana Republic, Bergdorf Goodman and Gap
Nicole Farhi: Resurrection Vintage
Nicole Miller: Sergio Rossi and Antique Boutique
Norma Kamali: Barneys
Ralph Lauren: Polo Ralph Lauren and Calypso St. Barths
Valentino: Malo
Vanessa Noel: Bergdorf Goodman and Bloomingdale's

Affordable Chic

Ann Taylor Loft
Banana Republic
Anthropologie
Eddie Bauer
Express
Find Outlet
Hennes & Mauritz
The Gap
Kenneth Cole
Klein's of Monticello
Pearl River
Nine West
Old Navy Clothing Co.
Ritz Furs

Best Designer Sample Sales

Bagley Mishka
Betsey Johnson
Diesel
Donna Karan
DKNY
Fendi
Michael Kors
Moschino
Miu Miu
Nicole Farhi
Prada
Theory
Tahari

Where Hollywood Shops

Andie MacDowell: Longchamp
Cameron Diaz : Tibet Arts & Crafts
Catherine Zeta-Jones: Louis Vuitton
Elle MacPherson: Thomas Pink
Gloria Estefan and Mariah Carey: Plein Sud
Gwyneth Paltrow: Dolce & Gabbana
Jewel: What Comes Around Goes Around
Jodi Foster: Armani
Kate Moss: Resurrection Vintage
Kelly Preston and Joan Cusack: Liz Lange Maternity
Lauryn Hill: Studio 109
Leonardo DiCaprio: Nova USA
Liz Hurley: Fendi
Madonna: Bond 07 and Manolo Blahnik
Martha Stewart: Vanessa Noel
Meryl Streep: Kinnu
Nicole Kidman and Tom Cruise: Nicole Farhi
Sarah Jessica Parker: La Petite Coquette
Sharon Stone: Lana Marks and Vera Wang
Uma Thurman: Alberta Ferretti

Penny Wise

Burlington Coat Factory
Easy Spirit
Forman's
Kleinberg & Sons
Loehmans
TJ Maxx
The Children's Place

Notable 2000 Closings

Alexander S. Kabbaz
Andrea Carrano
Aquascutum
Bijan
Classic Bodies
Gentryportofino
Guava
Kleinberg & Sherrill
Lulu
Patrick Cox

"Must-Haves"

A Eugenia Kim hat design
An Anya Hindmarch pony-skin handbag
Brunello Cucinelli cashmere
Bu and the Duck hand-crocheted children's sweaters
Clara Cottmann shirt from Leggiadro
Clarissa Hulse skirt from Language
Diesel jeans
Eres innerwear basics
Frederic Fekkai handbag
Furla coin purses and key chains
Hello Sari Indian embroidered coat jacket
I Golfini Della Nonna children's clothing from Erica Tanov
Jimmy Choo snakeskin mules
John Lobb men's shoes or boots
Joseph leather jacket
Leigh Bantivoglio lingerie from Le Corset
Levi's jean jacket
Louis Vuitton cashmere undergarments
Luci di Sole swimwear available at Barneys New York
Mark Schwartz python boots
Michael Stars T-shirt from Anthropologie
Scarpet a Porter printed chiffon sandals from Soco
Un Apres Midi de Chien utility handbag from TriBeCa
Luggage & Leather
Veronique Branquinho clothing
Vilebrequin swimtrunks

Unique Interiors

Christian Dior
Comme des Garçons
Costume National
Hermes
Jeffrey New York
Louis Vuitton SoHo
Nanette Lepore
Plein Sud

Polo Ralph Lauren
Stream
Su-zen
Tocca
Vanessa Noel
Ventilo
Vivienne Tam
Zao

Fashion Scoop

Abercrombie & Fitch: Prepares to launch both a store concept and a label called "Hollister Co," a lifestyle brand targeting high school boys and girls.

Alexander McQueen: Rumored to be giving up the design helm at Givenchy.

Barneys New York: Considering opening a chain of children's shops.

Daryl K: Introduces full-fledged menswear line for Fall 2001.

Kate Spade: Launches beauty products.

Steve Madden: Introduces a line of children's footwear and products for girls and teens under the new "Stevies" label.

Michael Kors: Rolls out his new fragrance "Michael."

Katayone Adeli: Introduces two new lower-priced lines called "2 by Katayone Adeli" and "2 Jeans."

Pamela Dennis: Launches full bridal line for 2001.

Gap: Goes online with its maternity collection.

Gap: expanded their size range in women's basics such as khakis and jeans up to size 24.

Narciso Rodriguez: Launches new accessories collection of shoes and handbags.

Galliano: Introduces a new line of handbags.

What's In

All accessories, especially retro-styled ones
Fur neck warmers
Cinched waists
Toe cleavage
Suits and blouses are back
Informal weddings
Anything crocodile (all other reptiles are OUT!)
Trenchcoats
Handbags worn on the wrist
Different shades of red
Fur embellishments on shoes, handbags and clothing
Belts
Pearls
Maternity chic
Jet set
Feathers
Lace
Romance
Cashmere treated as everyday essentials
Surf-inspired looks
Frame bags
Deco classics
Grosgrain ribbon trim
Gutsy glamour
Colored socks for men
Forties peep-toe pumps
Piping
Luxury classics
Floral prints
Beach towel chic
Custom-blended perfumes
Vintage
Denim
Pretty
Zippers
Mixing and matching
Beading and rhinestone embellishments
Fur-tied shawls
Leather

Where to Wear 2001

In-Store Restaurants

The Tea Box at Takashimaya
693 Fifth Avenue bet. 54/55th Street
212-350-0180

Nicole's at Nicole Farhi
10 East 60th Street bet. Madison/Fifth Avenue
212-223-2288

On Five at Bergdorf Goodman
754 Fifth Avenue bet. 57/58th Street
212-753-7300

Café 745 at Bergdorf Goodman Men
745 Fifth Avenue bet. 57/58th Street
212-753-7300

Showtime Café at Bloomingdale's
1000 Third Avenue bet. 59/60th Street
212-705-2000

Le Train Bleu at Bloomingdale's
1000 Third Avenue bet. 59/60th Street
212-705-2000

40 Karats at Bloomingdale's
1000 Third Avenue bet. 59/60th Street
212-705-2000

Blanche's Organic Café at DKNY
655 Madison at 60th Street
212-223-3569

Armani Café at Emporio Armani
601 Madison Avenue bet. 57/58th Street
212-317-0800

Café SFA at Saks Fifth Avenue
611 Fifth Avenue bet. 49/50th Street
212-753-4000

American Café at Lord & Taylor
424 Fifth Avenue bet. 38/39th Street
212-391-3344

Salon de The at Henri Bendel
712 Fifth Avenue bet. 55/56th Street
212-247-1100

Au Bon Pain at Macy's
Broadway at Herald Square bet. B'way/34th Street
212-695-4400

Fred's at Barneys
660 Madison Avenue at 61st Street
212-826-8900

Restaurants

The following is a compiled list of restaurants perfect for lunching during your shopping spree.

UPPER EAST SIDE (61st-96th Streets)

EAST 60'S

Amaranth (Bistro)
21 East 62nd Street bet. Madison/Fifth Avenue
212-980-6700

Bilboquet (French Bistro)
25 East 63rd Street bet. Madison/Park Avenue
212-751-3036

Ferrier (French Bistro)
29 East 65th Street bet. Madison/Park Avenue
212-772-9000

La Goulue (French Bistro)
746 Madison Avenue bet. 64/65th Street
212-988-8169

Le Charlot (French Bistro)
19 East 69th Street bet. Madison/Park Avenue
212-794-6419

Nello (Italian Bistro)
696 Madison Avenue bet. 62/63rd Street
212-980-9099

Serafina (Italian Pizzeria)
29 East 61st bet. Madison/Park Avenue
212-702-0118

EAST 70'S

The Gallery at The Carlyle Hotel
(Omelettes, Salads, and Sandwiches)
35 East 76th Street bet. 76/77th Street
212-570-7192

EJ's Lucheonette (Glorified Diner)
1271 Third Avenue at 73rd Street
212-472-0600

J.G. Melon (Hamburger Joint)
1291 Third Avenue at 74th Street
212-744-0585

Le Petit Hulot (French Bistro)
973 Lexington Avenue
212-794-9800

Where to Wear 2001

Mezzaluna (Pizzas and Pasta)
1295 Third Avenue bet. 73/74th Street
212-535-9600

Sant Ambroeus (Italian)
1000 Madison Avenue bet. 77/78th Street
212-570-2211

Swifty's (American Bistro)
1007 Lexington Avenue bet. 72/73rd Street
212-535-6000

EAST 80'S AND 90'S

E.A.T. (Gourmet Sandwiches and Salads)
1064 Madison Avenue bet. 80/81st Street
212-772-0022

Island (Italian Bistro)
1305 Madison Avenue bet. 92/93rd Street
212-996-1200

Jackson Hole (Hamburger Joint)
1270 Madison at 91st Street
212-427-2820

Sarabeth's (Tea Room)
1295 Madison at 92nd Street
212-410-7335

UPPER WEST SIDE

Café Luxembourg (French Bistro)
200 West 70th Street bet. Amsterdam/West End Avenue
212-873-7411

Blue Star (Glorified Diner)
329 Columbus bet. 75/76th Street
212-579-0505

Isabella's (Italian)
359 Columbus at 77th Street
212-724-2100

Nick & Toni (Mediterranean)
100 West 67th Street bet. B'way/Columbus
212-496-4000

Shun Lee Café (Chinese)
43 West 65th Street bet. Columbus/Central Park West
212-769-3888

Time Café (Brunch, Salads, Sandwiches)
2330 Broadway at 85th Street
212-579-5100

Vince & Eddie (American Bistro)
70 West 68th Street bet. Columbus/Central Park West
212-721-0068

MIDTOWN/FIFTH AVENUE (42nd-61st Streets)

California Pizza (Pizza, Pasta, and Salads)
201 East 60th Street on Third Avenue
212-755-7773

Cibi Cibi (Rustic Italian)
200 East 60th Street at Third Avenue
212-751-8615

Bice (Northern Italian)
7 East 54th Street bet. Madison/Fifth Avenue
212-688-1999

Fresco by Scotto on the Go (Italian)
40 E. 52nd Street bet. Madison/Park Avenue
212-754-2700

Le Taxi (French Bistro)
37 East 60th Street bet. Madison/Park Avenue
212-832-5500

Match Uptown (Asian Fusion)
33 East 60th Street bet. Madison/Park Avenue
212-906-9177

Mme. Romaine de Lyon (Omelettes)
132 East 61st Street bet. Park/Lexington Avenue
212-758-2422

Rue 57 (French Bistro)
60 West 57th Street bet. Fifth/Sixth Avenue
212-307-5656

FLATIRON/NOHO/CENTRAL VILLAGE

Borgo Antico (Tuscan Fare)
22 East 13th Street bet. Fifth/University Place
212-807-1313

Bricco (Italian)
46 West 22nd Street bet. Fifth/Sixth Avenue
212-727-3362

City Bakery (Salad, Sandwich, Pastry)
22 East 17th Street bet. B'way/Fifth Avenue
212-366-1414

Cosi Sandwich Bar (Great Sandwiches)
3 East 17th Street bet. B'way/Fifth Avenue
212-414-8468

Indochine (French Vietnamese)
430 Lafayette Street bet. Astor Place/4th Street
212-505-5111

Marquet Patisserie (Bistro)
15 East 12th Street bet. Fifth/University Place
212-229-9313

Where to Wear 2001

Time Café (Brunch, Salads, Sandwiches)
380 Lafayette bet. East 4th St./ Great Jones
212-533-7000

The Adore (Pastries, Salads, Sandwiches)
17 East 13th Street bet. Fifth/University Place
212-243-8742

T Salon (Soups, Salads, Sandwiches)
11 East 20th Street bet. B'way/Fifth Avenue
212-358-0506

CHELSEA

Amy's Bread (Sandwiches)
75 Ninth Avenue bet. 15/16th Street (Chelsea Market)
212-462-4338

Chelsea Bistro & Bar (French Bistro)
358 West 23rd Street bet. Eighth/Ninth Avenue
212-727-2026

Le Madri (Italian)
168 West 18th Street at Seventh Avenue
212-727-8022

Markt (Belgian Brasserie)
401 West 14th Street at Ninth Avenue
212-727-3314

O Padeiro (Portuguese)
641 Sixth Avenue bet. 19/20th Street
212-414-9661

Petite Abeille (Soups, Waffles, and Sandwiches)
107 West 18th Street bet. Sixth/Seventh Avenue
212-604-9350

SOHO

Balthazar (French Bistro)
80 Spring bet. Broadway/Lafayette
212-965-1414

Boom (Italian)
152 Spring bet. Wooster/Broadway
212-431-3663

Downtown (Harry Cipriani's Soho Location)
376 West Broadway at Broome
212-343-0999

Fanelli's Café (Burgers)
94 Prince at Mercer
212-431-5744

Felix (French Bistro)
340 West Broadway bet. Broome/Grand
212-431-0021

Match (Asian Fusion)
160 Mercer bet. Houston/Prince
212-343-0020

Mezzogiorno (Italian)
195 Spring at Sullivan
212-334-2112

TRIBECA/LOWER MANHATTAN

Bouley Bakery (New French)
120 W. Broadway at Duane Street
212-964-2525

Nobu Next Door (Japanese)
105 Hudson at Franklin
212-334-4445

The Odeon (Bistro)
145 Broadway bet. Duane/Thomas St.
212-233-0507

Rosemarie's (Italian)
145 Duane bet. Church/W. B'way
212-285-2610

Seaport Soup Company (Soups & Sandwiches)
76 Fulton at Gold St.
212-693-1371

Spartina (Mediterranean)
355 Greenwich at Harrison
212-274-9310

Tribeca Grill (New American)
375 Greenwich Street
212-941-3900

Clothing and Shoe Size Equivalents

Children's Clothing

American	3	4	5	6	6X
Continental	98	104	110	116	122
British	18	20	22	24	26

Children's Shoes

American	8	9	10	11	12	12	1	2	3
Continental	24	25	27	28	29	30	32	33	34
British	7	8	9	10	11	12	13	1	2

Ladies' Coats, Dresses, Skirts

American	3	5	7	9	11	12	13	14	15
Continental	36	38	38	40	40	42	42	44	44
British	8	10	11	12	13	14	15	16	17

Ladies' Blouses and Sweaters

American	10	12	14	16	18	20
Continental	38	40	42	44	46	48
British	32	34	36	38	40	42

Ladies' Hosiery

American	8	8.5	9	9.5	10	10.5
Continental	1	2	3	4	5	6
British	8	8.5	9	9.5	10	10.5

Ladies' Shoes

American	5	6	7	8	9	10
Continental	36	37	38	39	40	41
British	3.5	4.5	5.5	6.5	7.5	8.5

Men's Suits

American	34	36	38	40	42	44	46	48
Continental	44	46	48	50	52	54	56	58
British	34	36	38	40	42	44	46	48

Men's Shirts

American	14	15	15.5	16	16.5	17	17.5	18
Continental	37	38	39	41	42	43	44	45
British	14	15	15.5	16	16	17	17.5	18

Men's Shoes

American	7	8	9	10	11	12	13
Continental	39.5	41	42	43	44.5	46	47
British	6	7	8	9	10	11	12

Coming Soon—
Fall 2000/Spring 2001

"Shoes are like men. The one of the moment is
the favorite." —*Diane Von Furstenberg*

"The ruin of American fashion has been casual Friday.
It has led people to mix-and-match disasters with no taste."
—*Martino Scabbia Guerrini*

"Thank God we're living in a country where the sky's
the limit, the stores are open late and you can shop
in bed thanks to television." —*Joan Rivers*

Coming Soon—Fall 2000/Spring 2001

As *Where to Wear's 2001 Edition* goes to press, the following stores are planning to open between November 2000 and April 2001.

Bottega Veneta
114 Wooster Street

Type: A luxury Italian company selling ready-to-wear and leathergoods.

Chanel
139 Spring Street

Type: Luxury clothing and accessories by designer Karl Lagerfeld.

Christian Dior (jewelry)
17 East 57th Street

Type: Designer jewelry by Dior.

Club Monaco
699 Fifth Avenue

Type: A Canadian based company selling high fashion sportswear.

Coach
445 West Broadway

Type: An American leathergoods company.

Colette
356 West 58th Street in the Hudson Hotel

Type: Paris-based company selling high-end designer clothing and accessories.

Donna Karan Collection
819 Madison Avenue

Type: Donna Karan's men's and women's ready-to-wear collection.

Emporio Armani
436 West Broadway

Type: Italian designer Giorgio Armani's secondary line.

Eres
625 Madison Avenue

Type: A luxury French company famous for its feminine lingerie and swimwear.

H & M (Hennes & Martinez)
34th Street and Broadway

Type: A Swedish sportswear company selling trendy and high fashion clothing at incredibly low prices.

Coming Soon—Fall 2000/Spring 2001

Hogan
132 Spring Street

Type: A sporty Italian footwear and accessories company.

Holland & Holland
139 Spring Street

Type: Specializing in hunting gear and refined weekend wear.

Hugo Boss
132 Greene Street

Type: A German-based luxury company selling men's and women's apparel and accessories.

Hugo Boss
Flagship store on Fifth Avenue

Type: A German-based luxury company selling men's and women's apparel and accessories.

Intermix
210 Columbus Avenue

Type: Up-to-the-minute fashions by trendy designers.

J. Lindberg
126 Spring Street

Type: A Swedish retailer selling forward-thinking menswear, as well as golf gear.

John Varvatos
149 Mercer

Type: Men's fashions by Calvin Klein prodigy.

Kenneth Cole
610 Fifth Avenue

Type: A 17,000 sq. ft. flagship selling shoes, sweaters, outerwear, briefcases, and accessories.

Kenzo
80 Wooster

Type: Spirited ready-to-wear, sportswear and casual wear collection.

Louis Vuitton
Fifth Avenue at the St. Regis Hotel

Type: Luxury leathergoods, as well as a ready-to-wear collection by designer Marc Jacobs.

Max Mara
450 West Broadway

Type: An Italian company selling luxury basics.

Coming Soon—Fall 2000/Spring 2001

Olive & Bette's
158 Spring Street

Type: A boutique selling trendy designer labels favored by young fashionistas.

Onward Soho
172 Mercer Street

Type: Stocks women's collections by Matt Murphy, Peplum, Chuch Roaste, and others.

Tahari
510 Fifth Avenue

Tardini
142 Wooster

Type: Luxury Italian leathergoods and shoes.

Tommy Hilfiger
372 West Broadway

Type: All-American sportswear and casual wear.

Urban Outfitters
14th Street and Sixth Avenue

Type: Trendy sportswear and casual wear at reasonable prices. Favored by gen-xers.

Vanessa Noel
158 East 64th Street

Type: American shoe designer specializing in luxury footwear.

Victoria Secret
1981 Broadway

Type: Sexy lingerie at reasonable prices.

Alphabetical Store Directory

"It is admirable for a man to take his son fishing, but there's a special place in heaven for the father who takes his daughter shopping." —*John Sinor*

"If men liked shopping, they'd call it research." —*Cynthia Nelms*

"My Calvins." —*Alexander McQueen's reply to Elton John, when asked what he wore under his kilt to the VH1 Fashion Awards.*

Addison on Madison

Abercrombie & Fitch M/W/C
Abercrombie & Fitch has become iconic clothing for gen-x, a magnet for teens seeking trendy casualwear and the ubiquitous "A & F" logo. And why not? As last year's chart topping song says, "I like girls who wear Abercrombie & Fitch." Find looks that combine outdoor utilitarian with all-American spirit. Shop for cargo pants, T-shirts, tanks, hooded sweaters, parachute pants, knits, fleece vests and more. Check out their kid's division named "Abercrombie." Accessories also available. 800-432-0888
www.abercrombie.com

Lower Manhattan 212-809-9000
199 Water Street at South Street Seaport
NYC 10038 Mon.-Sat. 10-9, Sun. 11-8

A. Cheng W
Past terms of duty at retailing giants like the Gap, Tommy Hilfiger and the Limited have given designer Alice Cheng the experience and savvy she needed to open up her own shop. A. Cheng's collection caters predominately to modern day professionals who want easy-to-wear clothing with just the right amount of punch, i.e., casual work clothes with personality. Find skirts, pants, jackets and shirts in classic shapes with interesting details like chunky zippers, colors and soft prints. It's multi-purpose clothing with subtle attitude.

East Village 212-979-7324
443 East 9th Street bet. Ave. A/1st Ave.
NYC 10009 Mon.-Fri. 1-8, Sat. & Sun. 12-8

Add W
As every fashion magazine says, accessories are beyond hot and what better place to shop for them than at Add, one of New York's best sources for accessories. Add will definitely add the finishing touches to any wardrobe, be it everyday, evening or special occasion. Select from over 40 designers for the perfect hat, handbag, evening wrap, shawl, jewelry and belt. Find the latest fabric trends, from high fashion to quiet chic. Handbags include satin evening purses, whimsical patterned pokey bags and raffia totes with labels like Cerruti, Francesco Biasia, Franchi, Dollar Grand, Pibra and more. Hat styles include fancy dress toppers, adjustable straw boaters, madras caps, and Panamas by Kokin, Sylvia Richards, and Annabel Ingal. One of New York's best sources for accessories.

SoHo 212-539-1439
461 West Broadway bet. Houston/Prince
NYC 10012 Mon.-Sun. 11-8

Addison On Madison M
This is strictly a dress shirt shop for men. Choose from over 400 different styles at an average price of $75. Manufactured in Italian cotton, shirts come in a full cut with a relaxed fit.

Accessories include neckties, bow ties, pocket squares and cufflinks. Addison On Madison is great value for your money.

Upper East Side   212-308-2660
698 Madison Avenue   bet. 62/63rd St.
NYC 10021   Mon.-Sat. 10:30-6:30

A Détacher   W

Both an austere Japanese sensibility and a Jil Sanders minimalism influence owner/designer Monica Kowalska's collection. Think "art fashions for adults." Find a clean, simple line of monochromatic dresses, pants, skirts, blouses and more. She uses linear cuts (not form-fitting) and a basic color palette of black, white and gray. Perhaps best for the over 40 crowd.

SoHo   212-625-3380
262 Mott Street   bet. Houston/Prince
NYC 10012   Tues.-Sun. 12-7

Aerosoles   M/W

Aerosoles designs orthopedically correct shoes that cater more to comfort than fashion. Styles include sneakers, flats, sandals and casual shoes that emphasize stretch, movement and flexibility.   800-798-9478   www.aerosoles.com

Upper East Side   212-751-6372
1155 Second Avenue   at 61st St.
NYC 10021   Mon.-Sat. 10-8, Sun. 12-6

Upper West Side   212-579-8659
310 Columbus Avenue   bet. 74/75th St.
NYC 10023   Mon.-Sat. 10-8, Sun. 12-6

NoHo   212-358-7855
63 East 8th Street   bet. B'way/University Pl.
NYC 10003   Mon.-Sat. 10-8, Sun. 12-7

Lower Manhattan   212-577-9298
18 John Street   bet. B'way/Nassau
NYC 10038   Mon.-Fri. 9-7

Agnes B.   W

A line of chic French clothing that has long pleased New York's best-dressed women. Find a collection of contemporary ready-to-wear that's simple, snappy and feminine. Choose from suits, pants, jackets, skirts, sweaters and accessories. Don't leave without scooping up an Agnes B. T-shirt; they're fantastique. Faite Attention: sizes run itsy bitsy.

Upper East Side   212-570-9333
1063 Madison Avenue   bet. 80/81st St.
NYC 10028   Mon.-Sat. 11-7, Sun. 12-6

Chelsea   212-741-2585
13 East 16th Street   bet. Fifth/Union Sq. West
NYC 10003   Mon.-Sat. 11-7, Sun.12-6

SoHo   212-925-4649
116 Prince Street   bet. Wooster/Greene
NYC 10012   Mon.-Sun 11-7

Agnes B. Homme M
Find a ready-to-wear line for the fashion conscious shopper. From suits and dress pants to khakis and jeans, Agnes B. offers men a complete look, featuring simple clothes with snappy French attitude. Sizes run small.

SoHo 212-431-4339
79 Greene Street at Spring St.
NYC 10012 Mon.-Sun. 11-7

Akiue-Go W
We suppose the history of Akiue-Go is the retail equivalent of a movie star being discovered at the soda fountain counter. At a talent competition in Japan Akiue won first prize – an all expenses paid chance to open his own shop in New York City. Now comes the hard part for the lucky winner: surviving in Manhattan's dog-eat-dog retail world. The good news: find fun "girlie" denim skirts trimmed with checks and T-shirts with fringes and ruffles. The bad news: the collection is limited, and unless you happen to fit into their size 6 rack sample, you must custom order.

East Village 212-473-2720
445 East 9th Street bet. Ave. A/1st Ave.
NYC 10009 Tues.-Sun. 12-8

Alan Flusser M
You might say, "There will always be an England as long as Flusser is with us." Alan Flusser is not only the king of Saville Row tailoring, but also one of the world's foremost authorities on custom-made clothing. Wall Street types flock here to fit themselves with a look of English elegance just like famous Flusser clients Fred Astaire and the Duke of Windsor. Find a selection of shirts to complement your suit. In addition, shop for men's furnishings that include ties, hand-finished suspenders, hand-clocked socks, as well as bench-made shoes. Custom suits start at $2,000.

Fifth Avenue 212-888-7100
611 Fifth Avenue at Saks bet. 49/50th St.
NYC 10022 Mon.-Fri. 10-7, Sat.10-6:30, Sun. 12-6

Alberene Cashmere M/W
The pleasure of owning and wearing cashmere is usually an expensive one. However, thanks to Alberene's prices, cashmere is now more affordable, at least one third off department store prices. It all comes from Scotland in an abundance of colors. Find sweaters in a variety of styles, even hooded sweatshirts, as well as scarves, socks, capes and gloves. Pay $199 for a standard crew neck sweater.

Fifth Avenue 212-689-0151
435 Fifth Avenue, 3rd Fl. bet. 38/39th St.
NYC 10016 Mon.-Fri. 10-6, Sat. 10-5

Aldo M/W
Calling all gen-xers! Aldo's sells "street vibe" looks at attractive prices. Manufactured in Italy, Aldo's label features

Alexandre de Paris

chunky platforms and rubber soles packed with hip-hop attitude.

Upper East Side   212-828-3725
157 East 86th Street   bet. Third/Lexington Ave.
NYC 10028   Mon.-Sat. 10-8, Sun. 12-7

Midtown East   212-832-1692
730 Lexington Avenue   bet. 58/59th Street
NYC 10022   Mon.-Wed. 10-8, Thurs.-Sat. 10-9, Sun. 12-7

Midtown West   212-239-4045
29 West 34th Street   bet. Fifth/Sixth Ave.
NYC 10001   Mon.-Fri. 10-8, Sat. 11-8, Sun. 12-6

NoHo   212-982-0958
700 Broadway   at West 4th Street
NYC 10003   Mon.-Sat. 11-8, Sun. 12-7

SoHo   212-226-7974
579 Broadway   bet. Houston/Prince
NYC 10012   Mon.-Sat. 10-9, Sun. 11-7

Alexandre de Paris   W

A French retailer of hair accessories. Styles include chinois pins, snoods, hairnets, headbands, hair forks, combs and barrettes. Each item is hand-made to perfection. Styles run from simply beaded to fabulously bejeweled. Private line of hairbrushes and sunglasses also available.

Upper East Side   212-717-2122
971 Madison Avenue   bet. 75/76th St.
NYC 10021   Mon.- Fri. 10-6, Sat. 10-6

Alexandros Furs   M/W

At Alexandros Furs choose from a collection of quality avant-garde and classic fur coats — from sporty fox and raccoon to luxurious mink, sable or lynx by labels like Halston, Mark Montano and Ekso. Other outerwear includes cashmere overcoats and reversibles. Alexandros also offers storage, cleaning and remodeling. New this year: a fur handbag collection.

Midtown East   212-702-0744
5 East 59th Street, 2nd Fl.   bet. Madison/Fifth
NYC 10022   Mon.- Fri.10-6, Sat. 10-5

Chelsea   212-967-1222
213 West 28th Street   bet. 7/8th Ave.
NYC 10001   Mon.-Sun. 10-6

Alexia Crawford Accessories   W

Although this SoHo newcomer's main focus is jewelry, her accessories should not be missed. Find a great collection of silky, diaphanous scarves, shawls and wraps that coordinate with matched evening bags. Styles run from young and trendy to classic and sophisticated. Quality is outstanding and prices affordable.

SoHo   212-473-9703
199 Prince Street   bet. Sullivan/MacDougal
NYC 10012   Mon.-Sun. 11-7

Alfred Dunhill M
The Dunhill label is classic English luxury for the sophisticated man. The main floor features accessories, fragrances, jewelry and cigars. Saunter up to the second floor to find suits, shirts, ties, knitwear, sportswear and outerwear, all with the Dunhill label. Off-the-rack suits run from $900 to $1,700, while a custom suit goes from $1,900 to $5,000. Take it from us: the place positively reeks of taste and class.
800-860-8362

Upper East Side 212-879-8711
846 Madison Avenue bet. 69/70th St.
NYC 10021 Mon.-Sat. 10-6

Midtown East 212-753-9292
450 Park Avenue at 57th St.
NYC 10022 Mon.-Sat. 10-6:00

Alice Underground W
At Alice Underground, you'll discover secondhand clothing and other serendipitous goodies. Shop for vintage clothing from the 40's to the 60's, as well as accessories, jewelry and shoes. Don't overlook the bargain bins in the front and a variety of merchandise (from T-shirts and sweaters to leathers and dresses) in the back. Buyer beware: it doesn't necessarily come cheap.

SoHo 212-431-9067
481 Broadway bet. Broome/Grand
NYC 10012 Mon.-Sun. 11-7:30

Alicia Mugetti W
Alicia Mugetti carries a large selection of romantic dresses that are in rich velvets and crushed satins. Find them in beautiful colors and feminine, floor-length silhouettes. Lush fabrics and Renaissance looks define the Mugetti label.

Upper East Side 212-794-6186
999 Madison Avenue bet. 77/78th Street
NYC 10021 Mon.-Sat. 10-6

Alixandre W
Run by three generations of the Schulman family, Alixandre delivers honest, reliable and knowledgeable service, as well as an outstanding selection of fur coats. Find top quality shearlings, broadtails, minks and sables from designer labels that include Oscar de la Renta and Valentino.
www.alixandrefurs.com

Midtown West 212-736-5550
150 West 30th Street, 13th Fl. bet. 6/7th Ave.
NYC 10001 Mon.-Fri. 9-5, Sat. 9-1:30
by appointment only

Allan & Suzi M/W
Rummage through the over-stuffed racks at this secondhand shop and select a high-glam or outrageously fun little outfit that a famous model has, in many cases, worn only once or twice. Find designer garb by Jean Paul Gaultier,

Vivienne Westwood, Versace, Prada, Comme des Garcons, as well as shoes by Manolo Blahnik and Gucci. In addition, Allan & Suzi's features vintage pieces by Courreges, Pierre Cardin and others. The shop's environment and merchandise is sure to send tingles up and down your spine, but these gently-used designer duds don't always come cheap.

Upper West Side	**212-724-7445**
416 Amsterdam Avenue	at 80th Street
NYC 10024	Mon.-Fri. 12-8, Sat. 12-7, Sun. 12-6

Allen-Edmonds M

For over 75 years Allen-Edmonds has been designing with the customer's needs in mind. Find over 200 styles of dress and corporate classics, casual weekend shoes, as well as fashion forward lifestyle footwear. Great care has gone into obtaining the perfect balance between quality and price.
800-235-2348

Midtown East	**212-308-8305**
551 Madison Avenue	bet. 55/56th St.
NYC 10022	Mon.-Fri. 9-7, Sat. 9-6, Sun. 12-5
Midtown East	**212-682-3144**
24 East 44th Street	bet. Madison/5th
NYC 10017	Mon.-Fri. 9-7, Sat. 9-6, Sun. 12-5

Allure Lingerie W

A well-stocked neighborhood lingerie shop featuring brands like Only Hearts, Hanky Panky, Hanro, Cosabella and LeJaby. Find a great selection of seamless bras, panties and thongs, as well as hosiery by DKNY and Wolford. Robes and slippers also available.

Upper East Side	**212-860-7871**
1324 Lexington Avenue	bet. 88/89th St.
NYC 10128	Mon.-Fri. 11-7, Sat. 11-6

Alpana Bawa W

An Alpana Bawa design highlights color and decorative accents. Find a vibrant collection of coats, dresses, jackets, skirts, pants, tops and accessories made from hand-embroidered wools, silks, nylons and cottons, often featuring geometric and floral patterns. Also find cotton men's shirts, embellished with prints and embroidery, favored by actors like Willem Defoe.

SoHo	**212-965-0559**
41 Grand Street	bet. W. B'way/Thompson
NYC 10013	Mon.-Fri. 11-7, Sat. 12-7, Sun. 12-6

Alskling W/G

Alskling means "darling" in Swedish and, yes, the clothes are darling. This shop boasts an enormous collection of dresses, as well as pants, tops and skirts. Almost everything is washable and easy to care for. Their forte is the little slip dress featured in an array of prints. The look is soft, feminine and romantic, but maybe too precious for some. Adorable floral dresses for girls up to size 6.

Amy Downs Hats

Upper West Side   212-787-7066
228 Columbus Avenue   bet. 70/71st St.
NYC 10023   Mon.-Sun. 11-7

American Colors   W
Henry Lehr's private label line, "American Colors," features casual basics —all made in America and garment dyed in a rainbow of colors, hence the name. The merchandise is machine washable and dryable (i.e., low-maintenance). Find jeans by A. Gold E., Earl, and Levi's, as well as corduroys, khakis, shirts and plenty of T-shirts.

NoLiTa   212-334-2656
232 Elizabeth Street   bet. Prince/Houston
NYC 10012   Mon.-Sun. 11-7

American Eagle Outfitters   M/W
AEO targets the collegiate male and female shopper who desire affordable, all-American, casual lifestyle clothing. Find jeans, graphic T-shirts, pants, sweaters, khakis, outerwear, shoes and accessories. The look is wholesome and guaranteed not to offend parents. 888-232-4535.
www.ae.com

Lower Manhattan   212-571-5354
89 South Street   at the South Street Seaport
NYC 10038   Mon.-Sat. 10-9, Sun. 11-8

American Jean   M/W
More accurately, the name of this store should be Levi Jean, as this is the only label sold here. Choose from Levi 501's, 512's, 517's, 505's and 550's. Each pair is at a terrific price of $35. Sales staff is underwhelming.

Midtown West   212-258-2244
142 West 57th Street   bet. 6/7th Ave.
NYC 10019   Mon.-Sun. 9:30-8

Amy Chan   W
Fashionable girls shop here for designer Amy Chan's unique and delightful assortment of handbags, whether it's a party purse or a tote to carry all their "stuff" to the beaches. Chan's signature design is her distinctive mosaic bag that comes in all shapes, sizes, and fabrics (saris, pastel checks, stripes, oriental-like floral motifs, denim and so on). Small acrylic tiles are heat-sealed onto these marvelous, colorful fabrics and, voila, you've got an Amy Chan original. Prices run from $130 to $350. Other styles include clutches, brightly toned beach bags, and Moroccan print bags. A small clothing collection is also available.

NoLiTa   212-966-3417
247 Mulberry Street   bet. Prince/Spring
NYC 10012   Tues.-Sat. 12-7

Amy Downs Hats   W
Welcome to Amy Downs, one of New York's most creative milliners. Place your order from the overhead hat menu and

select a topper named Twister or Happy Family. This hat shop is filled with wry and whimsical designs in bright colors. Her styles feature a "downtown" look with eclectic and unusual designs. Find a collection of polar fleece and wool hats, hunting caps, straw boaters, funky felts, fun furs, bold berets, wool ski hats and more.

Lower East Side	212-598-4189
103 Stanton Street	bet. Orchard/Ludlow St.
NYC 10002	Wed.-Sun. 1-6

Andy's Chee-Pees M/W

A vintage and retro shop for the younger set in search of fun, one-of-a-kind "previously owned" items. Find collectible denim, swing clothes from the 40's and 50's, biker and bomber jackets, jeans, old police leather jackets, Hawaiian shirts, a complete line of unisex dickeys in bold brights, party wigs, vintage jewelry and more. For the 18 to 35 crowd.

West Village	212-420-5980
691 Broadway	bet. 3rd/4th St.
NYC 10012	Mon.-Sat. 11-9, Sun. 12-8

Anik W

Young, professional women shop here for fashionable career clothing that doesn't scream corporate. Find hip designers like Teflon, Chaiken, Theory, Bianca Nero and Easel with clean, simple lines and a contemporary feel that will have you looking stylish at the office and chic in the evening.

Upper East Side	212-861-9840
1355 Third Avenue	bet. 77/78th St.
NYC 10021	Mon.-Sat. 11-8, Sun. 12-7

Upper East Side	212-249-2417
1122 Madison Avenue	bet. 83/84th St.
NYC 10028	Mon.-Sat. 10-8, Sun. 11-7

Anna W

At Anna's, owner Kathy Ann Kemp has one goal: to provide her customer with a unique and distinctive clothing collection that she sees nowhere else. So for those of you looking for one-of-a-kind pieces, Anna's should be one of your stops. Much of Kemp's inspiration comes from the dance world, where the use of fabrics like silk jersey, that combine movement, texture and shape, play a vital role. Find girlish silk skirts, smocked tops, print dresses and carefully chosen vintage pieces that complement the rest of the collection. The look is fun, feminine and fashionable.

East Village	212-358-0195
150 East 3rd Street	bet. Ave. A/B
NYC 10009	Mon.-Fri. 1-8, Sat. & Sun. 1-7

Anna Sui W

At the heart of every Anna Sui collection comes "the celebration of the nouvelle hippie." This trendy Chinese designer sticks to what she does best: renounce minimalism, pile on the design elements of pattern, color and texture and top it off with a bit of Sui wit and imagination. The end result: vintage schoolgirl punk (trust us). Find clothes for day that happily slink into night. Choose from dresses, skirts tossed with a crochet piece, romantic blouses, chunky coats, an array of tops, jackets, pants, a patchwork piece accessorized with fringe, denim and even dainty underwear. All in unique fabrics and form-fitted silhouettes plus accessories like handbags and jewelry. A Sui design is about an eclectic mix of influences, from decades long past to '80's rock. Accessories include handbags and jewelry.

SoHo	**212-941-8406**
113 Greene Street	bet. Prince/Spring
NYC 10012	Mon.-Sat. 11:30-7:00, Sun. 12-7

Ann Crabtree W

This small two-story boutique is filled with classic clothing for the mature woman on her way to a chic luncheon or a weekend in the Hamptons. Find a selection of designer sportswear, suits and separates, as well as linen pants, silk tops and comfortable jeans. Prices can be daunting.

Upper East Side	**212-996-6499**
1310 Madison Avenue	at 93rd Street
NYC 10128	Mon.-Fri. 10:30-6:30, Sat. 10:30-6

Ann Taylor W

Gone are the days of the old Ann Taylor that catered predominately to young professionals; new and improved Ann Taylor is for everyone, from corporate women to chic urbanites of all ages. Find suits and separates for the office, sportswear for weekends and understated cocktail dresses for evening. In addition, shop a terrific selection of private label shoes, an extensive petite section, as well as accessories. Great sales! 800-677-0300

Upper East Side	**212-832-2010**
645 Madison Avenue	at 60th St.
NYC 10022	Mon.-Fri. 10-8, Sat. 10-7, Sun. 12-6
Upper East Side	**212-861-3392**
1320 Third Avenue	bet. 75/76th St
NYC 10021	Mon.-Fri. 10-8, Sat. 10-6, Sun. 12-6
Upper West Side	**212-721-3130**
2380 Broadway	at 87th St.
NYC 10024	Mon.-Sat. 10-8, Sun. 12-6
Upper West Side	**212-873-7344**
2015-17 Broadway	at 69th St.
NYC 10023	Mon.-Sat.10-8, Sun. 12-6
Midtown East	**212-308-5333**
850 Third Avenue	at 52nd St.
NYC 10022	Mon.-Fri. 10-8, Sat. 10-6, Sun. 12-5
Fifth Avenue	**212-922-3621**
575 Fifth Avenue	at 47th St.
NYC 10017	Mon.-Fri. 10-8, Sat. 10-7, Sun. 11-6

Ann Taylor Loft W

Ann Taylor keeps getting better and better and this year they've launched their new Loft stores featuring perfect weekend clothing. The Ann Taylor customer shops here for casual basics that include sweater sets, pants, cotton and silk shirts, dresses and accessories. It's about dependable, relaxed and practical fashions at lower price points.

Upper East Side 212-472-7281
1492 Third Avenue bet. 84/85th St.
NYC 10028 Mon.-Sat. 10-9, Sun. 11-6

Upper East Side 212-772-9952
1155 Third Avenue at 68th
NYC 10021 Mon.-Sat. 10-8, Sun. 11-7

Midtown East 212-883-8766
150 East 42nd Street at Lexington
NYC 10017 Mon.-Fri. 9-9, Sat.10-8, Sun. 11-6

Midtown East 212-308-1129
488 Madison Avenue at 52nd Street
NYC 10022 Mon.-Sat.10-8, Sun. 11-6

Anne Fontaine W

Talented 29-year-old French designer Anne Fontaine has turned the basic concept of a white shirt into a multimillion-dollar business. Her philosophy: "Feminize the traditional shirt so there is no need to hide it under a jacket anymore. It should be a piece of clothing itself." Fabrics include luxurious organdy, cotton gauze, pique, poplin and more. Choose simple button-down shirts to exquisitely detailed embroidered silhouettes and pin-front camisoles. Prices run from $65 to $125, and with each purchase discover a rose sachet tucked into your shirt. New this year: Fontaine has recently expanded her collection to include a few black styles.

Upper East Side 212-639-9651
791 Madison Avenue at 67th Street
NYC 10021 Mon.-Sat. 10-6, Sun. 12-5

SoHo 212-343-3154
93 Greene Street bet. Prince/Spring
NYC 10012 Mon.-Sat. 11-7, Sun. 12-6

Anthropologie W

An immense store packed with an eclectic and versatile selection of apparel and home furnishings. Find sportswear and casual basics with looks that run from fashion forward to ethnically inspired. Choose from slacks, dresses, shirts, sweaters, tees, shorts and accessories that are a combination of downtown artsy with urban sensibility. Labels include Anthroplogie, Liquid, Free People, Michael Stars, Tease tees and more. A vast selection of housewares.
800-309-2500   www.anthropologie.com

SoHo 212-343-7070
375 West Broadway bet. Broome/Spring
NYC 10012 Mon.-Sat. 11-8, Sun. 11-6

Flatiron   212-627-5885
85 Fifth Avenue   at 16th St.
NYC 10003   Mon.-Sat. 10-8, Sun. 10-6

Antique Boutique   M/W

Originally Antique Boutique sold vintage garb; however, in the last year "retro" takes a backseat to "new." Although you will still find an assortment of vintage clothing from the 60's and 70's (Levi's, polyester pieces, T-shirts, dresses and purses), their main focus is contemporary, edgy looks. Shop for fashionable clothing in high-tech fabrics from labels like All Saints, Cassandra Loomis, New York Industry, Alternate Sin, Jay Lindberg, Fake, UFO, Michelle Mason, Mandarina Duck, and Jurgi Persoons. A favorite among fashion thrill-seekers.

NoHo   212-995-5577
712-714 Broadway   bet. 4th/Astor Place
NYC 10003   Mon.-Thurs. 11-9, Fri. & Sat. 11-10, Sun. 12-8

Antoin   W

Your typical neighborhood shoe store that features a collection of generic shoe brands that follow the fashion trends. Blacks and browns are the predominant colors. High prices.

Upper East Side   212-249-6703
1110 Lexington Avenue   bet. 77/78th St.
NYC 10021   Mon.-Fri. 9-8, Sat. 10-8, Sun. 11-8

☆ Anya Hindmarch   W

Already with four stores in London, 31-year-old Anya Hindmarch is heating up the streets of New York with her sophisticated collection of handbags. Whether it's for day or evening, each bag is beautifully crafted (made in Italy) from the finest materials. Choose from everyday classics in scratch-free, luxurious leathers, ponyskins and tweeds. Evening stunners include couture satins, velvets and silks, while some of her amusing pieces include whimsical candy-box bags, velvet clutches trimmed in feathers and silk bags with photographic images of people and pets. So if you're in the market for a smart-looking shoulder bag or a playful creation, know that your Hindmarch will set you apart from everyone else. Pay anywhere from $100 to $1,200. Small leathergoods, jewelry, travel and make-up bags complete the assortment.

Upper East Side   212-750-3974
29 East 60th Street   bet. Park/Madison Ave.
NYC 10022   Mon.-Sat. 10-7, Sun. 12-5

A.P.C.   M/W

This typically French shop, A.P.C., an abbreviation for Atelier de Production et Creations, breaks all gender rules. At A.P.C. girls will be boys in mannish tailored clothes. A Jean Touitou design is functional, understated and wearable. Find that unisex look in button-down shirts, straight leg pants, sweaters and outerwear, all manufactured in natural fabrics.

The Apartment

SoHo   212-966-9685
131 Mercer Street   bet. Prince/Spring St.
NYC 10012   Mon.-Sat. 11-7, Sun. 12-6

The Apartment   M/W

Uber-hip Manhattanites have yet another venue to explore the latest trend in retailing: reality entertainment, where the customer plays the role of performer/observer and the shop and merchandise become the stage and props. As one would expect, The Apartment's primary focus is on furniture, kitchen equipment and bathroom fixtures; however, cutting-edge clothing and accessories from Gripo, Marithe and Francois Girbaud and Not Tom, Dick and Harry are creatively displayed amongst the housewares.

Soho   212-219-3661
101 Crosby Steet   bet. Prince/Spring St.
NYC 10012   Tues.-Fri. 11-7, Sat. & Sun. 11-8

April Cornell   W/G

While most people come to April Cornell for her lovely table and bed linens, she also features a clothing line for women and children. Find a collection of dresses, jackets, skirts, nighties and hats in delightful combinations of Indian inspired fabrics.

Upper West Side   212-799-4342
487 Columbus Avenue   bet. 83/84th St.
NYC 10024   Mon.-Sat. 10-8, Sun. 11-7

Arche   W

A popular French company known for comfortable, spongy leather shoes in a myriad of colors and styles. Refined they're not; however, these thick rubber soles and clunky heels continue to please younger customers.

Upper East Side   212-439-0700
995 Madison Avenue   at 77th St.
NYC 10021   Mon.-Fri. 10-7, Sat. 10-6, Sun. 12-5

Upper East Side   212-838-1933
1045 Third Avenue   bet. 61/62nd St.
NYC 10021   Mon.-Fri. 10-7, Sat. 10-6, Sun. 12-5

Midtown West   212-262-5488
128 West 57th Street   bet. 6/7th Ave.
NYC 10019   Mon.-Fri. 10-7, Sat. 10-6, Sun. 12-5

NoHo   212-529-4808
10 Astor Place   bet. B'way/Lafayette
NYC 10003   Mon.-Fri. 10-7, Sat. 10-6, Sun. 12-5

Arleen Bowman   W

Since 1987, Arleen Bowman has been selling casual sportswear boasting comfort, simplicity and color. Their best item is the "Arleen Bowman" two-pocket shirt, available in cotton, linen, silk charmeuse, seersucker, suede or velvet. In addition, find travelling suits by Alex Garfield, sweaters by DAR and Margaret O'Leary, sportswear pieces by Lileth, pants by Sanctuary, For Joseph jeans, 3 Dot T-shirts and Only Hearts. Accessories include jewelry and handbags.

West Village | 212-645-8740
353 Bleecker Street | bet. West 10th St./Charles
NYC 10014 | Mon.-Sat. 12-7, Sun. 1-6

Arthur Gluck Shirtmakers   M/W
Gluck specializes in custom shirts at reasonable prices ($200). Hand-sewn monograms and mother-of-pearl buttons are a Gluck trademark. Orders take approximately one month. www.shirtcreations.com

Midtown West | 212-755-8165
47 West 57th Street | bet. 5/6th Ave.
NYC 10019 | Mon.-Thurs. 9-5, Fri. 9-2

Artificial Life (Alife)   M/W
Opened by four friends from the graphic design business, Alife is not your typical shop. The store's eclectic mix includes footwear, T-shirts, graffiti paraphernalia, sneakers, Lacoste shirts and, yes, stuffed animals. The store's mission: to offer its customers the unconventional and the intriguing, and hope it sells. Footwear brands include Trippen, Gola, and Snipe, while the majority of the clothing collection is by young designers getting their first exposure.

Lower East Side | 646-654-0628
178 Orchard Street | bet. Houston/Stanton
NYC 10002 | Mon.-Sun. 12-8

Ascot Chang   M/W
Ranked as one of today's finest shirt-makers, Ascot Chang caters to some of the world's nattiest dressers. Chang specializes in custom and made-to-measure suits, shirts and overcoats. Choose from 2,000 luxurious fabrics and know with confidence that your purchase will wear forever. If wallets aren't flush, Chang also features off-the-rack shirts, sportcoats, blazers and overcoats. Furnishings, pajamas and silk robes available.

Midtown West | 212-759-3333
7 West 57th Street | bet. 5/6th Ave
NYC 10019 | Mon.-Sat. 9:30-6

Ashanti   W
Large-sized fashion for work or play. Find wool suits, silk blouses, day dresses, skirts and jackets, knit ensembles, evening pieces and accessories. Looks run from casual to dressy. Ashanti is for plus-sized women who adore color and pattern. Alterations done on premises. From size 14 to 32. www.ashanti-largersizes.com

Upper East Side | 212-535-0740
872 Lexington Avenue | bet. 65/66th St.
NYC 10021 | Mon.-Sat. 10-6, Thurs. 10-8

Assets London   W
This British knitwear company caters to the young and trendy. Assets London features hip designers like Anna Sui, Cynthia Rowley and Paul & Joe. Find career, club and weekend wear, as well as shoes and accessories. Think 7th floor Barneys with less expensive prices.

A. Testoni

Upper West Side   212-874-8253
464 Columbus Avenue   bet. 82/83rd St.
NYC 10024   Mon.- Sat. 11-8, Sun. 12-7

A. Testoni   M/W

An established footwear retailer from Bologna, Italy, A. Testoni features high-quality leather shoes that are classic, understated and modern in design. For men, find handmade and bench-made dress shoes, as well as slip-ons and loafers. For women, styles run from loafers and boots to pumps and evening wear. Handbags, briefcases, scarves, ties, belts and luggage also available. Expensive. 877-testoni.

Fifth Avenue   212-223-0909
665 Fifth Avenue   bet. 52/53rd St.
NYC 10022   Mon.- Fri. 10-7, Sat. 10-6:00, Sun. 12-5

AT Harris Formalwear, Ltd.   M

A good source for renting a tuxedo, especially for weddings. Find the AT Harris brand name and expect to pay $145 to $165 for a 24-hour rental. Shirts and the necessary black tie accoutrements also available.

Midtown East   212-682-6325
11 East 44th Street   bet. Madison/5th Ave.
NYC 10017   Mon.-Fri. 9-5:45, Sat. 10-3:45 by appointment

Athlete's Foot   M/W/C

Strictly sneakers for the sport of your choice, whether it's aerobics, tennis, running or basketball. Find every top brand, including Adidas, New Balance, Nike, Reebok and more. Children's sizes from 1 toddler to size 6.
www.theathletesfoot.com

Upper East Side   212-223-8022
1031 Third Avenue   at 61st St.
NYC 10021   Mon.-Sat. 10-8, Sun. 10:30-7

Upper West Side   212-579-2153
2265 Broadway   bet. 81/82nd St.
NYC 10024   Mon.-Sat. 10-8, Sun. 11-6

Upper West Side   212-961-9556
2563 Broadway   bet. 96/97th St.
NYC 10025   Mon.-Sat. 10-9, Sun. 11-6

Midtown East   212-317-1920
655 Lexington Avenue   at 55th St.
NYC 10022   Mon.-Fri. 9:30-8, Sat. 9:30-8, Sun. 10-6

Midtown East   212-867-4599
41 East 42nd Street   bet. Madison/Vanderbilt Ave.
NYC 10017   Mon.-Sat. 9-8, Sun. 12-6

Midtown West   212-768-3195
1568 Broadway   at 47th Street
NYC 10036   Mon.-Sat. 9-10, Sun. 10-9

Midtown West   212-629-8200
46 West 34th St.   bet. 5/6th Ave.
NYC 10001   Mon.-Sat. 9-9, Sun. 10-8

	August Max Women
NoHo	212-260-0360
60 East 8th St.	at Broadway
NYC 10003	Mon.-Sat. 10-9, Sun. 12-6

Athletic Style M
You won't find serious athletic gear here, but you will find stylized workout clothes. Clothing includes polar fleece, warm-up suits, sweats, polo shirts, jackets, sweaters and baseball caps by labels like Russell and Gear. Any item can be personalized with your name or favorite logo. Allow approximately two weeks for delivery. Find a good selection of sneakers by Nike, Reebok, Adidas and others.

Midtown East	212-838-2564
118 East 59th Street	bet. Lex./Park Ave.
NYC 10022	Mon.-Fri. 9-5

Atrium M/W
Atrium features just about every designer label from A to Z. Find sportswear and casual wear by Calvin Klein, Theory, Diesel, DKNY, Iceberg, Maharishi, Evisu, G-Star, Marithe & Francois Giraud, Polo Sport and more.

NoHo	212-473-9200
644 Broadway	at Bleecker St.
NYC 10012	Mon.-Sat. 10-9, Sun. 11-8

Atsuro Tayama W
Atsuro Tayama, once a disciple of Yohji Yamamoto, breaks out on his own with this SoHo shop. Women can choose from three diverse collections ranging from avant-garde designs with deconstructed looks to a classic approach providing well-tailored styles. Unlike some of today's Japanese designers, Tayama's creations are sensible, approachable and, yes, wearable.

SoHo	212-334-6002
120 Wooster Street	bet. Spring/Prince
NYC 10012	Mon.-Sat. 11-7, Sun. 12-6

Au Chat Botté B/G
A venerable East Side children's shop featuring top-of-the-line European brand names. Known for luxurious bassinets and crib furnishings. Au Chat Botte is also recognized for its fine quality traditional clothing. From hand-smocked dresses and dainty blouses to rompers and knit outfits, your child will be beautifully dressed. From newborn to 24 months.

Upper East Side	212-722-6474
1192 Madison Avenue	bet. 87/88th St.
NYC 10028	Mon.-Sat. 10-6

August Max Women W
August Max specializes in larger-sized clothing for women at work or play. Find career clothing, weekend wear, hosiery and accessories at affordable price points.

Lower Manhattan	212-432-0178
330 World Trade Center	bet. Church/Vesey
NYC 10048	Mon.-Fri. 7:30-8, Sat. 10-6, Sun. 12-5

Avitto M/W
Footwear styles that cover all the bases in the heart of SoHo. Find a collection of clean, modern classics by top designer footwear labels. Women can choose from mules, pumps, slingbacks, evening shoes and a large boot selection. Men can shop for business and casual shoes including everything from casual sandals to $800 alligator lace-ups. Labels include Calvin Klein, Cesare Paciotti, Trussardi, Yoriko Powel, Ferre, and Avitto.

SoHo   **212-219-7501**
424 West Broadway   bet. Prince/Spring
NYC 10012   Mon.-Sun. 11-8

A/X Armani Exchange M/W
This 10,000-sq. ft. emporium caters to the fashion conscious in search of casual basics with a designer label. Find jeans, T-shirts, pants, sweaters, jackets and outerwear that's relaxed and hip, and all with the Armani logo. Think an upscale designer Gap. Prices are surprisingly reasonable and quality is up to Armani standards.
www.armaniexchange.com

Fifth Avenue   **212-980-3037**
645 Fifth Avenue   at 51st St.
NYC 10022   Mon.-Sat. 10-8, Sun. 10-7

SoHo   **212-431-6000**
568 Broadway   at Prince
NYC 10012   Mon.-Sat. 10-8, Sun. 11-7

The Baby Collection B/G
This Upper East Side neighborhood children's shop is packed with European and American labels, emphasizing non-traditional, snazzy outfits. The selection includes casual clothing, hand-knit sweaters, dresses, outerwear, shoes and accessories. Labels include Absorba, Petit Bateau, Cozy Toes, and Molli. From newborn to 6X.

Upper East Side   **212-828-8633**
1384 Lexington Avenue   bet. 91/92nd St
NYC 10128   Mon.-Fri. 10:15-7, Sat. 11-6, Sun. 11-5

Bagutta W
A sleek, modern boutique with up-to-the-minute fashions from the world's top designers. Find ready-to-wear collections from McQueen, Demeulemeester, Dolce & Gabbana, Gaultier, Comme des Garcons, Dries Van Noten, Marni, Thimister and more. The atmosphere is relaxed and the sales staff knowledgeable. A good alternative to department store shopping.

SoHo   **212-925-5216**
402 West Broadway   at Spring
NYC 10012   Mon.-Fri. 11-7, Sat. 11-7:30, Sun. 12-6:30

Baldwin Formalwear M
Getting married? Need a tux? Well, make your way to Baldwin Formalwear and they'll take care of all your needs

(except, of course, finding you a bride). Specialists in tuxedos, they give you the option of buying or renting. Find top designer labels like Ralph Lauren, Christian Dior, Oscar de la Renta, Perry Ellis and more. Pay $100 to $175 to rent and $300+ to buy. In addition, find all necessary black tie amenities like neckwear, vests and cummerbunds, as well as shoes by Fredericko Deleon.

Midtown West   212-245-8190
52 West 56th Street, 2nd Fl.   bet. Fifth/Sixth Ave.
NYC 10019   Mon. & Thurs. 8:30-7,
Tues, Wed. & Fri. 8:30-6, Sat. 10-4

Bally M/W

Recently acquired by the Texas Pacific Group, this 150-year-old Swiss company now seeks a more youthful image and true luxury brand status. Only time will tell, but in the meantime, Bally's current look will have to do. This flagship store showcases an entire collection of shoes, handbags, leather clothing and small leathergoods. While the collection of dress and casual shoes is conservative and mature, Bally's line of handbags and leather clothing is refreshingly stylish and fashion forward. 800-332-2559
www.ballyswiss.com

Midtown East   212-751-9082
628 Madison Avenue   at 59th St.
NYC 10153   Mon.-Fri. 10-6:30, Thurs. 10-7,
Sat. 10-6, Sun. 12-5

Midtown East   212-986-0872
347 Madison Avenue   bet. 44/45th St.
NYC 10017   Mon.-Fri. 9-6:30, Sat. 10-6

Bambini B/G

Every child should be so lucky to be outfitted in one of Bambini's outfits. Find everything from casual and back-to-school basics to party and dress wear. Bambini is packed with Italian brand names featuring traditional looks. Choose from pants, dresses, shirts, sweaters, T-shirts, rompers and more. Highlights include their private label shoes and hand-knit sweaters. From newborn to 12 years.

Upper East Side   212-717-6742
1367 Third Avenue   at 78th St.
NYC 10021   Mon.-Sat. 10-6:30, Sun. 12-5

Banana Republic M/W

For the past four years Banana Republic's fashions have always been right on the money. Welcome to one-stop-shopping for a great-looking wardrobe. Banana Republic is the source for understated, affordable clothing that's more chic than trendy. Efficient tailoring, feel good fabrics and clean sensible shapes make up Banana Republic's label. Find suits, sportswear, casual basics, cashmeres, shoes and accessories with up-to-the-minute looks for dressing up or down. New this year: home furnishings. 888-277-8953
www.bananarepublic.com

Barami

Fifth Avenue (Flagship Store)   212-974-2350
626 Fifth Avenue   at Rockefeller Center
NYC 10022   Mon.-Fri. 10-9, Sat. 9-8, Sun. 11-7

Upper East Side   212-570-2465
1136 Madison Avenue   bet. 84/85th St.
NYC 10028   Mon.-Fri. 10-8, Sat. 10-7, Sun. 12-6

Upper East Side (W)   212-288-4279
1131 Third Avenue   at 67th St.
NYC 10021   Mon.-Sat. 10-8, Sun. 11-7

Upper West Side   212-787-2064
2360 Broadway   at 86th St.
NYC 10024   Mon.-Sat. 10-9, Sun. 11-7

Upper West Side   212-873-9048
215 Columbus Avenue   bet. 69/70th St.
NYC 10023   Mon.-Sat. 10-9, Sun. 10-7

Midtown East   212-751-5570
130 East 59th Street   at Lexington Ave.
NYC 10022   Mon.-Fri. 9-9, Sat. 9-8, Sun. 10-8

Midtown West (Flagship)   212-244-3060
17 West 34th Street   bet. 5/6th Ave.
NYC 10001   Mon.-Sat. 9:30-8:30, Sun. 11-7

Fifth Avenue (M)   212-644-6678
655 Fifth Avenue   at 52nd St.
NYC 10022   Mon.-Sat. 9:30-8, Sun. 10-7

Flatiron (M)   212-366-4691
122 Fifth Avenue   at 18th St.
NYC 10011   Mon.-Fri. 10-9, Sat. 10-8, Sun. 11-7

Flatiron (W)   212-366-4630
89 Fifth Avenue   bet. 16/17th St.
NYC 10003   Mon.-Fri. 10-9, Fri. & Sat. 10-8, Sun. 11-7

Chelsea (M)   212-645-1032
111 Eighth Avenue   bet. 15/16th St.
NYC 10011   Mon.-Sat. 10-9, Sun. 12-7

West Village   212-473-9570
205 Bleecker Street   at 6th Ave.
NYC 10012   Mon.-Sat. 10-9, Sun. 11-8

SoHo (W)   212-925-0308
552 Broadway   bet. Spring/Prince
NYC 10012   Mon.-Sat. 10-8, Sun. 11-7

SoHo (M)   212-334-3034
528 Broadway   at Spring
NYC 10012   Mon.-Sat. 10-8, Sun. 11-7

Barami   W

Barami is an excellent resource for cost-conscious corporate women seeking contemporary looks. Find suits with matching coordinates, tailored shirts, separates and accessories, all domestically manufactured. It comes in fashion forward styles and is well priced.

Upper East Side   212-988-3470
1404 Second Avenue   at 73rd St.
NYC 10021   Mon.-Fri. 10-8, Sat. 10-7, Sun. 12-6

Upper West Side 212-246-2930
1879 Broadway at 62nd St.
NYC 10023 Mon.-Fri. 8-8, Sat. 10-8, Sun. 11-6

Midtown East 212-980-9333
136 East 57th Street at Lexington Ave.
NYC 10022 Mon.- Fri. 9-9, Sat. 9-8, Sun. 11-7

Midtown West 212-308-0600
37 West 57th Street bet. 5/6th Ave.
NYC 10019 Mon.-Fri. 9-8, Sat. 10-8, Sun. 12- 6

Flatiron 212-529-2300
119 Fifth Avenue at 19th St.
NYC 10003 Mon.-Fri. 9-8, Sat. 10-8, Sun. 12-6

Lower Manhattan 212-321-2480
4 World Trade Center bet. Church/Vesey
NYC 10048 Mon.-Fri. 8-8, Sat. 11-6, Sun. 12-5

Barbara Bui W

This French designer has earned a reputation for creating classic shapes in luxury fabrics. Find it all in this enormous, minimalist shop which serves as the backdrop for her ready-to-wear collection. Bui's forte is her extensive collection of beautifully tailored pants, ranging from bootleg to man-tailored. In addition, choose from jackets, skirts, sweaters, dresses, form-fitted tees and outerwear—all designed with clean lines, flattering silhouettes, sleek looks and a European cut. Expensive.

SoHo 212-625-1938
117 Wooster Street bet. Prince/Spring
NYC 10012 Mon.-Sat. 11-7, Sun. 12-6

Barbara Feinman Millinery W

Don't breeze down 7th Street too quickly or you'll walk right past this special little hat shop. All of Barbara Feinman's toppers are made on the premises, and she is always happy to educate a customer in the art of hand-blocked hats or do a custom fitting. Find cloches, Panama's, cowboy hats and lampshade hats in fabrics like straw, raffia, canvas, denim, felt, velvet and velour. Accessories include straw and beaded handbags and jewelry.
Feinmanhats@mindspring.com

East Village 212-358-7092
66 East 7th Street bet. 1st/2nd Avenue
NYC 10003 Mon.-Sat. 12:30-8, Sun. 1-7

Barbara Shaum M/W

Although Barbara Shaum has been designing sandals since 1954, her current success is owed to Calvin Klein, who recently paired his men's collection with Shaum's sandals. Since then Shaum has hit the big leagues, with her sandals caressing the fabulous feet of model Iman, photographer Steve Meisel and designer Ralph Lauren. Prices run from $145 to $400. Belts also available.

East Village 212-254-4250
60 East 4th Street bet. Bowery/2nd Ave.
NYC 10003 Wed.-Fri. 1-8, Sat. 1-6

Barneys New York M/W/C
This terminally chic fashion emporium is where Hollywood loves to shop. Barneys has come a long way from the days when off-price suits were their stock in trade. Apart from excellent cosmetic and accessories departments, Barneys boasts five floors of ultra-hip clothing that has defined avant-garde retailing for the past 15 years. Find designer collections by Clements Ribeiro, Narciso Rodriguez, Prada, Hussein Chalayan, Ann Demeulemeester, Yohji Yamamoto, Richard Tyler, Armani, Dries Van Noten, Ralph Lauren, Jil Sander and more. Barneys' ability to spot trends just around the corner is nothing short of legendary, and is showcased on the 7th floor and 8th floor Co-op, their take on an upscale, indoor bazaar. Young fashionistas shop the high-energy atmosphere of these floors for contemporary and casual sportswear, denim, swimwear, lingerie, shoes and accessories. Choose from hip labels like Daryl K, Tocca, Jill Stuart, Future Ozbek, Paul & Joe and many others. Other departments include outerwear, designer shoes, lingerie, Barneys' private label, a new maternity line aptly named "Procreation," a newborn and toddler section and Chelsea Passage, a tabletop and gift department. Last but not least is Barneys' new vintage department, as well as a full-fledged bridal salon, featuring the crème de la crème of designer wedding gowns. Select from over 60 styles, whether it's an exquisite Richard Tyler design or a Yohji Yamamoto creation. By contrast the men's store is a quiet oasis that pays homage to the very finest menswear designers from around the world. Traditionalists will appreciate suits from makers such as Oxxford, Ralph Lauren Purple Label, Hickey-Freeman, Kilgour, French & Stanbury and Huntsman, while those on the cutting edge can choose from designers like Armani, Zegna, Dolce & Gabbana, John Bartlett, Prada, Yohji Yamamoto, Helmut Lang, Gucci and more. Other outstanding departments include men's furnishings, made-to-measure suits and dress shirts, designer shoes, sportswear, rainwear, outerwear, special sizes, casual wear, formalwear, shoes and accessories. Grab a bite at their in-store restaurant named Fred's. Shop Barneys' famous warehouse sale held twice a year.   888-222-7639
www.barneys.com

Upper East Side 212-826-8900
660 Madison Avenue at 61st St.
NYC 10021 Mon.-Fri. 10-8, Sat. 10-7, Sun. 11-6

Lower Manhattan (M/W) 212-945-1600
2 World Financial Center Mon.-Fri. 10-7,
NYC 10281 Sat. 11-5, Sun. 12-5

Barneys Co-op M/W
Located around the corner from the original Barneys New York, the Co-op features weekend oriented, night-on-the-town clothes that are found on the two Co-op floors of the Madison Avenue store. This is great news for die-hard downtowners who won't venture uptown for those cool,

trendy labels that Barneys is so well known for. Find jeans, pants, shirts, T-shirts, sweaters, dresses, outerwear and footwear from labels like Skim.com, Punk Empire, Levi's Red Label, Diane Von Furstenberg and Tocca as well as many others too cool to mention. Accessories and a Kiehl's skin care counter also available. www.barneys.com

Chelsea 212-593-7800
236 W. 18th Street bet. 7th/8th Ave.
NYC 10011 Mon.-Fri. 11-8, Sat. 11-7, Sun. 11-6

Basic Basic W

As the shop's name subtly hints, find basic contemporary junior clothing here. Choose from a great selection of T-shirts by Le Petit Bateau, 3 Dots and Juicy Couture, as well as jeans by Buffalo and Fiorucci. Cute skirts, dresses, sweaters and pants round out the assortment. Shoes by "Unlisted," a division of Kenneth Cole.

West Village 212-477-5711
710 Broadway bet. Washington Pl./4th St.
NYC 10003 Mon.-Sat. 11-8, Sun. 12-7

Bati W

A convenient neighborhood shoe store that features the latest in footwear designs. Shop European labels like Guiseppe Zanotti, Le Tini, L'Autre Chose and more. Styles include boots, flats, pumps, mules, sandals and wedges in trendy fabrications and shapes. Prices run from $60 to $500.

Upper West Side 212-724-7214
2323 Broadway bet. 84/85th St.
NYC 10024 Mon.-Sat. 11-8, Sun. 12-7

BCBG by Max Azria W

For years we idly wondered what the letters BCBG meant (if anything). Well, the answer is "bon chic, bon genre," Parisian slang for "good style, good attitude." On the other hand, we've never wondered what the secret to Azria's success was: the perfect balance between urban trend and classic styling, European sophistication and American spirit, clean lines, body loving shapes, and cutting-edge fabrics. Find sleek suits, fitted sweater sets, dresses, jackets and jazzy shoes at excellent prices. Best of all, the price is right!

Upper East Side 212-717-4225
770 Madison Avenue at 66th Street
NYC 10021 Mon.-Sat. 10-7, Sun. 12-6

Beau Brummel M

Beau Brummel is a destination shop for the busy executive. Find suits, furnishings, sportswear, casual wear, outerwear and accessories with European labels like Zegna, Hugo Boss and Canali, as well as private label. On the spot tailoring, excellent service and a relaxed atmosphere are all part of the Brummel experience.

Bebe

SoHo	212-219-2666
421 West Broadway	bet. Prince/Spring
NYC 10012	Mon.-Sat. 11-7, Sun. 12-7

Bebe W

If you're been searching for an outfit that will give you that calculated bare-all look and that will elicit oohs and aahs, you're in the right shop. Find a line of tight, sexy clothing that's in keeping with the latest fashion trends. Pant and skirt ensembles, form-fitted dresses, body-baring tops, tanks, tees and accessories make up Bebe's collection. Are they flattering? Depends on your hips, attitude and how you wear them. Best for the under 35 crowd.
www.bebe.com

Upper East Side	212-517-2323
1044 Madison Avenue	bet. 79/80th St.
NYC 10021	Mon.-Fri. 10-8, Sat. 10-7, Sun. 11-6

Upper East Side	212-935-2444
1127 Third Avenue	at 66th St.
NYC 10021	Mon.-Fri. 10-8, Sat. 10-7, Sun. 11-6

Midtown East	212-588-9060
805 Third Avenue	at 50th St.
NYC 10022	Mon.-Fri. 10-8, Sat. 10-7, Sun. 12-5

Flatiron	212-675-2323
100 Fifth Avenue	at 15th St.
NYC 10011	Mon.-Fri. 10-8, Sat. 10-7, Sun. 11-6

Bebesh W

If slinky long gowns are where it's at, then Bebesh is it. Designs feature a downtown "glam" look. Also find a selection of shoes, handbags, suits and separates. The look is contemporary and borderline funky.

SoHo	212-226-4969
425 West Broadway	bet. Prince/Spring
NYC 10012	Mon.-Sun. 11-8

Bebe Thompson B/G

Strictly irresistible is the name of the game at Bebe Thompson. Find casual basics and dress-up wear with designer labels like Claude Velle, Lili Gaufrette, Lily Pulitzer, Paul Smith, Bill Tornade, Charabia and more that will have your child looking adorably well-dressed. From newborn to 16.

Upper East Side	212-249-4740
1216 Lexington Avenue	bet. 82/83rd St.
NYC 10028	Mon.-Fri. 10-6, Sat. 11-6

Belgian Shoes M/W

Gone are the old digs, and buried with it, we hope, the famously snooty sales staff. The new millennium has ushered in a new and even better Belgian Shoes. Their soft, distinctive, handmade loafers continue to be waspy status symbols. Once hooked, you may end up collecting all their color

Bergdorf Goodman

combinations (over 50). Sizing is unusual and runs two to three sizes below normal. Expect to wait 12 to 18 months for special orders (roughly the same gestation as for elephants).

Midtown East 212-755-7372
110 East 55th Street bet. Park/Lex.
NYC 10022 Mon.-Fri. 9-4

Benetton M/W

Benetton's flagship store occupies the ground floor of the landmark Scribner Building, where the architecture alone is worth the visit. Best known for its sweaters, this Italian sportswear company features modern suits perfect for your first interview, and a colorful sportswear collection. Snappy clothing for the younger set. 800-535-4491
www.benetton.com

Fifth Avenue 212-317-2501
597 Fifth Avenue bet. 48/49th St.
NYC 10017 Mon.-Sat. 10-7, Sun. 11-5

West Village 212-533-0230
749 Broadway bet. 8th St./Astor Pl.
NYC 10003 Mon.-Sat. 10-9, Sun. 12-8

Ben Thylan Furs W

Ben Thylan's extensive fur collection features styles that run from sporty to dressy. Their specialty: fur-lined or fur-trimmed water-repellent coats. These all-weather classics can be lined in mink, fox, sable or any other fur of your choosing. Cashmere, wool and camel's hair coats also available. Services include color and fashion consultants, as well as storage and cleaning.

Chelsea 212-753-7700
345 Seventh Avenue, 24th Fl. bet. 29/30th St.
NYC 10001 Mon.-Fri. 9-5, Sat. 9-1
  by appointment only

Beretta M/W

Known the world over for their guns, Beretta also manufactures fine hunting, sporting and weekend wear—an Italian version of Holland & Holland if you like. Tweeds, lodens, fine cashmeres and wools make up their collection of classic sportswear. This is clothing fit for an Italian nobleman's hunting retreat, if you could only find one (an Italian nobleman that is).

Upper East Side 212-319-3235
718 Madison Avenue bet. 63/64th St.
NYC 10021 Mon.-Sat. 10-6

☆ Bergdorf Goodman W

This seven-story emporium is the epitome of luxury retailing, offering the finest fashions from around the world. From a first floor devoted to handbags, jewelry, hosiery and accessories to five floors of boutique settings stocked with the world's top designers, it's one of New York's premier

Bergdorf Goodman Men

shopping havens. From Richard Tyler, Valentino, Chloe to Courreges, Chanel and Calvin Klein, find fashions that are straight off the runways. The talk of the town continues to be Bergdorf's brand new "Level of Beauty," a lower level emporium featuring exclusive beauty and skincare treatments, fragrances, spa products, Michael George's flower shop, and Morganthal Federics' optical shop, and a manicure bar. Other departments include designer and trendy shoes, lingerie, eveningwear, suits, bridal, custom outerwear and a stellar gift and tabletop shop. John Barrett Hair Salon and Susan Ciminelli Day Spa are housed on the ninth floor. 800-964-8619

Fifth Avenue	**212-753-7300**
754 Fifth Avenue	bet. 57/58th St.
NYC 10019	Mon.-Fri. 10-7, Thurs. 10-8, Sat. 10-6

Bergdorf Goodman Men M

A 45,000-sq. ft. emporium with the feel of a gentleman's club, featuring the ultimate in menswear fashions. Find furnishings by Turnbull & Asser, Charvet, Ferragamo and more. Traditional suit collections by Oxxford, Canali, Hickey-Freeman and Luciano Barbera offer conservative elegance and a classic cut. Shop in boutique settings for trendy international designers like Armani, Versace, Jil Sander, Etro and Gucci. New custom lines include Saint Andrews, Kiton, Sartoria Attolini, as well as Domenico Spano and Oxxford. In short, a luxury fashion mecca for the sophisticated man. Great sales. 800-964-8619

Fifth Avenue	**212-753-7300**
745 Fifth Avenue	at 58th St.
NYC 10022	Mon-Wed., Fri. 10-7, Thurs. 10-8, Sat. 10-6

Berk M/W

Invest in one of Berk's cashmere sweaters and know with confidence that it will endure a lifetime of wear; their Ballantyne label is world renowned for quality and craftmanship. Choose from classic styles in 60 glorious shades. Find crew necks, turtlenecks, twin sets, and cardigans, as well as capes, stoles and accessories. Great velvet slippers.

Upper East Side	**212-570-0285**
781 Madison Avenue	bet. 66/67th St.
NYC 10021	Mon.-Fri. 10-6, Sat. 10-5

Best of Scotland M/W

A top floor hideaway that features cashmere sweaters at terrific values. Crew necks priced at $390 on Madison Avenue retail here for $190. It's well worth a look.

Fifth Avenue	**212-644-0403**
581 Fifth Avenue, Penthouse	bet. 47/48th St.
NYC 10017	Mon.-Sat. 10-5:30

Betsey Bunky Nini W

This attractive shop highlights expensive European designers. Find an extensive sportswear and sweater selection, jackets, suits and eveningwear by labels like Cividini, Anna Molinari, Dosa, Piazza Sempione, Ghost, Gunext, Alberta Ferretti, Paul Smith and others. The look is urban with an edge. Accessories include handbags and jewelry.

Upper East Side   212-744-6716
980 Lexington Avenue   bet. 71/72nd St.
NYC 10021   Mon.-Sat. 10:30-6,
Thurs. 10:30-7, Sun. 12-5

Betsey Johnson W

Earning the CFDA award in 1999 for timeless talent, Betsey Johnson keeps getting stronger and stronger with each collection. Known for turning out wild and sexy looks, her clothes are about an attitude, not an age. Although some looks may be over-the-top for some, remember, there's always something for everyone. For twenty years she's been thrilling women with her trademark slip dresses and coordinating cardigans. In addition, find slinky micro minis, biased skirts, form-fitted pants, velvet and animal print pieces, as well as fun holiday and special occasion dresses. So if you're in the market for a "meet-your-guy" kind of look, check out the fun at Betsey Johnson.

Upper East Side   212-734-1257
1060 Madison Avenue   bet. 80/81st St.
NYC 10028   Mon-Sat. 11-7, Sun. 11-6

Upper East Side   212-319-7699
251 East 60th Street   bet. 2/3rd Ave.
NYC 10022   Mon.-Sun. 12-7

Upper West Side   212-362-3364
248 Columbus Avenue   bet. 71/72 St.
NYC 10023   Mon.-Sat. 11-7, Sun. 12-7

SoHo   212-995-5048
138 Wooster Street   bet. Houston/Prince
NYC 10012   Mon.-Sat. 11-7, Sun. 12-7

Bicycle Habitat M/W/C

Bicycle Habitat features mountain, road and suspension bikes from manufacturers such as Specialized and Trek, priced from $250 to $3,000. High-end brands include Bontrager and Klein, with price tags that run from $1,000 to $4,000. Biking apparel is available, as well as a lifetime service guarantee on all their bikes.

SoHo   212-431-3315
244 Lafayette Street   bet. Prince/Spring
NYC 10012   Mon.-Thurs. 10-7,
Fri. 10-6:30, Sat. & Sun. 10-6

Bicycle Renaissance M/W/C

A selection of mountain, road and hybrid bikes from makers like Specialized, Cannondale, Trek and Klein. Price tags run from $330 to $4000. Clothing, accessories and workshops make this a full-service establishment.

Big Drop

Upper West Side	212-724-2350
430 Columbus Avenue	at 81st St.
NYC 10024	Mon.-Fri. 10-7:30, Sat. 10-6, Sun. 10-5

Big Drop   W

Find hip, urban clothing for the 18 to 35 crowd from a global mix of young designers worldwide. Big Drop is packed with casual, trendy and funky fashions. Find labels by Earl, Juicy, Rebecca Dannenberg, Vanessa Bruno, Big Drop, 3 Dot, Beautiful People, Tracy Reese, Easel, Inc and more. A good selection of fun handbags, too.

Upper East Side	212-988-3344
1321 Third Avenue	bet. 75/76th St.
NYC 10021	Mon.-Sat. 11-8, Sun. 12-7

SoHo	212-966-4299
174 Spring Street	bet. Thompson/W. B'way
NYC 10012	Mon.-Sat. 11-8, Sun. 12-8

Bill Amberg   M/W

After years of outfitting airport lounges with those ubiquitous leather and aluminum chairs, Bill Amberg has changed gears and landed in NoLiTa with a handsome collection of leather goods for men and women. His collection of constructed handbags, briefcases, desk accessories and small leathergoods are manufactured in fine English bridle leather and are available in a variety of colors. Prices run from $130 to $900.

NoLiTa	212-625-8556
230 Elizabeth Street	bet. Prince/Houston
NYC 10012	Mon. & Tues. by appt.
	Wed.-Fri. 12-7, Sat. 11-7, Sun. 12-6

Billy Martins   M/W

Yee haw! Round up your herd and ride on over to Billy Martin's for a Western fix. It's positively the best source for fancy Western belts. Find everything from cowboy boots to high-priced duds that will get you back to your Ponderosa. 800-888-8915

Upper East Side	212-861-3100
220 East 60th St	at Third Avenue
NYC 10022	Mon.-Fri. 10-7, Sat. 10-6, Sun. 12-5

Bis   W

Every other day there's a new delivery of designer merchandise that comes straight from the closets of well-dressed, well-heeled New Yorkers into Bis for resale. Women shop here for high-end labels in tip-top condition. At any given time you might come across eveningwear by Armani, Mary McFadden or Givenchy, a handbag by Fendi or Ferragamo, or a pair of shoes by Blahnik or Chanel. Expect to pay 30% less than retail, but remember, timing is everything when shopping consignment.

Upper East Side   212-396-2760
1134 Madison Avenue, 2nd Fl.   bet. 84/85th St.
NYC 10028   Mon.-Thurs. 10-7,
Fri. & Sat. 10-6, Sun. 12-5

Bisou-Bisou   W

The shop's name means Kiss-Kiss, but French designer Michele Bohbot explains her line of clothing as being "about a woman who is not a child, but not really a woman—she is somewhere in between." Find contemporary sportswear that includes stretch pants, tight tops, dresses, skirts, shoes and accessories. Best to buy as separates to coordinate with your wardrobe rather than top-to-bottom complete outfits. Pay $108 for pants, $165 to $299 for jackets and $38 to $120 for tops. Fashions for the young and lean.

SoHo   212-260-9640
474 West Broadway   bet. Houston/Prince
NYC 10012   Mon.-Sat. 11-8, Sun. 12-7

Blades Board and Skate   M/W/C

Out-of-towners and Gothamites alike can catch the rollerblading fever by checking out Blades, New York's best destination for in-line skates and other board sports. The selection includes rollerblades, skateboards, snowboards and ice skates, as well as the obligatory protective gear. Top it off with matching clothing and accessories and you're ready to go. In-line skate rentals are $27 a day with a $200 deposit. Helpful, nice sales staff.

Upper East Side   212-996-1644
160 East 86th Street   bet. 3rd/Lexington Ave.
NYC 10028   Mon.-Fri. 11-8, Sat. 10-8, Sun. 10-6

Upper East Side   212-249-3178
1414 Second Avenue   bet. 72/73rd Street
NYC 10021   Mon.-Sat. 11-7, Sun. 11-6

Upper West Side   212-787-3911
120 West 72nd Street   bet. Columbus/Broadway
NYC 10023   Mon.-Sat. 10-8, Sun. 10-6

Midtown West   212-563-2488
901 Sixth Avenue at Manhattan Mall   at 32nd Street
NYC 10001   Mon.-Sun. 10-8

NoHo   212-477-7350
659 Broadway   bet. 3rd St./Bleecker
NYC 10012   Mon.-Sat. 10-9, Sun.11-6

Bloomers   W

An upscale lingerie shop featuring high-end European labels. Find casual and sexy underpinnings, silk chemises, loungewear, sleepwear, robes, and slippers by labels like Aubade, LeJaby, Lou, Chantelle, Marie Jo and others. Children's clothing also available.

Upper East Side   212-570-9529
1042 Lexington Avenue   bet. 74/75th St.
NYC 10021   Mon.-Sat. 10-6:30, Thurs. 10-7

Bloomingdale's   M/W/C

Nearly everyone who comes to New York wants to experience Bloomingdale's, and he or she should, at least once anyway, for this can be an exhausting adventure for even the veteran shopper. The crush of people extends well past the first floor, and at any given moment you can easily get lost or confused. However, on a positive note, this store has historically been a fashion trendsetter with innovative merchandising concepts and sales extravaganzas. Clothing and shoes for men, women and children, from trendy to conservative, are available from every major designer. Boulevard Four showcases the latest designer fashions for women by Armani, Calvin Klein, Chanel, Donna Karan, Ralph Lauren and others. For contemporary looks, hipsters can choose from collections by Trina Turk, Theory, Helmut Lang, Daryl K, William B. and many more. Men's fashions run from designer suits and formal wear to sportswear and casual wear with names like Joseph Abboud, Canali, Donna Karan, Hugo Boss and Kenneth Cole, as well as their own private label. Also find one of the largest cosmetics and accessories departments, along with three floors of home furnishings and decorative accessories. With such an enormous selection, most customers feel that if they can't find it at Bloomies, it doesn't exist! An added plus is Bloomies' outstanding service departments that include personalized shopping, in-store TicketMaster, hotel delivery and bridal registry. For shoppers in need of a bite, choose from four eateries. 800-777-0000 www.bloomingdales.com

Midtown East   212-705-2000
1000 Third Avenue   bet. 59/60th St.
NYC 10022   Mon.-Fri.10-8:30, Sat. 10-7, Sun, 11-7

Blue Bag   W

One of the most refreshing handbag boutiques to sprout in New York's hip NoLiTa area. Husband and wife team Marnie and Pascal Legrand explore the entire realm of bag designs. Women can shop a unique selection of limited edition handbag styles from classic Herve Chapelier totes and beautifully decorated evening bags to whimsically shaped one-of-a-kinds. Textures range from nubuck and leather to flannel and velvet. Cute beaded evening bags and amusing feathered trim mini totes are perfect for club hopping. New arrivals constantly.

NoLiTa   212-966-8566
266 Elizabeth Street   bet. Houston/Prince
NYC 10012   Mon.-Sun. 11-8

Bolton's   W

With its convenient locations in Manhattan, Bolton's is always within easy reach. Find a selection of wardrobe staples that include career suits, blouses, sportswear, lingerie and accessories, all at discounted prices. Beware: you'll have to search high and low for that designer label.

Upper East Side   212-996-1006
161 East 86th Street   bet. Lex./Third
NYC 10028   Mon.-Sat. 10-8, Sun. 10-7

Upper East Side   212-223-3450
787 Lexington Avenue   bet. 61/62nd St.
NYC 10021   Mon.-Fri. 9:30-8:30, Sat. 10-7, Sun. 11-7

Upper East Side   212-722-4419
1180 Madison Avenue   at 86th St.
NYC 10028   Mon.-Sat. 10-7, Sun. 12-6

Midtown East   212-684-3750
4 East 34th Street   bet. 5th/Madison Ave.
NYC 10016   Mon., Tues. & Fri. 9-7,
Wed. & Thurs. 9-8, Sat. 10-7, Sun. 10-6

Midtown West   212-935-4431
27 West 57th Street   bet. 5/6th Ave.
NYC 10019   Mon.-Fri. 10-8, Sat. 10-7, Sun. 12-6

Midtown West   212-245-5227
110 West 51st Street   at 6th Ave.
NYC 10020   Mon.-Fri. 8-6:30, Sat. & Sun. 10-6

Midtown West   212-307-5089
1700 Broadway   at 54th St.
NYC 10019   Mon, Tues. & Fri. 10-7,
Wed. & Thurs. 9-8, Sat. 10-7, Sun. 10-8

☆ Bond 07   W

Owner Selima Salaun is the force behind this downtown success, as well as Selima Optique and Le Corset. This fashionable boutique is an "accessories wonderland," filled with an imaginative and colorful collection from around the world. Find everything and anything that screams "chic"—from children's wear, stylish eyewear, frilly lingerie, hats, handbags, vintage pieces, antiques, perfumes, jewelry, clothing and shoes. Clothing fashionistas will relish browsing the racks of new design talent, as well as hip downtown designer labels like Eugenia Kim, Bettye Muller, Anna Sui and others. Bond 07 is currently one of New York's most "in" shops.

NoHo   212-677-8487
7 Bond Street   bet. B'way/Lafayette
NYC 10012   Mon.-Sat. 11-7, Sun. 12-7

Bonpoint   B/G

Exclusive French clothes for the mother eager to have her child on the best-dressed list. Luxury fabrics, attention to detail and impeccable tailoring are the key to Bonpoint's well-earned reputation. If only they made clothing for adults! Although they do carry casual clothes, fancy dress-up is their forte (christenings, weddings, birthdays, etc.). Choose from beautiful hand-smocked dresses, traditional blouses, shirts, pants, outerwear, swimwear and accessories, all at haute couture prices! Newborn to size 16 girls/8 boys.

Upper East Side   212-722-7720
1269 Madison Avenue   at 91st St.
NYC 10128   Mon.-Sat. 10-6

Bostonian

Upper East Side	**212-879-0900**
811 Madison Avenue	at 68th St.
NYC 10021	Mon.-Sat. 10-6

Bostonian M

Men come here for the selection of affordable footwear which runs from business wear to weekend casual. Shop the Bostonian label for classic work shoes (lace-ups and dressy loafers), for sporty looks (brands like Kenneth Cole) and for casual styles (labels include Timberland, Ecco, Clarks and Rockport). Expect to pay anywhere from $89 to $189.

Midtown East	**212-758-7551**
515 Madison Avenue	at 53rd St.
NYC 10022	Mon.-Fri. 9-6:30, Thurs. 9-7, Sat. 9-6, Sun. 12-5

Midtown East	**212-949-9545**
363 Madison Avenue	at 45th St.
NYC 10017	Mon.-Fri. 9-6:30, Thurs. 9-7, Sat. 9-6, Sun. 12-5

Bottega Veneta M/W

This Italian company is all about quiet luxury. Cognoscenti have long shopped here for handbags, luggage, small leathergoods and shoes. Bottega Veneta hopes to reach a new breed of customer with the relaunch of their 1976 BV logo and the expansion of their relatively new ready-to-wear collection. Luxurious fabrics, tailored shapes and attention to detail define the Bottega Veneta label. Find lots of leather and suede, tweed and fitted pants, trenchcoats and even crocodile blazers. As for handbags and leathergoods, they're first-class, especially their trademark wovens and buttery soft leathers. Bottega Veneta combines sporty chic and understated elegance. 877-362-1715
www.bottegaveneta.com

Midtown East	**212-371-5511**
635 Madison Avenue	bet. 59/60th St.
NYC 10022	Mon.-Fri. 10-6, Sat. 11-6

Botticelli M/W

Located in the convenient Midtown area, Botticelli features Italian leather shoes under their own label. Find classic shoes for work, casual loafers for weekend wear and weatherproof boots for urban living or country getaways. Other styles include sandals, mules, sling-backs, fur-lined loafers, fashionable boots and evening shoes. Prices run from $195 to $595.

Fifth Avenue	**212-221-9075**
522 Fifth Avenue	bet. 43/44th St.
NYC 10036	Mon.-Fri. 10-7:30, Sat. 10-7, Sun. 11-5

Fifth Avenue	**212-586-7421**
666 Fifth Avenue (enter on 53rd St.)	bet. 5/6th Ave.
NYC 10103	Mon.-Sun. 10-7

Fifth Avenue (W) 212-582-6313
620 Fifth Avenue at Rockefeller Center
NYC 10020 Mon.-Sat. 10-7, Sun. 11-5

Boyd's Madison Avenue M/W
A good source for top-of-the-line European hair accessories. Find headbands, elaborate combs, clips, chinois pins, mink twisters, barrettes and more in simple and ornate designs. Brand names include Alexandre de Paris, Vuille and Francois Huchard. Excellent health and beauty products, including an extensive collection of cosmetics and perfumes. Other items include pashmina shawls selling for $250, jewelry and lingerie. Sales staff can be outright aggressive.

Upper East Side 212-838-6558
655 Madison Avenue bet. 60/61st St.
NYC 10021 Mon.-Fri. 8:30-7:30,
Sat. 9:30-7, Sun. 12-6

Bra Smythe W
A must for those in search of the perfect bra. Choose from over 1,500 styles with bra sizes that range from A to DDD cups. Custom fittings and alterations are their specialty. Also, find a good selection of undergarments from Hanro, Lise Charmel, Donna Karan, Chantelle and Wacoal. In addition, Bra Smythe features a nice collection of swimwear by makers like Karla Colletto, Rosa Ferrer and Domani.

Upper East Side 212-772-9400
905 Madison Avenue bet. 72/73rd St.
NYC 10021 Mon.-Sat. 10-7, Sun. 12-5

The Bridal Party-Dresses for Bridesmaids W
Owner Daphne Silverstein wants to dress your bridesmaids, whether your wedding is formal or informal. Although she stocks a full range of bridesmaid dresses, she loves the idea of using separates to outfit her clients, believing that "separates allow the bride to find clothes that flatter her bridesmaids no matter what body type." Looks range from full-length ballgown-styled skirts to knee-length skirts paired with a cashmere sweater.

Upper East Side 212-861-2318
243 East 82nd Street bet. 2/3rd Ave.
NYC 10028 Tues. & Wed. 11-7,
Thurs. 11-8, Fri. & Sat. 11-5

Bridge M/W
Bridge's leather collection is shown in two adjacent shops. One store sells lower priced merchandise, predominately leather jackets, while a slightly (and we do mean slightly) fancier one houses fashion forward looks in leather jackets, pants and coats. Labels include Red Kid, Ducksport and others. Prices are generally good.

Lower East Side 212-979-9777
98-100 Orchard Street bet. Broome/Delancey
NYC 10002 Sun.-Fri. 10-5:30

Brief Encounters W

Brief Encounters features a vast selection of American and European lingerie designers. Find everything from everyday basics to sexy, seductive underpinnings for evening. Labels include Lise Charmel, Kenzo, LeJaby, Gemma, Chantelle, Mystere, Natori and Calvin Klein. Custom fitting also available.

Upper West Side   **212-496-5649**
239 Columbus Avenue   at 71st St.
NYC 10023   Mon.-Fri. 10-7, Sat. 10-6, Sun. 1-6

Brioni M

For the past 50 years this Italian hand-tailored menswear house has dressed Hollywood's biggest stars, from Clark Gable and Gary Cooper to the latest James Bond, Pierce Brosnan. Classic sensibility, luxury fabrics and elegant European styling define the Brioni label. Choose from off-the-rack suits or custom order, then add an elegant, patterned dress shirt and lively tie. In addition, find sportswear, separates and outerwear. The look is tailored, sophisticated and stylish. Over-the-top prices. New this year: Brioni's newest suit silhouette "The Millennio". 800-444-1613

Midtown East   **212-376-5777**
57 East 57th Street   bet. Park/Madison Ave.
NYC 10022   Mon.-Sat. 10-6

Midtown East   **212-355-1940**
59 East 52nd Street   bet. Park/Madison Ave.
NYC 10022   Mon.-Sat. 9:30-6

☆ Brooks Brothers M/W/B

Brooks Brothers has made a quantum leap forward from the days when it outfitted prep school and Ivy League types. While this five-floor institution still features traditional, classic clothing for men, women, and boys, it has infused its line with sophistication and style. From men's furnishings, suits, formal wear, sportswear, shoes and accessories, the look is American, the cut classic, and the quality first-rate. Great for corduroy pants, cotton boxers, and dress shirts. Women will be pleasantly surprised by an entire department of updated classic clothing. While Brooks Brothers continues to satisfy their traditional customer, they are appealing to a younger, hipper clientele with casual clothing that is modern in color, cut, and style. Capri pants, cashmere sweater sets, T-shirts, and dresses in hot, vibrant colors are a big hit with this new generation of shoppers. Also find suits, shirts, skirts, pants, and jackets, as well as outerwear that is perfect for a "casual business" look. And for boys over age 5, tradition dictates a trip to Brooks Brothers for that first pair of gray flannels and navy blazer. www.brooksbrothers.com

Midtown East   **212-682-8800**
346 Madison Avenue   bet. 44/45th St.
NYC 10017   Mon.-Sat. 9-7, Thurs. 9-8, Sun. 12-6

Fifth Avenue   **212-261-9440**
666 Fifth Avenue   bet. 52/53rd St.
NYC 10103   Mon.-Fri. 10-8, Sat. 10-7, Sun. 11-7

Lower Manhattan 212-267-2400
One Liberty Plaza at Church St.
NYC 10006 Mon.-Fri. 8:30-6:30, Sat. 10-5,

Bruno Magli M/W

Catapulted to fame thanks to the O.J. Simpson trial, this quality Italian manufacturer is still basking in the limelight. Find a menswear collection of rubber-soled shoes, formal patent leather pumps, and lace-ups and loafer styles for business attire. For women, choose from classic feminine styles in supple leathers.

Fifth Avenue 212-752-7900
677 Fifth Avenue at 53rd St.
NYC 10022 Mon.-Fri. 10-6:30, Thurs. 10-7,
Sat. 10-6, Sun. 12-5

Bu and the Duck B/G

Inspired by American styles of the 30's, owner Susan Lane has created a clothing and toy collection that captures the innocence of children. Find wonderful crocheted sweaters from Peru, cotton dresses with crocheted tops, linen overalls and mini-skirts, and shirts made from kimonos. Accessories include shoes, delicately hand-embroidered quilts by Judy Boisson, stuffed animals, hair accessories, and vintage baby carriages. From newborn to 6 years.
www.buandtheduck.com

TriBeCa 212-431-9226
106 Franklin Street bet. W. B'way/Church
NYC 10013 Mon.-Sun. 10-7

Buffalo Chips USA M/W

Buffalo Chips specializes in custom, handmade western footwear from well-known Texas boot makers like Stallion, Ammons, Liberty and Tres Outlaw. In clothing, find leathers for rockers, cowboys, bikers and even Manhattan cliff dwellers. Ranch jackets, chaps, cowboy hats, silver belt buckles and alligator and lizard belts round out the assortment. Check out their table of bargain boots marked down 50%.

SoHo 212-625-8400
355 West Broadway bet. Broome/Grand
NYC 10013 Mon.-Wed. & Sat. 11-7,
Thurs. & Fri. 11-8, Sun. 12-6

Burberrys M/W

The sun is shining on this once stuffy, bland British design house whose claim to fame has always been its signature plaid-lined trenchcoat. Find career wear, sportswear and outerwear that combine English classic looks with Italian spirit. Burberrys has revitalized its image with a collection of wonderful tweeds, newly muted plaids and hipper design shapes. Designer Menichetti has successfully converted a once staid label into a promising chic brand. 800-284-8480

Midtown East 212-371-5010
9 East 57th Street bet. 5th/Madison Ave.
NYC 10022 Mon.-Fri. 9:30-7, Sat. 9:30-6, Sun. 12-5

Burlington Coat Factory M/W/C
One of retailing's unusual hybrids, off-price mass merchant and department store, Burlington Coat Factory continues to be a fast growing national chain. "More than just great coats," as their motto says, find career and sportswear, children's wear, maternity, plus sizes, shoes and baby furniture, all at discounted prices. Did we forget to mention a simply huge selection of coats? Carries all sizes including plus sizes. 800-444-2628

Chelsea   212-229-1300
707 Sixth Avenue   at 23rd St.
NYC 10011   Mon.-Sat. 9-9, Sun. 10-6

Caché W
More familiar to the suburban shopping mall set than confirmed city slickers, Caché is best for special-event eveningwear. Although Caché stocks the latest trends in its collection, expect most of its line to be manufactured in synthetic fabrics. Looks include spaghetti-strapped dresses, sequined little tops, and snug-fitting outfits perfect for club-hopping. A massive selection of coordinating jewelry rounds out their collection. 800-788-cache
www.cache.com

Midtown East   212-588-8719
805 Third Avenue   bet. 49/50th St.
NYC 10022   Mon.-Fri. 10-7, Sat. 10-6, Sun. 12-6

Calvin Klein M/W
Thirty-one years ago Calvin Klein started his company with an investment of $10,000, and today he has become both a commercial powerhouse and a respected designer. His secret: the marriage of design talent with provocative advertising campaigns. For years Klein has been a master at striking the perfect balance between uptown polish and downtown cool. Each collection presents updated fabric combinations, a neutral color palette and minimalist designs. Find a versatile line of ready-to-wear that includes sleek suits, fitted knits, shirts, dresses, skirts, relaxed sweaters, as well as eveningwear. Shoes and accessories round out the assortment. His fashions speak softly and simply, but are attention-grabbing nonetheless. Klein's secret: good things come in simple designs. 877-256-7373

Upper East Side   212-292-9000
654 Madison Avenue   at 60th St.
NYC 10021   Mon.-Sat. 10-6,
    Thurs. 10-8, Sun. 12-6

Calypso Enfants B/G
A delightful children's shop that carries top-of-the-line French clothing. Find an adorable layette selection with labels like Le Petit Bateau, as well as sailor outfits, jumpers, pleated skirts, dresses by Le Mona, knits with matching hats, outerwear, shoes and accessories. From newborn to size 8.

NoLiTa   212-965-8910
284 Mulberry Street   bet. Houston/Prince
NYC 10012   Mon.-Sat. 11-7, Sun. 12-6

☆ Calypso St. Barths   W/C

This French boutique opens new locations every year. One of New York's best shops for bright, spirited clothes by young French and American designers. Bursts of color (pinks, blues, reds, and oranges, but never black) and ethnic prints rule here. Find refreshing, feminine looks in bustle skirts, silk-sleeved shirts, cashmere sweaters, form-fitted tops, filmy blouses, T-shirts, swimwear, sarongs by Matilde, sandals, and accessories. Mix and match, dress up or down, and revel in all their colors. Fabulous accessories include beaded purses, boas and fun jewelry. These irresistible frocks also come for children. New this year: Calypso Beaute, a retail shop devoted to beauty and home products.

Upper East Side   212-535-4100
935 Madison Avenue   bet. 74/75th St.
NYC 10021   Mon.-Fri. 10-7, Sat. 10-6, Sun. 12-6

SoHo   212-274-0449
424 Broome Street   bet. Crosby/Lafayette
NYC 10013   Mon.-Sat. 11-7, Sun. 12-6

NoLiTa   212-965-0990
280 Mott Street   bet. Houston/Prince
NYC 10012   Mon.-Sat. 11-7, Sun. 11-8:30

NoLiTa   212-925-6544
280 Mulberry   bet. Houston/ Prince
NYC 10012   Mon.-Sat. 11-7, Sun. 12-6

Camouflage   M

Classic, contemporary and fashion forward all at once? Yes, a mix that works here. Find Dockers and Pendleton wool shirts among Helmut Lang, Mandarina Duck, Paul Smith, Armande Basi, Industria, Byblos, John Bartlett, C.P. Company and others. A door apart, one space offers casual, younger clothing, while the other carries more sophisticated, elegant items. Strong in outerwear, cashmere and accessories.

Chelsea   212-741-9118
139/141 Eighth Avenue   at 17th St.
NYC 10011   Mon.-Fri. 12-7, Sat. 11:30-6:30, Sun. 12-6

Camper   M/W

Since 1877, this Spanish company has been manufacturing shoes, and now they've opened a shop in the New World. The concept: develop shoes so pure that your every step feels as though you are walking barefoot. The result: ultra-hip, comfortable shoes that are scratch-resistant, equipped with light rubber soles and have special linings to absorb perspiration. Find modern sneakers similar to rugby shoes, clogs, sandals, and loafers.

SoHo   212-358-1841
125 Prince Street   at Wooster
NYC 10012   Mon.-Sat. 11-8, Sun. 12-6

Canal Jean Company M/W

Everyone should experience this 50,000-sq. ft store at least once. You name it, new or vintage, they've got it. A huge supply of Levi's, but also Calvin Klein, Union Bay, Silver and more. Prices range from $30 to $60. Casual wear includes T-shirts, denim shirts, vests, motorcycle jackets, outerwear and vintage clothing. The look is downtown and the price is right!

SoHo	**212-226-1130**
504 Broadway	bet. Spring/Broome
NYC 10012	Mon.-Sun. 9:30-9:30

☆ Canyon Beachwear W

This California institution has thankfully come East, and they've brought some super hot swimwear. Find a full range of styles and sizes in over a hundred different brand names. Shop for bikinis, thongs, one piece, tankinis and everything in between in the best color selection around. European and American brands include Manuel Canovas, Ann Cole, Calvin Klein, Delfina, Shan, Domani and more. Sarongs, matching cover-ups, sandals, beach totes and lotions complete the assortment. Sizes run from 0 to 22.

Upper East Side	**917-432-0732**
1136 Third Avenue	bet. 66/67th St.
NYC 10121	Mon.-Sat. 10-8, Sun. 11-6
Upper West Side	**212-441-4062**
311 Columbus Avenue	bet. 74/75th St.
NYC 10023	Mon.-Sat. 10-7, Sun. 11-6

Capezio M/W/C

Since 1887 the Capezio brand has caressed the feet of theatrical legends and dancers like Anna Pavlova, Fred Astaire and Bob Fosse. Today the company has expanded its horizons to include other dance-related items. Mothers can outfit their little girls in Capezio's pink leotards and ballet slippers, while ballerinas can shop for traditional dance apparel. Find leotards, leg warmers, leggings, tights, jazz pants, sweaters and more by makers like Danskin, City Lights, Marika, Baltog and, of course, Capezio. Footwear includes ballet slippers as well as tap, jazz and toe shoes. New this year: Tap sneakers and Capezio's line of fashion merchandise.

Upper East Side	**212-758-8833**
136 East 61st Street	bet. Lex./Park Ave.
NYC 10021	Mon.-Fri. 10-7, Sat. 11-6, Sun. 12-5
Upper East Side	**212-348-7210**
1651 Third Avenue, 3rd Fl.	bet. 92/93rd St.
NYC 10028	Mon.-Fri. 9-6, Sat. 9-4
Midtown West	**212-245-2130**
1650 Broadway, 2nd Fl.	at 51st St.
NYC 10019	Mon.-Fri. 9:30-7, Sat. 9:30-6:30, Sun. 11:30-5
Midtown West	**212-586-5140**
1776 Broadway, 2nd Fl.	at 57th St.
NYC 10019	Mon.-Fri. 10-7, Sat. 10-6

☆ Carolina Herrera   W

New Yorkers can rejoice now that Carolina Herrera has opened up shop. Occupying the former Givenchy space, Herrera brings a new level of sophistication to Madison Avenue. "Back to basics" is the underlying theme of her collection of traditional, feminine silhouettes. Her ready-to-wear line includes "the perfect suit" in form-fitted stretch wools, boucle jackets paired with flared lean skirts and tailored pants, cashmere sweater wraps, and silk crepe blouses. In eveningwear Herrera designs unapologetic "entrance-makers" that can be a richly embroidered dress or a simple crepe gown. Getting married soon? Look for the grand staircase that leads you to her bridal boutique. Accessories include handbags, sunglasses and scarves.

Upper East Side	212-249-6552
954 Madison Avenue	at 74th Street
NYC 10021	Mon.-Sat. 10-6

Cashmere Cashmere   M/W

A good source for Italian and Scottish cashmere. Find a collection of classic styles that include twin sets, turtlenecks, cardigans, crew necks, and pants. Accessories include socks, cape shawls, stoles, gloves, scarves and blankets.

Upper East Side	212-988-5252
965 Madison Avenue	bet. 75/76th St.
NYC 10021	Mon.-Sat. 10-6

Cashmere New York   M/W

With shops in all the jet set resorts, Cashmere New York is where the terminally chic shop for Scottish and Italian cashmere. Choose from an abundance of styles available in 53 glorious shades. From your basic turtleneck and twin set to a fashionable satin-trimmed sweater, find the highest standards in quality and design. This shop is the crème de la crème for cashmere seekers.

Upper East Side	212-744-3500
1100 Madison Avenue	bet. 82/83rd St.
NYC 10028	Mon.-Sat. 10-6

Catherine   W

Enter this cheery Soho shop and find an eclectic mix of clothing and "objets" for the home. Owner and designer Catherine Malandrino is known for her passion for color and flirtatious femininity. Browse a ready-to-wear line named "Catherine," featuring designs with elusive looks and feminine flair. Choose from knitted skirts, dresses, leathers, thick woven sweaters, camisoles, pants, fuzzy tops and more. Accessories include silk embroidered and beaded shawls and hats.

SoHo	212-925-6765
468 Broome Street	at Greene
NYC 10013	Mon.-Sat. 11-7, Sun. 12-7

Catimini   B/G
Catamini, a French import, brings to New York its playful collection of comfortable children's clothing. Screen-printed fabrics, full of whimsy and charm, great pants, jackets, separates and outerwear. It's fun, casual clothing that children will love wearing. From newborn to age 10.

Upper East Side   212-987-0688
1284 Madison Avenue   bet. 91/92nd St.
NYC 10128   Mon.-Sat. 10-6, Sun. 12-5

Celine   W
These days there's nobody busier than designer Michael Kors. He's taken over the helm of this venerable French retailer, moved it to Madison Avenue and launched his own collection—and yet it all seems to come naturally for one of today's most talented designers. Luxury fabrics, attention to detail and design subtleties define the Celine label, and it continues to attract women of all age groups, from the ladies who lunch crowd to young Park Avenue socialites on-the-go. Find a collection of ready-to-wear, leathergoods and accessories that combine looks of sleek practicality with urban chic. Kors' formula: enabling women to dress comfortably without "dressing down." Great sales.

Upper East Side   212-486-9700
667 Madison Avenue   bet. 60/61st Street
NYC 10021   Mon.-Sat. 10-6

Century 21   M/W/C
At this discount department store for the entire family, featuring sportswear, career wear, casual basics and shoes, you might just stumble across a boffo designer label like Armani, Versace or Ralph Lauren. Cosmetics, housewares, linens, appliances and electronics round out the assortment.

Lower Manhattan   212-227-9092
22 Cortland Street   bet. Church/B'way
NYC 10007   Mon.-Fri. 7:45-8, Thurs. 7:45-8:30,
                                       Sat. 10-7:30, Sun. 11-6

Cerruti   M/W
Leave it to this design house to dress today's modern man and woman in stylish, discreetly glamorous urban clothes. Shop a four-floor luxury boutique featuring ready-to-wear collections, "Arte" and "Cerruti 1881." Men can choose from classic and modern suits, sportswear, outerwear, tuxedos, shoes and accessories, styled in sensible shapes and luxurious fabrics. Designer Peter Speliopoulos' women's collection features girlish suits, pleated skirts and dresses, coats, knits, as well as a collection of shoes made exclusively for Cerruti by Manolo Blahnik. Think Prada meets Armani.

Upper East Side   212-327-2222
789 Madison Avenue   at 67th St.
NYC 10021   Mon.-Sat. 10-6, Thurs. 10-7

Cesare Paciotti
M/W

With their signature silver dagger logo stamped or affixed to many of their footwear styles, you'll always be reminded that you're wearing a pair of Cesare Paciotti shoes. Paciotti showcases a collection of sexy stiletto heeled shoes, pumps, flats and boots, with toes as pointed and sharp as their dagger. For men find a slightly tamer selection of shoes and boots better suited to artsy pursuits than Wall Street types.

Upper East Side 212-452-1222
833 Madison Avenue bet. 69/70th St.
NYC 10021 Mon.-Sat. 10:30-6:30

Champs
M/W/C

Whether it's golf, soccer, basketball, racquet sports, running, billiards or darts, Champs is happy to accommodate you. Find a large sneaker department for the whole family, as well as team logo'd jerseys and sweats. Best for boys and men. 800-991-6813

Midtown West 212-757-3638
1381-99 Sixth Avenue at 56th St.
NYC 10019 Mon.-Sat. 9-9, Sun. 11-6

Lower Manhattan 212-406-6944
89 South Street at South Street Seaport
NYC 10038 Mon.-Sat. 10-9, Sun. 11-8

Chanel
W

Chanel continues to be one of the world's top status symbols, and no wardrobe is apparently complete without a set of interlocking C's. Since 1999 designer Karl Lagerfeld, a/k/a the Kaiser of Couture, has pushed to modernize the house of Chanel for future generations. Find a ready-to-wear collection that epitomizes Lagerfeld's strict design standards. His clothes must be "beautiful, wearable, understandable and interesting all in one." Chanel features stylish suits, lean coats worn over dresses and skirts, jackets, blouses and separates, as well as elegant eveningwear and shoes. Although a Chanel design is classic, Lagerfeld never fails to give a hint of something trendier. The ne plus ultra is, of course, the Chanel handbags, true icons in the fashion world and the pride of every woman's wardrobe. Cosmetics and fragrances also available.   800-550-3638

Midtown East 212-355-5050
15 East 57th Street bet. 5th/Madison
NYC 10022 Mon.-Wed., Fri. 10-6:30,
Thurs. 10-7, Sat. 10-6

Charles Jourdan
W

Need to add a little kick to your wardrobe? Shop this French shoe retailer for its diverse collection of shoes. A Charles Jourdan design is about color, sex appeal and high heels. Find evening shoes, eye-catching pumps, platforms, wedges, flats, sandals and more. If you're in the market for a pair of "statement" shoes, step into Charles Jourdan. 800-997-2717

Cheo Tailors

Upper East Side   212-585-2238
777 Madison Avenue   bet. 66/67th St.
NYC 10021   Mon.-Sat. 10-7, Sun. 12-5

Cheo Tailors M/W
Favored by social register types, Cheo Tailors specializes in classic Saville-Row suits in luxurious European fabrics with excellent tailoring. Six to eight week delivery with an average cost of $3,000.

Upper East Side   212-980-9838
30 East 60th Street   bet. Madison/Park Ave.
NYC 10022   Mon.-Fri. 10-6

Cherry M/W
Cherry's features an eclectic mix of merchandise, from modernist furnishings to vintage apparel and accessories. Their vintage collection (spanning the 50's to the 80's) features leather jackets, denim, Pucci print shirts, suedes, shirts, belts and more. Labels include Gucci, Courreges, Missoni, Yves Saint Laurent and shoes by Joseph La Rose, a renowned 50's designer whose shoes were often worn by celebrities.

Lower East Side   212-358-7131
185 Orchard Street   bet. Houston/Stanton
NYC 10002   Mon.-Wed. 1-8,
Thurs.-Sat. 1-10, Sun. 1-8

The Children's Place B/G
This chain's new stores has been popping up all over New York. Find lots of casual basics like jeans, T-shirts, dresses, pants, shorts, sweats and more. It's all under The Children's Place label at bargain prices. Fabric and quality aren't built to last. From newborn to size 16.

Upper East Side   212-831-5100
173 East 86th Street   bet. Lexington/Third Ave.
NYC 10028   Mon.-Sat. 9-9, Sun.11-6

Upper West Side   917-441-9807
2187 Broadway   at 77th St.
NYC 10024   Mon.-Sat. 9-8, Sun. 9-6

Upper West Side   917-441-2374
2039 Broadway   bet. Amsterdam/70th St.
NYC 10023   Mon.-Fri. 9-8, Sat.11-6, Sun. 12-5

Midtown West   212-398-4416
1460 Broadway   bet. 41/42nd St.
NYC 10035   Mon-Fri. 9:30-7, Sat. 10-7, Sun 11-6

Midtown West   212-268-7696
901 Sixth Avenue   bet. 32/33rd Street
at Manhattan Mall   Level C2
NYC 10001   Mon.-Sat. 9-8, Sun. 11-6

Lower Manhattan   212-432-6100
400 World Trade Center   bet. Liberty/Church
Concourse Level
NYC 10048   Mon.-Fri. 7:30-8, Sat. 11-6

Flatiron   212-529-2201
36 Union Square East   at 16th St.
NYC 10003   Mon.-Sat. 10-7, Sun. 11-6

Chloe   W

At the age of 25, Stella McCartney (Sir Paul's daughter) took the helm at this legendary French couture house, and rejuvenated its image. Women shop here for fashions that fuse femininity and wearability with edgy attitude. Find trouser suits with Saville Row tailoring, dresses, halter tops, knitwear, coats, jeans and eveningwear that are designed to be mixed and matched for the workplace or a glam night out. A Chloe creation is about accentuating the body (sexy, but not aggressive), attention to detail, and a mix of color and fabric combinations. Accessories include shoes, handbags, sunglasses and perfume.

Upper East Side   212-717-8220
850 Madison Avenue   at 70th St.
NYC 10021   Mon.-Sat. 10-6

Christian Dior   W

At the base of the new LVMH tower sits the new, glamorous digs of Christian Dior. This 6,000-sq. ft. interior is modern and clean. The first floor is devoted to handbags, small leathergoods, scarves, eyeglasses, cosmetics and fragrances, as well as an elegant shoe salon at the back. A dramatic, angular staircase leads up to the ready-to-wear floor. Find casual items like denim and knitwear, formal day attire, beautiful eveningwear and furs. Each collection expresses Galliano's passion for design. Inspired by the history of costume, John Galliano has mastery of fabric and complex cutting methods. Ultra feminine, romantic and slightly decadent is the mood of Dior's sophisticated designs.
www.dior.com

Midtown East   212-931-2950
19 East 57th St.   bet. 5th/Madison Ave.
NYC 10022   Mon.-Sat. 10-6, Thurs. 10-7, Sun. 11-5

Christian Louboutin   W

This Parisian designer's arrival in New York is sure to send the girls running for a pair of his fanciful shoes. Christian Louboutin says he aspires to looks that run from "stateside chic" to "frivolous sleek," and that his trademark red soles give women "an invitation to flirt." Shop for mules, embroidered flats, moccasins trimmed in mink, gray flannel spectator pumps, pony skin boots and evening stunners made from Charvet tie fabrics. Louboutin's ultra feminine collection runs from sensible day shoes to fantastic designs with offbeat detailing. Prices range from $350 to $650. And if you're really ready to splurge, check out Louboutin's classic crocodile pumps for a mere $2,000.

Upper East Side   212-396-1884
941 Madison Avenue   bet. 74/75th St.
NYC 10021   Mon.-Sat. 10-6

Christie Brothers Furs W
A discount retailer of luxury fur coats. Find a selection of mink, shearling, Russian sable, as well as cashmere and microfiber coats that can be custom-lined and fitted with the fur of your choosing. In-house storage facilities also available.

Chelsea 212-736-6944
333 Seventh Avenue, 11th Fl. bet. 28/29th St.
NYC 10001 Mon.-Fri. 9-5 and by appointment

Christine Ganeaux W
Christine Ganeaux attracts all sorts of chic New Yorkers to her streamlined downtown shop. In fact, she's giving ultra-hip, downtown designer Daryl K some serious competition with her bootleg cut pants. Her collection stresses casual, urban chic with modern sensibility. Find silk dresses, slinky knits, leather trenchcoats, pants that fit like a dream, waxed motor cross jackets and more. It's uncomplicated clothing in body skimming shapes with a dash of sex appeal. Best Bet: leathers.

SoHo 212-431-4462
45 Crosby Street bet. Spring/Broome
NYC 10012 Mon.-Sat. 11-6,
Sun. 12-6 or by appointment

Christopher Totman M/W
Christopher Totman successfully brings New Yorkers a clothing collection infused with a strong South American flavor. Find fashions in colorful Guatemalan stripes, hand-loomed fabrics, circular crochets and alpaca knits. Choose from his trademark single-seam long skirt ("LaLunaskirt"), gauze shirts, dresses, hand-knit pima cotton sweaters and more. It's clothing that involves an extensive use of handwork with ethnic flavor.

NoLiTa 212-925-7495
262 Mott Street bet. Houston/Prince
NYC 10012 Mon.-Sat. 11-7, Sun. 12-7

Chuckies W
A small boutique featuring up-to-the-minute footwear fashions that will have you walking the streets in high style. Find designer labels by Jimmy Choo, Sergio Rossi, Casadei, Miu Miu, L'Autre Chose, Cynthia Rowley and more. An excellent source for fun, funky and glamorous shoes that you won't find anywhere else.

Upper East Side 212-593-9898
1073 Third Avenue bet. 63/64th St.
NYC 10021 Mon.-Fri. 10:45-7:45,
Sat. 11-6:30, Sun. 12:30-5:30

SoHo 212-343-1717
399 West Broadway bet. Spring/Broome
NYC 10012 Mon.-Sat. 11-7:30, Sun. 12-8

Chuck Roaste M/W

Japanese designer Toshi Hosogai, who earned the moniker Chuck Roaste in the 80's from his good friend Andy Warhol, has opened his eponymous shop. Find his signature reversible jean collection retailing at $135, as well as jackets, vests, capri and stretch jeans, graphic T-shirts, baseball caps and canvas tote bags.

Lower East Side 212-375-8655
49 Clinton Street bet. Rivington/Stanton
NYC 10002 Wed.-Sun. 12-7,
Mon. & Tues. by appt. only

Church's English Shoes M

When it comes to men's shoes, no one does it better than the English. For 125 years, Church's has been recognized the world over for classic, bench-made shoes. (Last year, Prada, Italy's trendiest fashion house, purchased the company; let's hope that they preserve Church's tradition of quality.) The sophisticated executive shops here for footwear. Choose from two collections with styles that include plain-toe oxfords, banker shoes, slip-ons, tie-up wingtips, traditional five-eyelet bluchers, loafers and moccasins. Prices run from $180 to $800. Six-month delivery for custom orders. Great sales. 800-221-4540 www.churchsshoes.com

Midtown East 212-755-4313
428 Madison Avenue at 49th St.
NYC 10017 Mon.-Fri. 9-7, Sat. 9-6, Sun. 12-5

Cinco W

Owned by the ultra-hip boutique Precision, Cinco features a similar collection and is packed to the rafters with American and European hip labels like Michael Stars, Tark, Momba, 3 Dot, Diab'less and more. Mix and match different labels and create a look that will have you running with New York's young trendsters.

Upper East Side 212-794-3826
960 Lexington Avenue at 70th St.
NYC 10021 Mon.-Fri. 10-7, Sat. 11-7, Sun. 12-6:30

Citishoes M

Citishoes is popular with midtown executives, as well as tourists staying at neighboring hotels. Packed with every brand name dress shoe imaginable, including Cole-Haan, Alden, Allen-Edmonds, Bally, Bruno Magli and Rockport. We simply defy you to leave empty handed.

Midtown East 212-751-3200
445 Park Avenue bet. 56/57th St.
NYC 10022 Mon.-Fri. 9:30-6:30, Sat. 10:30-5:30

CK Calvin Klein Shoes and Bags M/W

Welcome to Calvin Klein's SoHo shop devoted to shoes and bags. The up-to-the-minute selection will appeal to gen-xers and baby boomers alike. Find affordably priced loafers, lace-ups, sandals, mules, boots and pumps in leather, suede, patent leather and plastic. Accessories include leather jackets, belts, handbags and socks.

SoHo   **212-505-3549**
133 Prince Street   bet. Wooster/W.B'way
NYC 10012   Mon.-Thurs. 11-8,
Fri. & Sat. 10-8, Sun. 11-7

Claire Blaydon   W

This bright, sunny shop is filled with Blaydon's signature collection of restructured knitwear, jersey tops, lacy dresses, skirts and accessories. She uses delicate trimmings and silk embroidered borders to enhance the fronts, collars and cuffs of all her tops and sweaters making each a one-of-kind piece. While some may balk at the price of a trimmed T-shirt ($95), it's hard to resist adding one of her sweaters to your closet. Accessories include jewelry, handbags, hats and gloves.

NoLiTa   **212-219-1490**
202A Mott Street   bet. Spring/Kenmare
NYC 10012   Mon.-Sat. 11-7, Sun. 12-6

Clifford Michael Design   W

Clifford Michael specializes in silk dressings for special occasions and mothers-of-the-bride. Find simple and elaborate gowns, long flowing taffeta skirts with matching tops, tuxedo and dressy evening suits, as well as coordinating handbags and silk scarves. Upstairs choose from a collection of leathers and shearlings.

Upper East Side   **212-888-7665**
45 East 60th Street   bet. Madison/Park
NYC 10022   Mon.-Fri. 10-6:30, Thurs. 10-7,
Sat. 10-6, Sun. 12-5

Club Monaco   M/W

Yes, you'd rather have designer labels in your closet, but let's face it, you're about maxed out on your credit cards. So let Club Monaco, a Canadian-based company owned by fashion tycoon Ralph Lauren, come to your rescue. Find high-fashion pieces and the latest runway trend looks mixed with sportswear that includes pants, jackets, tees, dresses, shirts and more. Club Monaco is a consistently good source for fresh young looks at affordable prices.
www.clubmonaco.com

Upper East Side   **212-355-2949**
1111 Third Avenue   at 65th St.
NYC 10021   Mon.-Sat. 11-7, Sun. 12-5

Upper West Side   **212-579-2587**
2376 Broadway   at 87th St.
NYC 10024   Mon.-Sat. 10-8, Sun. 12-6

Fifth Avenue   **opening in September**
699 Fifth Avenue   bet. 54/55th St.
NYC 10022   Mon.-Sat. 10-6 Sun. 12-5

Fifth Avenue (W)   212-582-6313
620 Fifth Avenue   at Rockefeller Center
NYC 10020   Mon.-Sat. 10-7, Sun. 11-5

Boyd's Madison Avenue   M/W

A good source for top-of-the-line European hair accessories. Find headbands, elaborate combs, clips, chinois pins, mink twisters, barrettes and more in simple and ornate designs. Brand names include Alexandre de Paris, Vuille and Francois Huchard. Excellent health and beauty products, including an extensive collection of cosmetics and perfumes. Other items include pashmina shawls selling for $250, jewelry and lingerie. Sales staff can be outright aggressive.

Upper East Side   212-838-6558
655 Madison Avenue   bet. 60/61st St.
NYC 10021   Mon.-Fri. 8:30-7:30,
          Sat. 9:30-7, Sun. 12-6

Bra Smythe   W

A must for those in search of the perfect bra. Choose from over 1,500 styles with bra sizes that range from A to DDD cups. Custom fittings and alterations are their specialty. Also, find a good selection of undergarments from Hanro, Lise Charmel, Donna Karan, Chantelle and Wacoal. In addition, Bra Smythe features a nice collection of swimwear by makers like Karla Colletto, Rosa Ferrer and Domani.

Upper East Side   212-772-9400
905 Madison Avenue   bet. 72/73rd St.
NYC 10021   Mon.-Sat. 10-7, Sun. 12-5

The Bridal Party-Dresses for Bridesmaids   W

Owner Daphne Silverstein wants to dress your bridesmaids, whether your wedding is formal or informal. Although she stocks a full range of bridesmaid dresses, she loves the idea of using separates to outfit her clients, believing that "separates allow the bride to find clothes that flatter her bridesmaids no matter what body type." Looks range from full-length ballgown-styled skirts to knee-length skirts paired with a cashmere sweater.

Upper East Side   212-861-2318
243 East 82nd Street   bet. 2/3rd Ave.
NYC 10028   Tues. & Wed. 11-7,
          Thurs. 11-8, Fri. & Sat. 11-5

Bridge   M/W

Bridge's leather collection is shown in two adjacent shops. One store sells lower priced merchandise, predominately leather jackets, while a slightly (and we do mean slightly) fancier one houses fashion forward looks in leather jackets, pants and coats. Labels include Red Kid, Ducksport and others. Prices are generally good.

Lower East Side   212-979-9777
98-100 Orchard Street   bet. Broome/Delancey
NYC 10002   Sun.-Fri. 10-5:30

Brief Encounters W

Brief Encounters features a vast selection of American and European lingerie designers. Find everything from everyday basics to sexy, seductive underpinnings for evening. Labels include Lise Charmel, Kenzo, LeJaby, Gemma, Chantelle, Mystere, Natori and Calvin Klein. Custom fitting also available.

Upper West Side	**212-496-5649**
239 Columbus Avenue	at 71st St.
NYC 10023	Mon.-Fri. 10-7, Sat. 10-6, Sun. 1-6

Brioni M

For the past 50 years this Italian hand-tailored menswear house has dressed Hollywood's biggest stars, from Clark Gable and Gary Cooper to the latest James Bond, Pierce Brosnan. Classic sensibility, luxury fabrics and elegant European styling define the Brioni label. Choose from off-the-rack suits or custom order, then add an elegant, patterned dress shirt and lively tie. In addition, find sportswear, separates and outerwear. The look is tailored, sophisticated and stylish. Over-the-top prices. New this year: Brioni's newest suit silhouette "The Millennio". 800-444-1613

Midtown East	**212-376-5777**
57 East 57th Street	bet. Park/Madison Ave.
NYC 10022	Mon.-Sat. 10-6
Midtown East	**212-355-1940**
59 East 52nd Street	bet. Park/Madison Ave.
NYC 10022	Mon.-Sat. 9:30-6

★ Brooks Brothers M/W/B

Brooks Brothers has made a quantum leap forward from the days when it outfitted prep school and Ivy League types. While this five-floor institution still features traditional, classic clothing for men, women, and boys, it has infused its line with sophistication and style. From men's furnishings, suits, formal wear, sportswear, shoes and accessories, the look is American, the cut classic, and the quality first-rate. Great for corduroy pants, cotton boxers, and dress shirts. Women will be pleasantly surprised by an entire department of updated classic clothing. While Brooks Brothers continues to satisfy their traditional customer, they are appealing to a younger, hipper clientele with casual clothing that is modern in color, cut, and style. Capri pants, cashmere sweater sets, T-shirts, and dresses in hot, vibrant colors are a big hit with this new generation of shoppers. Also find suits, shirts, skirts, pants, and jackets, as well as outerwear that is perfect for a "casual business" look. And for boys over age 5, tradition dictates a trip to Brooks Brothers for that first pair of gray flannels and navy blazer. www.brooksbrothers.com

Midtown East	**212-682-8800**
346 Madison Avenue	bet. 44/45th St.
NYC 10017	Mon.-Sat. 9-7, Thurs. 9-8, Sun. 12-6
Fifth Avenue	**212-261-9440**
666 Fifth Avenue	bet. 52/53rd St.
NYC 10103	Mon.-Fri. 10-8, Sat. 10-7, Sun. 11-7

Lower Manhattan   212-267-2400
One Liberty Plaza   at Church St.
NYC 10006   Mon.-Fri. 8:30-6:30, Sat. 10-5,

Bruno Magli   M/W

Catapulted to fame thanks to the O.J. Simpson trial, this quality Italian manufacturer is still basking in the limelight. Find a menswear collection of rubber-soled shoes, formal patent leather pumps, and lace-ups and loafer styles for business attire. For women, choose from classic feminine styles in supple leathers.

Fifth Avenue   212-752-7900
677 Fifth Avenue   at 53rd St.
NYC 10022   Mon.-Fri. 10-6:30, Thurs. 10-7,
    Sat. 10-6, Sun. 12-5

Bu and the Duck   B/G

Inspired by American styles of the 30's, owner Susan Lane has created a clothing and toy collection that captures the innocence of children. Find wonderful crocheted sweaters from Peru, cotton dresses with crocheted tops, linen overalls and mini-skirts, and shirts made from kimonos. Accessories include shoes, delicately hand-embroidered quilts by Judy Boisson, stuffed animals, hair accessories, and vintage baby carriages. From newborn to 6 years.
www.buandtheduck.com

TriBeCa   212-431-9226
106 Franklin Street   bet. W. B'way/Church
NYC 10013   Mon.-Sun. 10-7

Buffalo Chips USA   M/W

Buffalo Chips specializes in custom, handmade western footwear from well-known Texas boot makers like Stallion, Ammons, Liberty and Tres Outlaw. In clothing, find leathers for rockers, cowboys, bikers and even Manhattan cliff dwellers. Ranch jackets, chaps, cowboy hats, silver belt buckles and alligator and lizard belts round out the assortment. Check out their table of bargain boots marked down 50%.

SoHo   212-625-8400
355 West Broadway   bet. Broome/Grand
NYC 10013   Mon.-Wed. & Sat. 11-7,
    Thurs. & Fri. 11-8, Sun. 12-6

Burberrys   M/W

The sun is shining on this once stuffy, bland British design house whose claim to fame has always been its signature plaid-lined trenchcoat. Find career wear, sportswear and outerwear that combine English classic looks with Italian spirit. Burberrys has revitalized its image with a collection of wonderful tweeds, newly muted plaids and hipper design shapes. Designer Menichetti has successfully converted a once staid label into a promising chic brand. 800-284-8480

Midtown East   212-371-5010
9 East 57th Street   bet. 5th/Madison Ave.
NYC 10022   Mon.-Fri. 9:30-7, Sat. 9:30-6, Sun. 12-5

Burlington Coat Factory   M/W/C

One of retailing's unusual hybrids, off-price mass merchant and department store, Burlington Coat Factory continues to be a fast growing national chain. "More than just great coats," as their motto says, find career and sportswear, children's wear, maternity, plus sizes, shoes and baby furniture, all at discounted prices. Did we forget to mention a simply huge selection of coats? Carries all sizes including plus sizes. 800-444-2628

Chelsea 212-229-1300
707 Sixth Avenue at 23rd St.
NYC 10011 Mon.-Sat. 9-9, Sun. 10-6

Caché   W

More familiar to the suburban shopping mall set than confirmed city slickers, Caché is best for special-event eveningwear. Although Caché stocks the latest trends in its collection, expect most of its line to be manufactured in synthetic fabrics. Looks include spaghetti-strapped dresses, sequined little tops, and snug-fitting outfits perfect for club-hopping. A massive selection of coordinating jewelry rounds out their collection.   800-788-cache
www.cache.com

Midtown East 212-588-8719
805 Third Avenue bet. 49/50th St.
NYC 10022 Mon.-Fri. 10-7, Sat. 10-6, Sun. 12-6

Calvin Klein   M/W

Thirty-one years ago Calvin Klein started his company with an investment of $10,000, and today he has become both a commercial powerhouse and a respected designer. His secret: the marriage of design talent with provocative advertising campaigns. For years Klein has been a master at striking the perfect balance between uptown polish and downtown cool. Each collection presents updated fabric combinations, a neutral color palette and minimalist designs. Find a versatile line of ready-to-wear that includes sleek suits, fitted knits, shirts, dresses, skirts, relaxed sweaters, as well as eveningwear. Shoes and accessories round out the assortment. His fashions speak softly and simply, but are attention-grabbing nonetheless. Klein's secret: good things come in simple designs.   877-256-7373

Upper East Side 212-292-9000
654 Madison Avenue at 60th St.
NYC 10021 Mon.-Sat. 10-6,
 Thurs. 10-8, Sun. 12-6

Calypso Enfants   B/G

A delightful children's shop that carries top-of-the-line French clothing. Find an adorable layette selection with labels like Le Petit Bateau, as well as sailor outfits, jumpers, pleated skirts, dresses by Le Mona, knits with matching hats, outerwear, shoes and accessories. From newborn to size 8.

NoLiTa 212-965-8910
284 Mulberry Street bet. Houston/Prince
NYC 10012 Mon.-Sat. 11-7, Sun. 12-6

☆ Calypso St. Barths W/C

This French boutique opens new locations every year. One of New York's best shops for bright, spirited clothes by young French and American designers. Bursts of color (pinks, blues, reds, and oranges, but never black) and ethnic prints rule here. Find refreshing, feminine looks in bustle skirts, silk-sleeved shirts, cashmere sweaters, form-fitted tops, filmy blouses, T-shirts, swimwear, sarongs by Matilde, sandals, and accessories. Mix and match, dress up or down, and revel in all their colors. Fabulous accessories include beaded purses, boas and fun jewelry. These irresistible frocks also come for children. New this year: Calypso Beaute, a retail shop devoted to beauty and home products.

Upper East Side 212-535-4100
935 Madison Avenue bet. 74/75th St.
NYC 10021 Mon.-Fri. 10-7, Sat. 10-6, Sun. 12-6

SoHo 212-274-0449
424 Broome Street bet. Crosby/Lafayette
NYC 10013 Mon.-Sat. 11-7, Sun. 12-6

NoLiTa 212-965-0990
280 Mott Street bet. Houston/Prince
NYC 10012 Mon.-Sat. 11-7, Sun. 11-8:30

NoLiTa 212-925-6544
280 Mulberry bet. Houston/ Prince
NYC 10012 Mon.-Sat. 11-7, Sun. 12-6

Camouflage M

Classic, contemporary and fashion forward all at once? Yes, a mix that works here. Find Dockers and Pendleton wool shirts among Helmut Lang, Mandarina Duck, Paul Smith, Armande Basi, Industria, Byblos, John Bartlett, C.P. Company and others. A door apart, one space offers casual, younger clothing, while the other carries more sophisticated, elegant items. Strong in outerwear, cashmere and accessories.

Chelsea 212-741-9118
139/141 Eighth Avenue at 17th St.
NYC 10011 Mon.-Fri. 12-7, Sat. 11:30-6:30, Sun. 12-6

Camper M/W

Since 1877, this Spanish company has been manufacturing shoes, and now they've opened a shop in the New World. The concept: develop shoes so pure that your every step feels as though you are walking barefoot. The result: ultra-hip, comfortable shoes that are scratch-resistant, equipped with light rubber soles and have special linings to absorb perspiration. Find modern sneakers similar to rugby shoes, clogs, sandals, and loafers.

SoHo 212-358-1841
125 Prince Street at Wooster
NYC 10012 Mon.-Sat. 11-8, Sun. 12-6

Canal Jean Company M/W

Everyone should experience this 50,000-sq. ft store at least once. You name it, new or vintage, they've got it. A huge supply of Levi's, but also Calvin Klein, Union Bay, Silver and more. Prices range from $30 to $60. Casual wear includes T-shirts, denim shirts, vests, motorcycle jackets, outerwear and vintage clothing. The look is downtown and the price is right!

SoHo 212-226-1130
504 Broadway bet. Spring/Broome
NYC 10012 Mon.-Sun. 9:30-9:30

☆ Canyon Beachwear W

This California institution has thankfully come East, and they've brought some super hot swimwear. Find a full range of styles and sizes in over a hundred different brand names. Shop for bikinis, thongs, one piece, tankinis and everything in between in the best color selection around. European and American brands include Manuel Canovas, Ann Cole, Calvin Klein, Delfina, Shan, Domani and more. Sarongs, matching cover-ups, sandals, beach totes and lotions complete the assortment. Sizes run from 0 to 22.

Upper East Side 917-432-0732
1136 Third Avenue bet. 66/67th St.
NYC 10121 Mon.-Sat. 10-8, Sun. 11-6

Upper West Side 212-441-4062
311 Columbus Avenue bet. 74/75th St.
NYC 10023 Mon.-Sat. 10-7, Sun. 11-6

Capezio M/W/C

Since 1887 the Capezio brand has caressed the feet of theatrical legends and dancers like Anna Pavlova, Fred Astaire and Bob Fosse. Today the company has expanded its horizons to include other dance-related items. Mothers can outfit their little girls in Capezio's pink leotards and ballet slippers, while ballerinas can shop for traditional dance apparel. Find leotards, leg warmers, leggings, tights, jazz pants, sweaters and more by makers like Danskin, City Lights, Marika, Baltog and, of course, Capezio. Footwear includes ballet slippers as well as tap, jazz and toe shoes. New this year: Tap sneakers and Capezio's line of fashion merchandise.

Upper East Side 212-758-8833
136 East 61st Street bet. Lex./Park Ave.
NYC 10021 Mon.-Fri. 10-7, Sat. 11-6, Sun. 12-5

Upper East Side 212-348-7210
1651 Third Avenue, 3rd Fl. bet. 92/93rd St.
NYC 10028 Mon.-Fri. 9-6, Sat. 9-4

Midtown West 212-245-2130
1650 Broadway, 2nd Fl. at 51st St.
NYC 10019 Mon.-Fri. 9:30-7, Sat. 9:30-6:30, Sun. 11:30-5

Midtown West 212-586-5140
1776 Broadway, 2nd Fl. at 57th St.
NYC 10019 Mon.-Fri. 10-7, Sat. 10-6

☆ Carolina Herrera   W

New Yorkers can rejoice now that Carolina Herrera has opened up shop. Occupying the former Givenchy space, Herrera brings a new level of sophistication to Madison Avenue. "Back to basics" is the underlying theme of her collection of traditional, feminine silhouettes. Her ready-to-wear line includes "the perfect suit" in form-fitted stretch wools, boucle jackets paired with flared lean skirts and tailored pants, cashmere sweater wraps, and silk crepe blouses. In eveningwear Herrera designs unapologetic "entrance-makers" that can be a richly embroidered dress or a simple crepe gown. Getting married soon? Look for the grand staircase that leads you to her bridal boutique. Accessories include handbags, sunglasses and scarves.

Upper East Side 212-249-6552
954 Madison Avenue at 74th Street
NYC 10021 Mon.-Sat. 10-6

Cashmere Cashmere   M/W

A good source for Italian and Scottish cashmere. Find a collection of classic styles that include twin sets, turtlenecks, cardigans, crew necks, and pants. Accessories include socks, cape shawls, stoles, gloves, scarves and blankets.

Upper East Side 212-988-5252
965 Madison Avenue bet. 75/76th St.
NYC 10021 Mon.-Sat. 10-6

Cashmere New York   M/W

With shops in all the jet set resorts, Cashmere New York is where the terminally chic shop for Scottish and Italian cashmere. Choose from an abundance of styles available in 53 glorious shades. From your basic turtleneck and twin set to a fashionable satin-trimmed sweater, find the highest standards in quality and design. This shop is the crème de la crème for cashmere seekers.

Upper East Side 212-744-3500
1100 Madison Avenue bet. 82/83rd St.
NYC 10028 Mon.-Sat. 10-6

Catherine   W

Enter this cheery Soho shop and find an eclectic mix of clothing and "objets" for the home. Owner and designer Catherine Malandrino is known for her passion for color and flirtatious femininity. Browse a ready-to-wear line named "Catherine," featuring designs with elusive looks and feminine flair. Choose from knitted skirts, dresses, leathers, thick woven sweaters, camisoles, pants, fuzzy tops and more. Accessories include silk embroidered and beaded shawls and hats.

SoHo 212-925-6765
468 Broome Street at Greene
NYC 10013 Mon.-Sat. 11-7, Sun. 12-7

Catimini   B/G
Catamini, a French import, brings to New York its playful collection of comfortable children's clothing. Screen-printed fabrics, full of whimsy and charm, great pants, jackets, separates and outerwear. It's fun, casual clothing that children will love wearing. From newborn to age 10.

Upper East Side   212-987-0688
1284 Madison Avenue   bet. 91/92nd St.
NYC 10128   Mon.-Sat. 10-6, Sun. 12-5

Celine   W
These days there's nobody busier than designer Michael Kors. He's taken over the helm of this venerable French retailer, moved it to Madison Avenue and launched his own collection—and yet it all seems to come naturally for one of today's most talented designers. Luxury fabrics, attention to detail and design subtleties define the Celine label, and it continues to attract women of all age groups, from the ladies who lunch crowd to young Park Avenue socialites on-the-go. Find a collection of ready-to-wear, leathergoods and accessories that combine looks of sleek practicality with urban chic. Kors' formula: enabling women to dress comfortably without "dressing down." Great sales.

Upper East Side   212-486-9700
667 Madison Avenue   bet. 60/61st Street
NYC 10021   Mon.-Sat. 10-6

Century 21   M/W/C
At this discount department store for the entire family, featuring sportswear, career wear, casual basics and shoes, you might just stumble across a boffo designer label like Armani, Versace or Ralph Lauren. Cosmetics, housewares, linens, appliances and electronics round out the assortment.

Lower Manhattan   212-227-9092
22 Cortland Street   bet. Church/B'way
NYC 10007   Mon.-Fri. 7:45-8, Thurs. 7:45-8:30,
                                   Sat. 10-7:30, Sun. 11-6

Cerruti   M/W
Leave it to this design house to dress today's modern man and woman in stylish, discreetly glamorous urban clothes. Shop a four-floor luxury boutique featuring ready-to-wear collections, "Arte" and "Cerruti 1881." Men can choose from classic and modern suits, sportswear, outerwear, tuxedos, shoes and accessories, styled in sensible shapes and luxurious fabrics. Designer Peter Speliopoulos' women's collection features girlish suits, pleated skirts and dresses, coats, knits, as well as a collection of shoes made exclusively for Cerruti by Manolo Blahnik. Think Prada meets Armani.

Upper East Side   212-327-2222
789 Madison Avenue   at 67th St.
NYC 10021   Mon.-Sat. 10-6, Thurs. 10-7

Cesare Paciotti
M/W

With their signature silver dagger logo stamped or affixed to many of their footwear styles, you'll always be reminded that you're wearing a pair of Cesare Paciotti shoes. Paciotti showcases a collection of sexy stiletto heeled shoes, pumps, flats and boots, with toes as pointed and sharp as their dagger. For men find a slightly tamer selection of shoes and boots better suited to artsy pursuits than Wall Street types.

Upper East Side   **212-452-1222**
833 Madison Avenue   bet. 69/70th St.
NYC 10021   Mon.-Sat. 10:30-6:30

Champs
M/W/C

Whether it's golf, soccer, basketball, racquet sports, running, billiards or darts, Champs is happy to accommodate you. Find a large sneaker department for the whole family, as well as team logo'd jerseys and sweats. Best for boys and men. 800-991-6813

Midtown West   **212-757-3638**
1381-99 Sixth Avenue   at 56th St.
NYC 10019   Mon.-Sat. 9-9, Sun. 11-6

Lower Manhattan   **212-406-6944**
89 South Street   at South Street Seaport
NYC 10038   Mon.-Sat. 10-9, Sun. 11-8

Chanel
W

Chanel continues to be one of the world's top status symbols, and no wardrobe is apparently complete without a set of interlocking C's. Since 1999 designer Karl Lagerfeld, a/k/a the Kaiser of Couture, has pushed to modernize the house of Chanel for future generations. Find a ready-to-wear collection that epitomizes Lagerfeld's strict design standards. His clothes must be "beautiful, wearable, understandable and interesting all in one." Chanel features stylish suits, lean coats worn over dresses and skirts, jackets, blouses and separates, as well as elegant eveningwear and shoes. Although a Chanel design is classic, Lagerfeld never fails to give a hint of something trendier. The ne plus ultra is, of course, the Chanel handbags, true icons in the fashion world and the pride of every woman's wardrobe. Cosmetics and fragrances also available.   800-550-3638

Midtown East   **212-355-5050**
15 East 57th Street   bet. 5th/Madison
NYC 10022   Mon.-Wed., Fri. 10-6:30,
    Thurs. 10-7, Sat. 10-6

Charles Jourdan
W

Need to add a little kick to your wardrobe? Shop this French shoe retailer for its diverse collection of shoes. A Charles Jourdan design is about color, sex appeal and high heels. Find evening shoes, eye-catching pumps, platforms, wedges, flats, sandals and more. If you're in the market for a pair of "statement" shoes, step into Charles Jourdan. 800-997-2717

Cheo Tailors

Upper East Side   **212-585-2238**
777 Madison Avenue   bet. 66/67th St.
NYC 10021   Mon.-Sat. 10-7, Sun. 12-5

Cheo Tailors   M/W

Favored by social register types, Cheo Tailors specializes in classic Saville-Row suits in luxurious European fabrics with excellent tailoring. Six to eight week delivery with an average cost of $3,000.

Upper East Side   **212-980-9838**
30 East 60th Street   bet. Madison/Park Ave.
NYC 10022   Mon.-Fri. 10-6

Cherry   M/W

Cherry's features an eclectic mix of merchandise, from modernist furnishings to vintage apparel and accessories. Their vintage collection (spanning the 50's to the 80's) features leather jackets, denim, Pucci print shirts, suedes, shirts, belts and more. Labels include Gucci, Courreges, Missoni, Yves Saint Laurent and shoes by Joseph La Rose, a renowned 50's designer whose shoes were often worn by celebrities.

Lower East Side   **212-358-7131**
185 Orchard Street   bet. Houston/Stanton
NYC 10002   Mon.-Wed. 1-8,
    Thurs.-Sat. 1-10, Sun. 1-8

The Children's Place   B/G

This chain's new stores has been popping up all over New York. Find lots of casual basics like jeans, T-shirts, dresses, pants, shorts, sweats and more. It's all under The Children's Place label at bargain prices. Fabric and quality aren't built to last. From newborn to size 16.

Upper East Side   **212-831-5100**
173 East 86th Street   bet. Lexington/Third Ave.
NYC 10028   Mon.-Sat. 9-9, Sun.11-6

Upper West Side   **917-441-9807**
2187 Broadway   at 77th St.
NYC 10024   Mon.-Sat. 9-8, Sun. 9-6

Upper West Side   **917-441-2374**
2039 Broadway   bet. Amsterdam/70th St.
NYC 10023   Mon.-Fri. 9-8, Sat.11-6, Sun. 12-5

Midtown West   **212-398-4416**
1460 Broadway   bet. 41/42nd St.
NYC 10035   Mon-Fri. 9:30-7, Sat. 10-7, Sun 11-6

Midtown West   **212-268-7696**
901 Sixth Avenue   bet. 32/33rd Street
at Manhattan Mall   Level C2
NYC 10001   Mon.-Sat. 9-8, Sun. 11-6

Lower Manhattan   **212-432-6100**
400 World Trade Center   bet. Liberty/Church
Concourse Level
NYC 10048   Mon.-Fri. 7:30-8, Sat. 11-6

Christian Louboutin

Flatiron 212-529-2201
36 Union Square East at 16th St.
NYC 10003 Mon.-Sat. 10-7, Sun. 11-6

Chloe W

At the age of 25, Stella McCartney (Sir Paul's daughter) took the helm at this legendary French couture house, and rejuvenated its image. Women shop here for fashions that fuse femininity and wearability with edgy attitude. Find trouser suits with Saville Row tailoring, dresses, halter tops, knitwear, coats, jeans and eveningwear that are designed to be mixed and matched for the workplace or a glam night out. A Chloe creation is about accentuating the body (sexy, but not aggressive), attention to detail, and a mix of color and fabric combinations. Accessories include shoes, handbags, sunglasses and perfume.

Upper East Side 212-717-8220
850 Madison Avenue at 70th St.
NYC 10021 Mon.-Sat. 10-6

Christian Dior W

At the base of the new LVMH tower sits the new, glamorous digs of Christian Dior. This 6,000-sq. ft. interior is modern and clean. The first floor is devoted to handbags, small leathergoods, scarves, eyeglasses, cosmetics and fragrances, as well as an elegant shoe salon at the back. A dramatic, angular staircase leads up to the ready-to-wear floor. Find casual items like denim and knitwear, formal day attire, beautiful eveningwear and furs. Each collection expresses Galliano's passion for design. Inspired by the history of costume, John Galliano has mastery of fabric and complex cutting methods. Ultra feminine, romantic and slightly decadent is the mood of Dior's sophisticated designs.
www.dior.com

Midtown East 212-931-2950
19 East 57th St. bet. 5th/Madison Ave.
NYC 10022 Mon.-Sat. 10-6, Thurs. 10-7, Sun. 11-5

Christian Louboutin W

This Parisian designer's arrival in New York is sure to send the girls running for a pair of his fanciful shoes. Christian Louboutin says he aspires to looks that run from "stateside chic" to "frivolous sleek," and that his trademark red soles give women "an invitation to flirt." Shop for mules, embroidered flats, moccasins trimmed in mink, gray flannel spectator pumps, pony skin boots and evening stunners made from Charvet tie fabrics. Louboutin's ultra feminine collection runs from sensible day shoes to fantastic designs with offbeat detailing. Prices range from $350 to $650. And if you're really ready to splurge, check out Louboutin's classic crocodile pumps for a mere $2,000.

Upper East Side 212-396-1884
941 Madison Avenue bet. 74/75th St.
NYC 10021 Mon.-Sat. 10-6

Christie Brothers Furs W
A discount retailer of luxury fur coats. Find a selection of mink, shearling, Russian sable, as well as cashmere and microfiber coats that can be custom-lined and fitted with the fur of your choosing. In-house storage facilities also available.

Chelsea 212-736-6944
333 Seventh Avenue, 11th Fl. bet. 28/29th St.
NYC 10001 Mon.-Fri. 9-5 and by appointment

Christine Ganeaux W
Christine Ganeaux attracts all sorts of chic New Yorkers to her streamlined downtown shop. In fact, she's giving ultra-hip, downtown designer Daryl K some serious competition with her bootleg cut pants. Her collection stresses casual, urban chic with modern sensibility. Find silk dresses, slinky knits, leather trenchcoats, pants that fit like a dream, waxed motor cross jackets and more. It's uncomplicated clothing in body skimming shapes with a dash of sex appeal. Best Bet: leathers.

SoHo 212-431-4462
45 Crosby Street bet. Spring/Broome
NYC 10012 Mon.-Sat. 11-6,
  Sun. 12-6 or by appointment

Christopher Totman M/W
Christopher Totman successfully brings New Yorkers a clothing collection infused with a strong South American flavor. Find fashions in colorful Guatemalan stripes, hand-loomed fabrics, circular crochets and alpaca knits. Choose from his trademark single-seam long skirt ("LaLunaskirt"), gauze shirts, dresses, hand-knit pima cotton sweaters and more. It's clothing that involves an extensive use of handwork with ethnic flavor.

NoLiTa 212-925-7495
262 Mott Street bet. Houston/Prince
NYC 10012 Mon.-Sat. 11-7, Sun. 12-7

Chuckies W
A small boutique featuring up-to-the-minute footwear fashions that will have you walking the streets in high style. Find designer labels by Jimmy Choo, Sergio Rossi, Casadei, Miu Miu, L'Autre Chose, Cynthia Rowley and more. An excellent source for fun, funky and glamorous shoes that you won't find anywhere else.

Upper East Side 212-593-9898
1073 Third Avenue bet. 63/64th St.
NYC 10021 Mon.-Fri. 10:45-7:45,
  Sat. 11-6:30, Sun. 12:30-5:30

SoHo 212-343-1717
399 West Broadway bet. Spring/Broome
NYC 10012 Mon.-Sat. 11-7:30, Sun. 12-8

CK Calvin Klein Shoes and Bags

Chuck Roaste M/W
Japanese designer Toshi Hosogai, who earned the moniker Chuck Roaste in the 80's from his good friend Andy Warhol, has opened his eponymous shop. Find his signature reversible jean collection retailing at $135, as well as jackets, vests, capri and stretch jeans, graphic T-shirts, baseball caps and canvas tote bags.

Lower East Side 212-375-8655
49 Clinton Street bet. Rivington/Stanton
NYC 10002 Wed.-Sun. 12-7,
Mon. & Tues. by appt. only

Church's English Shoes M
When it comes to men's shoes, no one does it better than the English. For 125 years, Church's has been recognized the world over for classic, bench-made shoes. (Last year, Prada, Italy's trendiest fashion house, purchased the company; let's hope that they preserve Church's tradition of quality.) The sophisticated executive shops here for footwear. Choose from two collections with styles that include plain-toe oxfords, banker shoes, slip-ons, tie-up wingtips, traditional five-eyelet bluchers, loafers and moccasins. Prices run from $180 to $800. Six-month delivery for custom orders. Great sales. 800-221-4540 www.churchsshoes.com

Midtown East 212-755-4313
428 Madison Avenue at 49th St.
NYC 10017 Mon.-Fri. 9-7, Sat. 9-6, Sun. 12-5

Cinco W
Owned by the ultra-hip boutique Precision, Cinco features a similar collection and is packed to the rafters with American and European hip labels like Michael Stars, Tark, Momba, 3 Dot, Diab'less and more. Mix and match different labels and create a look that will have you running with New York's young trendsters.

Upper East Side 212-794-3826
960 Lexington Avenue at 70th St.
NYC 10021 Mon.-Fri. 10-7, Sat. 11-7, Sun. 12-6:30

Citishoes M
Citishoes is popular with midtown executives, as well as tourists staying at neighboring hotels. Packed with every brand name dress shoe imaginable, including Cole-Haan, Alden, Allen-Edmonds, Bally, Bruno Magli and Rockport. We simply defy you to leave empty handed.

Midtown East 212-751-3200
445 Park Avenue bet. 56/57th St.
NYC 10022 Mon.-Fri. 9:30-6:30, Sat. 10:30-5:30

CK Calvin Klein Shoes and Bags M/W
Welcome to Calvin Klein's SoHo shop devoted to shoes and bags. The up-to-the-minute selection will appeal to gen-xers and baby boomers alike. Find affordably priced loafers,

lace-ups, sandals, mules, boots and pumps in leather, suede, patent leather and plastic. Accessories include leather jackets, belts, handbags and socks.

SoHo   **212-505-3549**
133 Prince Street   bet. Wooster/W.B'way
NYC 10012   Mon.-Thurs. 11-8,
Fri. & Sat. 10-8, Sun. 11-7

Claire Blaydon   W

This bright, sunny shop is filled with Blaydon's signature collection of restructured knitwear, jersey tops, lacy dresses, skirts and accessories. She uses delicate trimmings and silk embroidered borders to enhance the fronts, collars and cuffs of all her tops and sweaters making each a one-of-kind piece. While some may balk at the price of a trimmed T-shirt ($95), it's hard to resist adding one of her sweaters to your closet. Accessories include jewelry, handbags, hats and gloves.

NoLiTa   **212-219-1490**
202A Mott Street   bet. Spring/Kenmare
NYC 10012   Mon.-Sat. 11-7, Sun. 12-6

Clifford Michael Design   W

Clifford Michael specializes in silk dressings for special occasions and mothers-of-the-bride. Find simple and elaborate gowns, long flowing taffeta skirts with matching tops, tuxedo and dressy evening suits, as well as coordinating handbags and silk scarves. Upstairs choose from a collection of leathers and shearlings.

Upper East Side   **212-888-7665**
45 East 60th Street   bet. Madison/Park
NYC 10022   Mon.-Fri. 10-6:30, Thurs. 10-7,
Sat. 10-6, Sun. 12-5

Club Monaco   M/W

Yes, you'd rather have designer labels in your closet, but let's face it, you're about maxed out on your credit cards. So let Club Monaco, a Canadian-based company owned by fashion tycoon Ralph Lauren, come to your rescue. Find high-fashion pieces and the latest runway trend looks mixed with sportswear that includes pants, jackets, tees, dresses, shirts and more. Club Monaco is a consistently good source for fresh young looks at affordable prices.
www.clubmonaco.com

Upper East Side   **212-355-2949**
1111 Third Avenue   at 65th St.
NYC 10021   Mon.-Sat. 11-7, Sun. 12-5

Upper West Side   **212-579-2587**
2376 Broadway   at 87th St.
NYC 10024   Mon.-Sat. 10-8, Sun. 12-6

Fifth Avenue   **opening in September**
699 Fifth Avenue   bet. 54/55th St.
NYC 10022   Mon.-Sat. 10-6 Sun. 12-5

Coach

Flatiron   **212-352-0936**
160 Fifth Avenue   bet. 20/21st St.
NYC 10010   Mon.-Sat. 10-8, Sun. 12-7

SoHo   **212-533-8930**
121 Prince Street   bet. Wooster/Greene
NYC 10012   Mon.-Sat. 11-7, Sun. 12-6

SoHo   **212-941-1511**
520 Broadway   at Spring
NYC 10012   Mon.-Sat. 11-8, Sun. 12-7

Clyde's on Madison   M/W/C

In a city packed with cosmetic/drug/beauty stores, Clyde's is a standout. This redesigned luxury emporium features the finest American and European brands of cosmetics, fragrances, hair and skin care products, aromatherapy as well as toys, giftbaskets, candles, Alixandre de Paris hair accessories and more. Services they offer include a pharmacy, as well as an on-premise herbalist and nutritionist.   800-792-5933
www.clydesonmadison.com

Upper East Side   **212-744-5050**
926 Madison Avenue   bet. 73/74th St.
NYC 10021   Mon.-Fri. 9-7, Sat. 9-6

☆ Coach   M/W

With their newly redesigned stores, Coach is successfully redefining their image and attracting a new breed of younger and hipper customers. Shop for briefcases, handbags, travel bags and small leathergoods, manufactured in Coach's signature durable leather. Find shoulder bags, sleek clutches, cotton-twill travel totes and a collection of canvas bags trimmed in leather. Looks run from sporty chic to urban sleek. In addition, find a selection of leather jackets, wallets, belts, gloves, watches and umbrellas. Coach's designs have clean lines, can go anywhere and complement both casual and professional attire.   800-444-3611
www.coach.com

Upper West Side   **212-799-1624**
2321 Broadway   at 84th St.
NYC 10024   Mon.-Fri. 10-8, Sat. 10-7, Sun. 11-6

Midtown East   **212-754-0041**
595 Madison Avenue   at 57th St.
NYC 10022   Mon.-Sat. 10-8, Sun. 11-6

Midtown East   **212-599-4777**
342 Madison Avenue   bet. 43/44th St.
NYC 10017   Mon.-Fri. 8:30-7:30, Sat. 10-6, Sun. 11-5

Fifth Avenue   **212-245-4148**
620 Fifth Avenue   at Rockefeller Ctr.
NYC 10020   Mon.-Sat. 10-8, Sun. 11-7

Lower Manhattan   **212-488-0080**
5 World Trade Center   bet. Church/Vesey
NYC 10048   Mon.-Fri. 7:30-7:30, Sat. 11-6, Sun. 12-5

Coco & Z B/G
Affordable, adorable and an absolute must if you're shopping for children's wear on the West Side. Find casual and dress-up styles with upbeat looks. Fabrics often feature floral and animal motifs. From newborn to size 7.

Upper West Side   212-721-0415
222 Columbus Avenue   bet. 70/71st St.
NYC 10023   Mon.-Sat. 11-7, Sun. 12-6

Cole-Haan M/W
Cole-Haan specializes in quality career and weekend footwear. Styles are classic and timeless. Find a collection of loafers, rubber-soled shoes, boots, Italian dress shoes, sandals and more. Socks and belts also available.
800-488-2000   www.colehaan.com

Upper East Side   212-421-8440
667 Madison Avenue   at 61st St.
NYC 10021   Mon.-Sat. 10-7, Thurs. 10-8, Sun. 12-6

Fifth Avenue   212-765-9747
620 Fifth Avenue   at 50th St.
NYC 10020   Mon.-Sat. 10-7, Thurs. 10-8, Sun. 12-6

Comme des Garçons M/W
Previously occupied by an auto-body shop, this retail space has been transformed into a somewhat "trippy and disconcerting" space featuring an aluminum tunnel and foam covered walls. Designer Rei Kawakubo presents a ready-to-wear line long on intellectual and artistic interest, but short on comfort and wearability. Find shapes from the basic to the absurd, looks that will flatter and unflatter, and textiles that are wondrous in color and quality. Fabrics are used for one season only, making each collection a one-of-a-kind creation. This is avant-garde fashion taken to the extreme.

Chelsea   212-604-9200
520 West 22nd Street   bet. 10/11th Ave.
NYC 10011   Tues.-Sat. 11-7, Sun. 12-6

Conrad's Bike Shop M/W
Conrad's is for the elite cyclist who takes his biking seriously. Find everything from clothing, shoes, accessories, components and bicycles from top brand labels like Colnago, Serotta, Seven, DeRosa and Eddy Merckx. Price points range from $1,200 to $7,000. Best for pro-racing bikes.

Midtown East   212-697-6966
25 Tudor City Place   at 41st St.
NYC 10017   Mon.-Sat. 11-7

Cose Bella W
Located in a penthouse showroom, Cose Bella features a collection of sportswear, eveningwear and bridal attire. Designer Shannon McLean continues to please New Yorkers with her selection of clean, simple designs manufactured in luxury fabrics. Find pants, dresses, sweaters, as well as evening and bridal gowns. It's classic clothing with sporty elegance. Think a 90's Audrey Hepburn.

Couture by Jennifer Duke

Upper East Side   212-988-4210
7 East 81st St., 4th Fl.   bet. 5th/Madison Ave.
NYC 10028   Mon.-Fri. 10-6 by appointment only

Costume National   M/W

Costume National's dark interior of black walls serves as an ominous backdrop for designer Ennio Capasa's collection. Welcome to an androgynous world of retailing where the same design fabrications apply to both men and women. Find a ready-to-wear collection that is tailored, fitted and utilitarian. Like Prada, Costume National's use of high-tech fabrics creates looks that are modern, unconventional and always functional.

SoHo   212-431-1530
108 Wooster Street   bet. Prince/Spring
NYC 10012   Mon.-Sat. 11-7, Sun. 12-6

Country Road Australia   M/W

An Australian company that features career, sportswear and weekend wear. It's lifestyle-based clothing designed to give men and women a sense of ease and security. Find a collection of suits, coordinating separates, shirts, sweaters and pants in high-performance fabrics. Shoes and accessories round out the assortment. A good source for wardrobe essentials featuring classic urban looks. Great sales.
800-666-6677

Upper East Side   212-744-8633
1130 Third Avenue   bet. 66/67th St.
NYC 10021   Mon.-Wed., Fri. 9:30-7,
Thurs. 9:30-8, Sat. 10-6, Sun. 12-5

Midtown East   212-949-7380
335 Madison Avenue   bet. 43/44th St.
NYC 10017   Mon.-Fri. 9:30 -7, Thurs. 9:30-8,
Sat. 10-6, Sun. 12-5

Flatiron   212-366-6999
156 Fifth Avenue   bet. 20/21st St.
NYC 10010   Mon.-Fri. 10-8, Sat. 12-6, Sun. 12-5

SoHo   212-343-9544
411 West Broadway   bet. Prince/Spring
NYC 10012   Mon.-Sat. 10-8, Sun. 12-6

Lower Manhattan (Clearance Center)   212-248-0810
199 Water Street   at South Street Seaport
NYC 10038   Mon.-Sat. 10-7, Sun. 12-6

Couture by Jennifer Dule   W

Designer Jennifer Dule specializes in women's custom tailoring for "after five" and special occasion dressing, and bridal attire. Bring a photograph from a magazine and she'll copy it to a "T" or change it to your specifications. Pants average $350, while suits start at $1,200. An elaborate satin evening gown with lavish detailing will run you $3,000+.

Flatiron   212-777-2100
133 Fifth Avenue, 3rd Fl.   at 20th St.
NYC 10003   By appointment only

C. P. Shades   W

Carefree and comfortable defines C.P. Shades merchandise. Find dresses, skirts, pants and separates manufactured in easy-care fabrics. The C.P. Shade label is guaranteed to withstand the rigors of wash and wear. It's simple clothing designed with down-to-earth practicality. 800-900-9581

Upper East Side 212-759-5710
1119 Third Avenue bet. 65/66th St.
NYC 10021 Mon.-Sat. 11-7, Sun. 12-6

Upper West Side 212-724-9474
300 Columbus Avenue at 74th St.
NYC 10023 Mon.-Sat. 11-7, Sun. 12-6

SoHo 212-226-4434
154 Spring Street bet. Wooster/W. B'way
NYC 10012 Mon.-Sat. 11-7, Sun. 12-6

Crouch & Fitzgerald   M/W

Since opening its doors in 1939, Crouch and Fitzgerald has sold brand name leathergoods. Find a selection of handbags, luggage, small leathergoods, briefcases and belts. Labels include Ghurka, Longchamps, Goldpfeil, Tumi, Hartman, Dakota and private label. Their $69 handbag sale, held every August, is a must.

Midtown East 212-755-5888
400 Madison Avenue bet. 47/48th St.
NYC 10017 Mon.-Sat. 9-6

Crunch   M/W

This fitness facility also has its own shop packed with the "Crunch" workout wear label. Find fleece jackets, lycra outfits, leggings, mesh hockey jerseys, sweats, hats, unisex jazz pants, as well as bodywear and sportswear.

Upper West Side 212-875-1902
162 West 83rd St. bet. Columbus/Amsterdam
NYC 10024 Mon.-Fri. 5:30-11, Sat. & Sun. 8-9

Midtown East 212-758-3434
1109 Second Avenue bet. 58/59th St.
NYC 10022 Mon.-Thurs. 5-11, Fri. 5-10, Sat. 8:30-9

Midtown West 212-869-7788
144 West 38th St. bet. 7th/Broadway
NYC 10018 Mon.-Fri. 5:30-10, Sat. & Sun. 8-6

Midtown West 212-594-8050
560 West 43rd Street at 11th Ave.
NYC 10036 Mon.-Fri. 6-10, Sat. & Sun. 9-7

Flatiron 212-475-2018
54 East 13th Street bet. B'way/Univ. Pl.
NYC 10003 Mon.-Fri. 6-10, Sat. & Sun. 8-8

West Village 212-366-3725
152 Christopher Street bet. Washington/Greenwich
NYC 10014 Mon.-Fri. 6-11, Sat. & Sun. 8-9

SoHo 212-420-0507
623 Broadway at Houston St.
NYC 10012 Mon.-Fri. 6-12, Sat. 8-8, Sun. 9-8

	Daang Goodman
NoHo	212-614-0120
404 Lafayette	bet. Astor/E. 4th St.
NYC 10003	Mon.-Fri. open 24 hrs., Sat. to 9, Sun. 8-9

Custom Shop M/W

Who knew that custom could be so affordable? Since 1937 the Custom Shop has been making shirts for men and women, boasting prices from $80 to $140. Expect a six-week delivery with a four-shirt minimum. Also available: custom suits at $795. www.customshop.com

Midtown East	212-867-3650
338 Madison Avenue	at 44th St.
NYC 10173	Mon.-Fri. 9-7, Sat. 9-6
Midtown East	212-231-7701
599 Lexington Avenue	at 52nd St.
NYC 10022	Mon.-Fri. 9-7, Sat. 9-6
Fifth Avenue	212-245-2499
618 Fifth Avenue	at 49th St.
NYC 10020	Mon.-Fri. 9-6, Thurs. 9-8, Sat. 9-6
Lower Manhattan	212-480-2954
60 Wall Street	bet. Pine/Williams St.
NYC 10002	Mon.-Fri. 8:30-5:30

Cynthia Rowley W

The whimsical interior walls of Rowley's shop (decorated with slender, blushing girls making banal statements such as "Never share a dress!") carries the same sense of playfulness into her collections of "clothes full of spirited girlish antics." Find pants, dresses in floral prints, skirts, cozy separates, coats, shoes and accessories. Designs are fun, colorful and girlish. Rowley has a genius for combining feminine fantasy (sweet and flirtatious, not racy or trendy) with simple wearability.

SoHo	212-334-1144
112 Wooster Street	bet. Prince/Spring
NYC 10012	Mon.-Wed. & Sat. 11-7,
	Thurs. & Fri. 11-8, Sun. 12-6

Daang Goodman M/W

Daang Goodman offers a diversified collection of European lines that scream trend and funk. However, you will stumble across the occasional basic like a cotton T-shirt. Labels include M Collection, Tark, Wilson, E-play, Mandarina Duck, as well as Thai designer Daang Goodman's own line called Tripp. Choose from dresses, pants, funky tops made from silicon, bleached and dirty denim, animated cartoon T-shirts and more. It's a combination of street and clubwear for those whose fashion sense is "way out there!"

SoHo	212-226-7465
68 Greene St.	bet. Broome/Spring
NYC 10012	Mon.-Wed. 11-7, Thurs. 11-7:30, Sun. 12-6

Daffy's   M/W/C

One of New York's largest discount chains, Daffy's carries clothing for the entire family with discounts up to 80%. Find sportswear, outerwear, workout apparel, underwear, accessories and shoes. And if you're lucky, you might even come across a designer label like Hilfiger, Versace or Guess. Daffy's claims their prices are so low that "you'll be tempted to haggle them up."

Midtown East 212-376-4477
135 East 57th Street bet. Lex./Park
NYC 10022 Mon.-Fri. 10-8, Sat. 10-7, Sun. 11-6

Midtown East 212-557-4422
335 Madison Avenue at 44th St.
NYC 10017 Mon.-Fri. 8-8, Sat. 10-6, Sun. 12-6

Midtown West 212-736-4477
1311 Broadway bet. 33/34th St.
NYC 10013 Mon.-Fri. 10-9, Sat. 10-8, Sun. 11-7

Flatiron 212-529-4477
111 Fifth Avenue at 18th St.
NYC 10003 Mon.-Sat. 10-9, Sun. 12-7

SoHo 212-334-7444
462 Broadway at Grand
NYC 10012 Mon.-Thurs. 10:30-7:30,
Fri. & Sat. 10:30-8, Sun. 12-7

Dana Buchman   W

Dana Buchman is the bridge division of Liz Claiborne—a collection that caters to the executive woman in search of professional, polished looks. Shop three separate lines: "Luxe," featuring top-of-the-line dressy looks that have desk-to-dinner versatility; "Dana Buchman," devoted to careerwear and suitings; and "Casual," offering dress-down Friday and weekend wear. Mix and match from the different collections and give yourself endless dress combinations. Prices run higher than your standard Liz Claiborne lines.

Midtown East 212-319-3257
65 East 57th Street bet. Madison/Park
NYC 10022 Mon.-Fri. 10-7, Sat. 10-6, Sun. 12-5

Midtown East—Dana Buchman Petites 212-308-6429
57 East 57th Street bet. Madison/Park Ave.
NYC 10022 Mon.-Fri. 10-7, Sat. 10-6, Sun. 12-5

Danskin   W/C

Exclusively Danskin is the name of the game here. Find exercise, dance and active apparel that include leotards, leggings, unitards, tanks, sweatpants, as well as ballet and jazz shoes. In addition, choose from Danskin's selection of fashionable street-wear such as short skirts, slim-fitted dresses and slinky tops.

Upper West Side 212-724-2992
159 Columbus Avenue bet. 67/68th St.
NYC 10023 Mon.-Sat. 10-9, Sun. 11-8

Barbara Gee Danskin Center (outlet) W
Upper West Side 212-769-2923
2282 ½ Broadway bet. 82/83rd St.
NYC 10024 Mon.-Sat. 10:30-7:30, Sun. 1-6

Barbara Gee Danskin Center (outlet) W
Upper West Side 212-769-1564
2487 Broadway bet. 92/93rd St.
NYC 10025 Mon.-Sat. 10:30-7:30, Sun. 1-6

Darryl's W
Darryl's is a convenient Upper West Side source for your day-to-day wardrobe staples. From career and eveningwear to casual and relaxed basics, find suits, separates, pants, knit outfits, twin sets and accessories. Labels include Encore, Zanella and Studio by Ferre.

Upper West Side 212-874-6677
492 Amsterdam Avenue bet. 83/84th St.
NYC 10024 Mon.-Fri. 11-7, Sat. 11-6, Sun. 12-6

Daryl K W
Daryl Kerrigan, one of New York's hottest designers, has built a successful business around her coveted hip huggers and streetwise aesthetics. As WWD reports, "No one catches the pulse of the streets better than Daryl Kerrigan." Labels Daryl K and K-189 target a hip, young audience in search of trendsetting fashions. Designs feature simple silhouettes with sleek looks for the well-toned body. Find hip-huggers, slim-fitting pants, jackets, shirts, skirts and dresses. The look is sexy and modern.

East Village 212-475-1255
208 East 6th Street bet. 2/3rd Ave.
NYC 10003 Mon.-Sat. 12-7, Sun. 12-6

NoHo 212-777-0713
21 Bond Street bet. Lafayette/Bowery
NYC 10012 Mon.-Sat. 11-7, Sun. 12-6

David Aaron W
It's hard to believe that the fashionable David Aaron and funky Steve Madden footwear lines are designed by the same team. For Prada looks without Prada prices, a stop at David Aaron will satisfy anyone in search of a pair of stylish shoes. Find ponyskin mules, driving moccasins, fun sandals, slip-ons, evening pumps and boots. Best of all, pay anywhere from $79 to $169 for a slice of urban chic and have everyone think you're wearing designer when you're not.

SoHo 212-431-6022
529 Broadway bet. Spring/Prince
NYC 10012 Mon.-Thurs. 11-8,
Fri. & Sat. 11-8:30, Sun. 11-7

Davide Cenci M/W
Davide Cenci features classic Italian clothing. His credo: comfort, warmth, lightness and balance. Find a collection of suits, sportswear, shirts, sweaters, outerwear, accessories, as well as a

DDC Lab

made-to-measure department. Luxurious fabrics, impeccable tailoring and subtle colors make up the Cenci label. Off-the-rack suits begin at $1,200 and made-to-measure start at $1,600. Also find Tod's footwear line. www.davidecenci.com

Upper East Side   **212-628-5910**
801 Madison Avenue   bet. 67/68th St.
NYC 10021   Mon.-Sat. 10-6:30, Thurs. 10-7:30

DDC Lab   M/W

DDC Lab's shopping atmosphere is quite an experience. Find a coffee bar, a magazine section and blaring rock music in the background. Amidst all this is DDC Lab's clothing collection, a combination of avant-garde and hip-hop looks. Find lots of denim in a variety of finishes, (stretch, raw and tie-dyed), as well as T-shirts, jackets, corduroys, futuristic sunglasses and watches, comfort shoes, fragrances and more. It's all about a cool, artsy image for gen-xers.

Lower East Side   **212-375-1647**
180 Orchard Street   bet. Stanton/Houston
NYC 10002   Mon.-Wed. 11-7,
    Thurs. & Sat. 11-9, Sun. 12-6

Deborah Moorfield   W

This New York designer has developed a cult-like following of fashionistas who covet her classic pieces. Her collection features dressy suits, dresses, skirts, feminine shirts and camisoles, as well as fashionable coats. New Yorkers shop here to add a touch of exclusivity to their wardrobe.

SoHo   **212-226-2647**
466 Broome Street   bet. Mercer/Greene
NYC 10013   Mon.-Sat. 11:30-7, Sun. 12-6

Deco Jewels, Inc.   W

Shop owner Janice Berkson lovingly restores Lucite handbags from the 40's and 50's to pristine perfection. She travels far and wide in search of these beauties, making them prized possessions. Prices start at $200. Vintage costume jewelry and cufflinks from the 1800s to the 1960s round out the assortment.

SoHo   **212-253-1222**
131 Thompson Street   bet. Prince/Houston
NYC 10012   Mon.-Sun. 12-8

Detour   W

A rather pricey shop for a younger set in search of hip, tight-fitting outfits. Trend seekers can choose from a selection of casual basics that includes tight tees, jeans, skirts, dresses, leather jackets, and racy ensembles perfect for "club hopping" nights out.

SoHo   **212-979-6315**
472 West Broadway   bet. Houston/Prince
NYC 10012   Mon.-Sun. 11-8

SoHo   **212-966-3635**
154 Prince Street   bet. W. B'way/Thompson
NYC 10012   Mon.-Sun. 11-8

SoHo (M)   212-219-2692
425 W. Broadway   bet. Prince/Spring
NYC 10012   Mon.-Sun. 11-8

D & G   M/W

Welcome to D & G, Dolce & Gabbana's secondary line. This 5,000-sq. ft. shop is packed with attitude and boasts a sophisticated, hip collection of clothing. Discover two floors of sportswear, eveningwear and casual wear. Find fitted suits, jackets, shirts, pants, outerwear, shoes and accessories, as well as a complete jeans line. The D & G image: funky, sexy and young.

SoHo   212-965-8000
434 West Broadway   bet. Prince/Spring
NYC 10012   Mon.-Sat. 11-7, Sun. 12-6

Denimax   M/W

Denimax showcases three floors dedicated to outerwear. Find coats and jackets manufactured in fur, shearling, leather, cashmere and microfiber in a variety of looks and fabrics, from leather jackets to luxury rabbit and mink coats. You can spend as little as $300 or as much as $100,000 if your heart is set on sable.

Midtown East   212-207-4900
444 Madison Avenue   bet. 49/50th St.
NYC 10022   Mon.-Fri. 10-7, Sat. 10-6, Sun. 11-5

Diana & Jeffries   W

Despite the unalluring exterior of the shop, it's worth taking a peek inside to check out their up-to-the-minute fashions. Shop for trendy labels like Theory, Nanette Lepore, Carol Horn, Catherine, Juicy, Vivienne Tam and more. Mix and match from the hip with street-wise collections.

Upper East Side   212-249-1891
1145 Madison Avenue   at 85th St.
NYC 10028   Mon.-Sat. 11-7, Sun. 12-6

Upper West Side   212-874-2884
2062 Broadway   bet. 70/71st St.
NYC 10023   Mon.-Sat. 11-8, Sun. 12-7

Diesel   M/W/C

Diesel caters to the "youth culture." Industrial dryers filled with jeans serve as Diesel's exterior window displays, while a futuristic décor sets the stage for the company's edgy collection of high-energy clothing. Find sportswear, jeans and casual clothing, as well as a small children's section, all heavily logo'd with the Diesel name. It's modern-styled basics with urban looks and Italian flair.

Upper East Side   212-308-0055
770 Lexington Avenue   at 60th St.
NYC 10022   Mon.-Sat. 10-8, Sun. 12-6

☆ DieselStyleLab   M/W

"The name 'StyleLab' originates from the desire to research and experiment with style, cuts, materials and ideas," say

DKNY

the folks at Diesel. Find a collection of high-end sportswear for the trendy urbanite that includes pants, jackets, shirts, sweaters, outerwear and accessories, all in innovative and high-tech fabric treatments and creative design concepts.

SoHo   212-343-3863
416 West Broadway   bet. Prince/Spring
NYC 10012   Mon.-Sat. 11-8, Sun. 11-7

DKNY   W

Donna Karan understands the beat of the streets and what consumers want when it comes to lifestyle clothing. Welcome DKNY, a high performance sportswear collection for today's modern man and woman. At DKNY, it's not about high fashion; it's about hip, sporty looks that are wearable and affordable. Shop a color coordinated collection of pants, tops, shirts, sweaters, knits and jackets that can be mixed and matched to create any mood, whether for day or evening. Casual wear includes jeans, vintage pieces, sweaters and outerwear. In addition, find handbags, shoes, accessories, a home collection, as well as Blanche's Organic Café for the health-conscious crowd.

Upper East Side   212-223-3569
655 Madison Avenue   at 60th St.
NYC 10021   Mon.-Sat. 10-7, Thurs. 10-9, Sun. 12-6

D/L Cerney   M/W

D/L Cerney is for those who believe that the novelty of trend-setting fashion wears thin. Husband and wife team of Linda St. John and Duane Cerney feature a collection of classic retro-inspired clothing. From simple gabardine shirts and straight skirts to fitted shift dresses and stretch pants, it's all in natural fabrics and hand-finished right down to the last button and stitch.

East Village   212-673-7033
13 East 7th Street   bet. 2/3rd Ave.
NYC 10003   Mon.-Sun. 12-8

TriBeCa   212-941-0530
222 West Broadway   bet. Franklin/White
NYC 10013   Sun.-Wed. 12-8, Thurs.-Sat. 12-9

Do Kham   W

Treasures from the Himalayas are beautifully displayed in this elegant SoHo shop. Choose from traditional Tibetan styled dresses, skirts and tops, as well as a collection of richly brocaded, fur-trimmed, silk hats. Worth a trip just to see their fabulous selection of Pashmina shawls ($175 to $395), scarves, boas and handbags. Find them plain or embroidered in a myriad of colors and fabrics.

SoHo   212-966-2404
51 Prince Street   bet. Mulberry/Lafayette
NYC 10012   Mon.-Sun. 10-8

East Village   212-358-1010
304 East 5th Street   bet. 1st/2nd Avenue
NYC 10003   Mon.-Sun. 11-8

Dolce & Gabbana   M/W

Here's your chance to get a first glimpse of what Hollywood is wearing. Dolce & Gabbana takes Manhattan by storm with its glitzy and glamorous label defined by lean lines, bra-styled straps and the perfect snug fit. Enter this 7,000-sq. ft. flagship store and find a modern collection for both men and women. This duo team, Dolce and Stefano, designs in sync with the hottest film and recording stars' fashion rhythms. Find a ready-to-wear collection, as well as some couture pieces featuring looks that run from pinstriped suits and seductive leopard dresses to gowns with elaborate finishing touches. Under the Dolce & Gabbana label, you can dress sexy one day and with a sense of humor the next. It all depends on your mood.

Upper East Side   212-249-4100
825 Madison Avenue   bet. 68/69th St.
NYC 10021   Mon.-Sat. 10-6, Thurs. 10-7

Doll House   G

Cool fashions with a little attitude for the junior set. Doll House features a casual wear collection perfect for trend-craving teenagers. Find jeans, T-shirts, mini-skirts, dresses, tube tops, cargo pants, capri pants and more.

NoHo   212-539-1800
400 Lafayette Street   at E. 4th St.
NYC 10003   Mon.-Sat. 11-8, Sun. 12-7

Donna Karan Collection   M/W

Which major designer has two flagship stores just six blocks from each other? Hint: You're reading the Donna Karan Collection entry. Scheduled to open in January of 2001, word is out that this flagship store will be an immense 10,000-sq. ft. space boasting three floors of lifestyle products, from men's and women's collections to accessories and home products.

Upper East Side   Opening Spring 2001
819 Madison Avenue   bet. 68/69th St.
NYC 10021   Mon.-Sat. 10-7, Sun. 12-6

Dooney and Burke   W

Find an extensive collection of handbags, leathergoods and luggage crafted in durable wide grained cowhide. These all-weather classics come in an abundance of colors and feature signature leather trim and saddle stitching. Another alternative is Dooney and Burke's lightweight collection of stain resistant, maintenance-free canvas bags.
800-347-5000

Upper East Side   212-439-1657
759 Madison Avenue   bet. 65/66th St.
NYC 10021   Mon.-Sat. 10-6

Fifth Avenue   212-308-0520
725 Fifth Avenue at Trump Tower   bet. 56/57th St.
NYC 10022   Mon.-Sat. 10-6

Dosa   W

A shop that sells a unique selection of women's clothing. From simple cut dresses and pants to Tibetan-inspired tops, the Dosa label uses an impressive mix of fabrics, including silks, linens and cashmeres.

SoHo   212-431-1733
107 Thompson Street   bet. Spring/Prince
NYC 10012   Mon.-Sat. 12-7, Sun. 12-6

D. Porthault & Co.   W

Long recognized for luxurious bed and bath linens, D. Porthault also features a small, enticing sleepwear department. Nighties are feminine and romantic, while nightshirts and robes come in all the Porthault prints.
www.porthault.fr.com

Upper East Side   212-688-1660
18 East 69th Street   bet. Madison/5th
NYC 10021   Mon.-Fri. 10-5:30, Sat. 10-5

The Dressing Room   W

What women love about The Dressing Room is an ever-changing selection of merchandise. Their private label line "DR" changes weekly and always gives the customer a good reason to come back. Other young designer labels include United Bamboo, Minimum and Troy Smith, as well as vintage designs by Albert Chan. Find pants, tank tops, sweaters, ponchos, shirts, handbags, beaded slippers and accessories. It's hip and colorful. Best for the under 35 crowd.

NoLiTa   212-431-6658
49 Prince Street   bet. Lafayette/Mulberry
NYC 10012   Mon.-Sat. 1-7, Sun. 1-6

East Side Kids   B/G

An uptown neighborhood children's shop featuring back-to-school basics, party shoes, weekend casual wear and fashion forward trendsetters. Brand names include Sam & Libby, Skechers, Stride Rite, Capezio, Enzo, Jumping Jack, Nike, Keds and more. From newborn to size 9/10.

Upper East Side   212-360-5000
1298 Madison Avenue   bet. 91/92nd St.
NYC 10128   Mon.-Fri. 9:30-6, Sat. 9-6

Eastern Mountain Sports   M/W

This shop specializes in apparel and equipment for the outdoor sports of mountaineering, backpacking, hiking, skiing and camping. Brand names include Columbia, Northface, Patagonia, as well as private label. 888-463-6367

NoHo   212-505-9860
611 Broadway   at Houston
NYC 10012   Mon.-Fri. 10-9, Sat. 10-8, Sun. 12-6

Upper West Side   212-397-4860
20 West 61st Street   bet. B'way/9th Ave.
NYC 10023   Mon.-Fri. 10-9, Sat. 10-6, Sun. 12-6

Eileen Fisher

Easy Spirit W

A patented, multi-layer cushioning support system guarantees Easy Spirit's comfortable fit. Styles range from career and fitness to fun and casual. It's footwear that protects your feet from shock and stress without denting your wallet. 800-284-9955

Upper East Side 212-828-9593
1518 Third Avenue bet. 85/86th St.
NYC 10028 Mon.-Fri. 10-8, Sat. 11-7, Sun. 11-6:30

Upper West Side 212-875-8146
2251 Broadway bet. 80/81st St.
NYC 10024 Mon.-Sat. 10-7, Sun. 11-6:30

Midtown East 212-715-0152
555 Madison Avenue at 56th St.
NYC 10022 Mon.-Fri. 9-7:30, Sat. 10-6, Sun. 12-5

Midtown West 212-398-2761
1166 Sixth Avenue at 46th St.
NYC 10036 Mon.-Fri. 9-8, Sat. 10-6, Sun. 12-5

Lower Manhattan 212-406-8159
182 Broadway bet. John/Maiden Lane
NYC 10038 Mon.-Wed. 8-6:45, Thurs. & Fri. 8-7:45,
Sat. 11-5:45, Sun. 12-4:45

Eddie Bauer M/W

Expanding from a single store in Seattle to 600 stores nationwide, Eddie Bauer continues to be one of America's top purveyors of casual lifestyle clothing. A well-organized display of merchandise and a friendly sales staff makes shopping at Eddie Bauer a pleasure. Shop the A/K/A, a dress/casual line of office clothing. In addition, find weekend wear for the indoors and out. Choose from wrinkle-resistant khakis, polo shirts, jeans, sweaters, outerwear, underwear and eyewear. You can even pack it all in one of their sport duffels. The look is classic, sporty and all-American. Terrific value. 800-426-6253

Upper East Side 212-737-0002
1172 Third Avenue bet. 68/69th St.
NYC 10021 Mon.-Sat. 10-8, Sun. 11-6

Upper West Side 212-877-7629
1978 Broadway at 67th St.
NYC 10023 Mon.-Thurs. 10-9,
Fri. & Sat. 10-11, Sun. 11-9

Midtown East 212-808-0820
711 Third Avenue bet. 44/45th St.
NYC 10017 Mon.-Fri. 10-8, Sat. 11-6, Sun. 12-5

SoHo 212-925-2179
578 Broadway bet. Houston/Prince
NYC 10012 Mon.-Thurs. 10-8, Fri. & Sat. 10-9, Sun. 11-7

Eileen Fisher W

Eileen Fisher features a collection of coordinated separates that are sporty, comfortable and easy to wear. Find jackets,

Eisenberg and Eisenberg

skirts, pants (with elastic waistlines) and T-shirts designed in a relaxed fit. A solid color palette makes mixing and matching a cinch. Fischer's claim to fame: casual, maintenance-free clothing that travels anywhere. 800-345-3362

Upper East Side 212-879-7799
1039 Madison Avenue bet. 79/80th St.
NYC 10021 Mon.-Sat. 10-7, Sun. 12-5

Upper West Side 212-362-3000
341 Columbus Avenue bet. 76/77th St.
NYC 10024 Mon.-Sat. 10-7, Sun. 12-6

Midtown East 212-759-9888
521 Madison Avenue bet. 53/54th St.
NYC 10022 Mon.-Sat. 10-7, Sun. 12-6

Flatiron 212-924-4777
103 Fifth Avenue bet. 17/18th St.
NYC 10003 Mon.-Sat. 10-8, Sun. 12-6

SoHo 212-431-4567
395 West Broadway bet. Broome/Spring
NYC 10012   Mon.-Thurs. 11-7, Fri. & Sat. 12-8, Sun. 12-6

East Village (outlet) 212-529-5715
314 East 9th Street bet. 1st/2nd Ave.
NYC 10003 Mon.-Sat. 12-8, Sun. 12-7

Eisenberg and Eisenberg   M

Since 1898, Eisenberg and Eisenberg has been one of New York's sources for inexpensive formal wear. Don't let the unglamorous façade deter you from venturing inside. Find suits, slacks, sportcoats, blazers, shirts and men's furnishings, as well as a full range of tuxedos. Pay an average price of $450 for suits and anywhere between $190 to $550 for tuxedos. Extra for alterations.

Chelsea 212-627-1290
16 West 17th Street bet. 5/6th St.
NYC 10011 Mon.-Fri. 9-5:30,
Thurs. 9-6:30, Sat. 9-5, Sun. 10-4

Emanual Ungaro   W

A French designer whose collection turns on color and fabric combinations. If you're wild about florals, paisleys and assorted prints, then you'll love Ungaro. Find a ready-to-wear line that includes dress suits, dresses and beautifully tailored jackets. An Ungaro is sophisticated, feminine and timeless. Accessories include shoes, belts, bags and shawls.

Upper East Side 212-249-4090
792 Madison Avenue at 67th St.
NYC 10021 Mon.-Sat. 10-6

Emilio Pucci   W

Now that LVMH has acquired Pucci, you better believe that big plans, i.e., expansion, lie ahead for this Italian fashion house. Since 1949, Pucci has been designing clothes inspired by the Italian art world. The end result: their signature looks of colorful, graphic motifs derived from abstract drawings. Today these prints continue to flourish, both as a current fashion trend and selling in vintage shops. Find dresses, skirts, pants, swimsuits and accessories in the latest Pucci prints. In vogue today and tomorrow, Pucci lives on.

Upper East Side   212-752-4777
24 East 64th Street   bet. 5th/Madison
NYC 10021   Mon.-Sat. 10-5

Emporio Armani   M/W

A multitude of elements create this lifestyle brand guaranteed to meet all your fashion expectations. From swimwear to eveningwear (and everything in between), men and women can shop for sporty, casual and dressy looks. Find suits, sportswear, knockout eveningwear, coats, jeans, T-shirts, shoes and accessories. Emporio features luxury merchandise for 50% less than Armani's signature collection. It's the same look without boutique prices.

Midtown East   212-317-0800
601 Madison Avenue   bet. 57/58th St.
NYC 10022   Mon.-Fri. 10-8, Sat. 10-7, Sun. 12-6

Flatiron   212-727-3240
110 Fifth Avenue   at 16th St.
NYC 10011   Mon.-Sat. 11-8, Sun. 12-6

SoHo   Opening Fall 2000
436 West Broadway   bet. Spring/Prince
NYC 10012   Mon.-Fri. 11-8, Sat. 11-7, Sun. 12-6

Encore   W

Perhaps one of New York's best consignment shops, selling high-end designer labels in mint condition. Unlike the "rummage-sale" environment found in most resale shops, Encore's collection is well-organized, and best known for its Chanel suits, Blahnik shoes and Yves Saint Laurent blouses. Other coveted labels include Celine, Yohji Yamamoto, Prada, Chloe, and Fendi, all at least 1/3 off original prices.

Upper East Side   212-879-2850
1132 Madison Avenue, 2nd Fl.   bet. 84/85th St.
NYC 10028   Mon.-Fri. 10:30-6:30,
  Sat. 10:30-6, Sun. 12-6

Enerla Lingerie   W

For twenty years this East Village shop has been pleasing customers with their collection of sexy, romantic lingerie and good selection of basics. The assortment includes sleepwear, robes, foundations, bustiers, swimwear, and hosiery from labels like Lu, La Mystere, Cosabella, Hanro, Tony Schiesser, Claire Pettibone, Chiarigi, Orablu, and Hue.

East Village   212-473-2454
48 East 7th Street   bet. 1st/2nd Avenue
NYC 10003   Sun.-Wed. 12-8:30, Thurs.-Sat. 12-9:30

Enrique Martinez   W

Enrique Martinez is perhaps the only Mexican designer to make it to Madison Avenue, and with a well-received ready-

En Soie

to-wear line to boot. Enter this sleek shop and find a classic, feminine collection designed to be mixed and matched. Choose from jackets in simple tweeds, solids and cashmeres (from the Loro Piana mills), pants, textured cashmere knits in wonderful shades of aubergines, olives and pastels, a collection of black evening dresses, as well as luxurious scarves. A Martinez design is about quality fabrics, clean cuts and sophisticated looks. For the over 30 crowd who are willing to spend.

Upper East Side   **212-734-5776**
785 Madison Avenue   bet. 66/67th St.
NYC 10021   Mon.-Sat. 10-6

En Soie   W

En Soie, once the manufacturer of beautiful silks for the great European couture houses, has now redirected its focus to include an eclectic selection of merchandise. Find a clothing collection manufactured in En Soie's exclusive silks, as well as accessories and ceramics, all designed with a dash of whimsy. You can also purchase their unique fabrics by the yard. Best for printed silk scarves.

Upper East Side   **212-717-7958**
988 Madison Avenue   bet. 76/77th St.
NYC 10021   Mon.-Sat. 10-6

★ Entre Nous   W

Just between us—or as the French say, *Entre Nous*—this shop is one of New York's best kept secrets for the mature urbanite. Entre Nous is about luxury European labels. Choose from Luciano Barbera's complete collection of pants, tweed jackets, cashmeres and shirts. In addition, find Guy Rover shirts, Sunspel T-shirts from England that feel like one-ply cashmere when worn, rainwear by Allegri, evening dresses and gowns by Sylvia Heisel and Melinda Eng and accessories including vintage jewelry and belts. Classic fashions for the sophisticated woman who demands impeccable quality.

Upper East Side   **212-249-2225**
1124 Third Avenue   bet. 65/66th St.
NYC 10021   Mon.-Fri. 10-6, Sat. 11-6

Enzo Angiolini   W

Enzo Angiolini is Nine West's better footwear division. Find hip, up-to-the-minute styles that include basic comfort flats, man-tailored loafers, trendy sandals, platforms, boots and more. It's about fashion forward shoes that look expensive, but aren't.

Midtown East   **212-688-0955**
714 Lexington Avenue   bet. 57/58th St.
NYC 10022   Mon.-Fri. 10-8, Thurs. 10-9,
    Sat. 10-7, Sun. 12-6

Midtown East   **212-339-8921**
551 Madison Avenue   at 55th St.
NYC 10022   Mon.-Fri. 9:30-7:30, Sat. 10-6, Sun. 12-5

Midtown East   212-286-8726
331 Madison Avenue   at 43rd St.
NYC 10017   Mon.-Fri. 8-8, Sat. 10-6, Sun. 12-5

Midtown West   212-695-8903
901 Sixth Avenue in Manhattan Mall   bet. B'way/33rd St.
NYC 10001   Mon.-Sat. 10-8, Sun. 11-6

Episode   W

Career women shop here in search of designer looks without designer prices. Episode features a collection of suits, sportswear, dresses, eveningwear and coats that follow the fashion trends. Take advantage of their VIP program: spend $1,000 in any two-month period and get 10% off any future purchases.

Midtown East   212-755-6061
625 Madison Avenue   bet. 58/59th St.
NYC 10022   Mon.-Fri. 10-7, Sat. 10-6

Epperson Studio   W

Husband-wife team Epperson and Lisha are the talents behind this transcultural clothing collection. Inspired by the cultures of China, India and Africa, their mixture of elements makes each piece unique. An Epperson design is defined by deconstructed shapes, patchwork, raw edges, and plenty of color. Find long dresses, capes, shirts, hats, and head wraps—mix and match them and add a touch of downtown fantasy to your wardrobe. Celebrities Erykah Badu and Lauryn Hill are customers.

SoHo   212-226-3181
25 Thompson Street   bet. Watts/Grand
NYC 10013   Tues.-Sat. 1-8

Equipment   W

Perhaps New York's best source for basic silk shirts that go with anything. It's feminine styling with classic looks. Find hand-washable silk shirts in a sea of colors and an array of styles at an average price of $178. Also, choose from a collection of casual separates that include pants, cashmere sweaters, boat-neck T-shirts and more.

Upper East Side   212-249-2083
872 Madison Avenue   at 71st St.
NYC 10021   Mon.-Sat. 10-6, Thurs. 10-7

Eres   W

With the financial backing of Chanel, this French luxury intimate apparel and swimwear manufacturer prepares to open their first US store. Shop a 1,000-sq. ft. space devoted to beautifully made lingerie, emphasizing everyday basics and feminine silhouettes. The Eres label is defined by "ethereal, lace-free, understated looks, microfiber blends, incredible fit, and, unfortunately, eye-popping prices." Panties start at $80, bras are priced from $160 to $180, and swimwear will run you anywhere from $180 to $280.

Eric Shoes

Midtown East | **Opening Fall 2000**
625 Madison Avenue | bet. 58/59th St.
NYC 10022 | Mon.-Sat. 10-6

Eric Shoes W
This popular Upper East Side shoe shop features fashion classics from top footwear designers. Women-on-the-go shop here for casual basics, career and evening shoes that feature edgy heel and toe treatments. Labels include Stuart Weitzman, Nicole Miller, Pancaldi, Johnny Bravo and Eric's private label collection.

Upper East Side | **212-289-5762**
1222 Madison Avenue | at 88th St.
NYC 10128 | Mon.-Fri. 10-7, Sat. 10-6, Sun. 12-6

Upper East Side | **212-288-8250**
1333 Third Avenue | at 76th St.
NYC 10021 | Mon-Fri. 10-7, Thurs. 11-8,
Sat. 10-6, Sun. 12-6

Erica Tanov W/C
This large, clean space is the perfect backdrop for Erica Tanov's collection of sophisticated women's wear, bed linens, baby clothes, lingerie and accessories. Elegant fabrics, classic styling, fine craftsmanship and careful attention to detail define her line of dresses, skirts, tops and pants. Find knitwear from John Smedley, dresses by Megan Parks and lingerie by Ripcosa. In addition, children can be turned out in I Golfini della Nonna's collection of cheerful printed rompers, bloomers and smocks that make perfect outfits for play or dress up. www.ericatanov.com

NoLiTa | **212-334-8020**
204 Elizabeth Street | bet. Spring/Prince
NYC 10012 | Tues.-Sat. 11-7, Sun. 12-6

Ermenegildo Zegna M
Zegna is in a class of its own when it comes to luxury suits and menswear. Sumptuous fabrics are the name of the game here—caress them and crave them! Find high-powered tailored styles and deconstructed suits with modern looks. Expect to pay an average price of $2,100 (and much more for custom). Shirts, ties, sportswear, outerwear, shoes and accessories complete the Zegna collection.
www.ezegna.com

Fifth Avenue | **212-421-4488**
743 Fifth Avenue | bet. 57/58th St.
NYC 10022 | Mon.-Fri. 10-7, Sat. 10-6, Sun. 12-5

Escada W
The designers at Escada cultivate women who love luxury, especially luxury that begs to be noticed. Shop three separate collections: Escada Couture, Escada Ready-to-Wear and Escada Sport. Find dressy day looks, evening separates, tuxedos and cocktail dresses, as well as ballgowns. For a more relaxed look women can choose from a selection of

sporty knits, flannel pants, leather parkas, denim and more. Opulent fabrics, bold colors and racy detailing are the trademarks of an Escada design.

Midtown East   212-755-2200
7 East 57th Street   bet. 5th/Madison Ave.
NYC 10022   Mon.-Sat. 10-6, Thurs. 10-7

Etro   M/W

At Etro it's about seasoning your wardrobe with color, pattern and texture. This six-floor fashion house features ready-to-wear, elegant weekend wear, home furnishings, shoes, accessories, luggage and fragrances. Exclusive materials, modern designs and expert craftsmanship personify Etro's vision of class and style. Men can shop English tailored suits, shirts, paisley ties galore, sportswear and outerwear, while women can select from a ready-to-wear line of skirts, slacks, shirts, cashmeres, classic riding styled jackets, outerwear and more. Classic fashions with Etro's unique mix of fabric and texture make an Etro design a one-of-a-kind. So embrace the world of Etro and add a little Italian pizzazz to your wardrobe.

Upper East Side   212-317-9096
720 Madison Avenue   bet. 63/64th St.
NYC 10021   Mon.-Sat. 10-6

☆ Eugenia Kim   W

Fashionable shops like Barneys and Bond 07 were the first to carry hat designer Eugenia Kim's wonderful creations, but it's worth a trip to her eponymous millinery shop to see firsthand her colorful toppers that run from conservative to downright decadent. Her clientele runs from uptown socialites to East Village hipsters. According to Kim, "Hats are the ultimate cosmetic, and the focal point of any look." Find styles like classic cloches, fedoras, cowboy hats in leopard prints, as well designs in beaver fur, ostrich feathers, and unusual straws. Prices run from $90 to $400.

East Village   212-673-9787
203 East 4th Street   bet. Ave. A/B
NYC 10009   Mon.-Sun. 1-8
    best to make an appointment

Express   W

Express is getting back on track by revamping its stores and restructuring its image. This is a good destination for younger shoppers who are making the transition from school to the workplace. Express will satisfy those on limited budgets with its collection of casual, fashionable basics at moderate price points. Find dresses, pants, skirts, T-shirts, leggings and accessories, in the latest color forecasts and trends. 877-657-2292

Upper West Side   212-580-5833
321 Columbus Avenue   bet. 75/76th St.
NYC 10023   Mon.-Fri. 10-8, Sat. 10-8, Sun. 11-7

Façonnable

Midtown East　　　　　　　　　　**212-421-7246**
722-28 Lexington Avenue　　　　　bet. 58/59th St.
NYC 10022　　　　　　　　　　　Mon.-Sat. 10-8,
　　　　　　　　　　Thurs. & Fri. 10-9, Sun. 12-7

Midtown East　　　　　　　　　　**212-644-4453**
477 Madison Avenue　　　　　　　bet. 51/52nd St.
NYC 10021　　　　　　　　Mon.-Sat. 10-8, Sun. 12-7

Midtown East　　　　　　　　　　**212-949-9784**
733 Third Avenue　　　　　　　　　　at 46th St.
NYC 10017　　　　　　　　Mon.-Sat. 10-8, Sun. 12-7

Midtown West　　　　　　　　　　**212-629-6838**
7 West 34th Street　　　　　　　　　bet. 5/6th Ave.
NYC 10001　　　　　　　Mon.-Fri. 10-8, Sat. 10-7, Sun. 12-6

Midtown West　　　　　　　　　　**212-971-3280**
901 Sixth Avenue　　　　　　　　bet. B'way/33rd St.
NYC 10001　　　　　　　　Mon.-Sat. 10-8, Sun. 11-6

Flatiron　　　　　　　　　　　　**212-633-9414**
130 Fifth Avenue　　　　　　　　　　at 18th St.
NYC 10011　　　　　　　Mon.-Fri. 10-8, Sat. 10-7, Sun. 12-6

Façonnable　　　　　　　　　　　　　　M

A destination for the well-dressed man who enjoys accessorizing. No wardrobe is complete without a Façonnable tie or button-down spread-collar shirt. Suits come in classic silhouettes, while their sportswear makes perfect weekend attire. Outerwear is simply a must, particularly ultra-fab micro-fiber bomber jackets in spring and winter weights. A stylish French version of Ralph Lauren. One quibble however: the Façonnable label is visible, ubiquitous and annoying (but can be removed upon request).

Fifth Avenue　　　　　　　　　　**212-319-0111**
689 Fifth Avenue　　　　　　　　　　at 54th St.
NYC 10022　　　　　Mon.-Sat. 10-7, Thurs. 10-8, Sun. 12-6

Fan Club　　　　　　　　　　　　　　W

Veteran TV host Gene London and his partner John Thomas' fascination with movie stars led them to acquire one of the most extensive collections of show biz wardrobes and memorabilia and inspired them to open their consignment shop, the Fan Club. Find sequined evening gowns, couture by Bob Mackie, wedding gowns and other glittery apparel once worn by soap, movie and theatre stars.

Chelsea　　　　　　　　　　　　**212-929-3349**
22 West 19th Street　　　　　　　　bet. 5/6th Ave.
NYC 10011　　　　　　　　　　　Tues.-Sat. 12-5

February Eleventh　　　　　　　　　　W

Women who love an artistic approach to fashion will appreciate the intricate handwork on display here—lots of crocheted dresses, separates and shawls, as well as embroidered, lace and hand-dyed pieces. Handbags and jewelry also available. (So what's up with the store's name? It's the owner's birthday.)

Final Home

East Village   212-529-1175
315 East 9th Street   bet. 1/2nd Ave.
NYC 10003   Mon.-Sun. 1-8

Fendi   M/W

These days multi-faceted designer Karl Lagerfeld couldn't be any hotter. One minute he's turning out polished Chanel haute couture and the next he's designing flash, dash and glitter for Fendi's jet-set audience. Welcome to the world of double F's, where most of the clothing and accessories is embossed with the Fendi logo. Find ready-to-wear, sportswear, handbags, shoes, accessories and luggage. However, a true "Fendinista" flocks here for the collection of furs. Wear one of these beauties (a mink bomber or a fur in a graphic, eye-popping pattern) and make a statement that leaves a lasting impression, As for handbags, the Fendi baguette is the current rage. It comes in a variety of textures and colors, from black nylon ($450) to crocodile with turquoise buckles ($6,000) to sequined and embroidered. So if you're in the market for a lavish fur or an outfit accessorized to the hilt, shop the international status symbol of Fendi's inverted FF logo. 800-336-3469

Fifth Avenue   212-767-0100
720 Fifth Avenue   at 56th St.
NYC 10019   Mon.-Sat. 10-6

Filene's Basement   M/W

This famous Boston institution now has two locations in Manhattan stocked with reasonably priced designer overruns. Find career wear, sportswear, shoes, luggage, accessories and fragrances. If you're lucky, you might even come across an outfit by Valentino, Donna Karan, Scassi or Liz Claiborne. However, like all discounters, it can be hit or miss.

Upper West Side   212-873-8000
2222 Broadway   at 79th St.
NYC 10024   Mon.-Sat. 10-9, Sun. 11-6

Chelsea   212-620-3100
620 Sixth Avenue   bet. 18/19th St.
NYC 10011   Mon.-Sat. 9:30-9, Sun. 11-7

Final Home   M/W

Final Home, a subsidiary of Issey Miyake, showcases Japanese designer Kosuke Tsumura's conceptual clothing collection. Tsumura believes clothes should adapt to their environment so the wearer can better survive urban living. The result: his signature nylon raincoat with 44 pockets(!) that can be accessorized with layers of down insulation. Also find peel-away high-tech shirts, nylon vests that convert to backpacks, and other unisex pieces made of futuristic rubberized fabrics. Is he a visionary or plain absurd? You be the judge.

NoLiTa   212-966-0202
241 Lafayette Street   bet. Prince/Spring
NYC 10012   Mon.-Sat. 11-7, Sun. 12-6

Fine & Klein W

The allure of Fine & Klein's is certainly not its ambiance, but rather its well-priced selection of 1,000 handbag styles. New Yorkers on limited budgets flock here for brand names like Pierre Cardin and Sharif. Enjoy the great prices, but watch out for huge crowds on Sundays and holidays.

Lower East Side 212-674-6720
119 Orchard Street at Delancey
NYC 10002 Sun.-Fri. 9-4:30, closed Sat.

Find Outlet W

Just blocks from Chelsea's art galleries and chic new restaurants comes Find Outlet, a fun and hip shop featuring racks of one-of-a-kind designer samples and over-stocks. Shop to your heart's desire for edgy clothing that's 50%-80% off retail. Find labels like Ankh, P.A.K., Built by Wendy, Intermix, Cashmere Studio, How & Wen, Anna Sui, Alice & Trixie, Lotta, Paul & Joe, Stephane Kelian and Tufi Duek. www.findoutlet.com

NoLiTa 212-243-3177
229 Mott Street bet. Prince/Spring
NYC 10012 Mon.-Sun. 12-7

Chelsea 212-243-3177
361 West 17th Street bet. Eighth/Ninth Ave.
NYC 10011 Thurs.-Sun. 12-7

Fiona Walker W

When department stores informed Fiona Walker that her clothes were too expensive to put into the young designer section, she opened her own digs located in Hell's kitchen. Having grown up studying textile and fabrics in Ireland, Fiona is at home in the world of knitting: yarn-fringed tops, popcorn-stitched turtlenecks, tweedy sweaters and more. Custom also available.

Midtown West 212-664-9699
451 West 46th Street bet. 9/10th Ave.
NYC 10036 Mon.-Fri. 1-7:30, Sat 12-7

Fisch for the Hip M/W

Anyone in search of a gently used Hermès handbag in perfect condition should hurry down to Fisch for the Hip, the new "luxe" consignment shop (and sister store to "Out of Our Closet"). In addition to three showcases packed with all the popular Hermès styles, owners Pamela and Terin Fisch do a bang-up job at bringing in the "best of the best" of high-end designer clothing. Find coveted labels like Gucci, Calvin Klein, Zegna, Prada, Dolce & Gabbana and more. The merchandise is in mint condition and one-half of retail. Also, find shoes by Manolo Blahnik, Prada, Chanel and others. Check out their new line Bardo, designed by the owners themselves.

Chelsea 212-633-9053
153 West 18th Street bet. 6/7th Ave.
NYC 10011 Mon.-Sat. 12-7, Sun. 12-6

Fogal
W

As Wolford is known for comfort and quality, Fogal is famous for its fabulous color selection. Treat your legs to over 100 different styles and 84 sumptuous colors. From sheer and opaque hose at $25 to Fogal's "UNA" collection of seamless pantyhose at $50, find five different sizes for a perfect fit. If you really want to splurge, invest in Fogal's "Tuxedo" hose, which will set you back a mere $395. Swimwear, bodysuits and lingerie round out the assortment. Good personalized service.

Upper East Side   **212-759-9782**
680 Madison Avenue   bet. 61/62nd St.
NYC 10021   Mon.-Sat. 10-6:30, Thurs. 10-8

Midtown East   **212-355-3254**
510 Madison Avenue   at 53rd St.
NYC 10022   Mon.-Sat. 10-6:30, Thurs., 10-8

Foley + Corinna
W

Flea-market queens Dana Foley and Anna Corinna bring New Yorkers one-of-a-kind looks, some vintage, some "pretty girl." Find hand-knit sweaters, skirts, T-shirts, coats, and pants, as well as funky totes and bags.

Lower East Side   **212-529-2338**
108 Stanton Street   bet. Ludlow/Essex St.
NYC 10002   Mon.-Sun. 1-8

Foot Locker
M/W/C

Foot Locker features athletic wear and footwear for the entire family. Find workout clothes for fitness and basketball, as well as a range of footwear lines suitable for running, tennis, basketball or cross training. Brand names include Nike, Reebok, Adidas, Fila and New Balance.
800-991-6681 www.footlocker.com

Upper East Side   **212-348-8652**
159 East 86th Street   bet. Third/Lex.
NYC 10028   Mon.-Sat. 9-8, Sun. 11-6

Upper East Side   **212-794-9082**
1345 First Avenue   at 72nd St.
NYC 10021   Mon.-Sat. 10-8, Sun. 11-6

Upper East Side   **212-472-5996**
1187 Third Avenue   at 69th St.
NYC 10021   Mon.-Sat. 9-8, Sun. 11-6

Midtown East   **212-856-9411**
150 East 42nd Street   bet. Lex./Third
NYC 10017   Mon.-Sat. 9-8, Sun. 12-6

Midtown West   **212-629-4419**
120 West 34th Street   bet. 6/7th Ave.
NYC 10001   Mon.- Fri. 8-9, Sat. 9-9, Sun. 11-7

Midtown West   **212-971-9449**
43 West 34th Street   bet. 5/6th Ave.
NYC 10001   Mon.-Fri. 8-9, Sat. 9-9, Sun. 11-7

Forman's

Flatiron	**212-254-9187**
252 First Avenue	at 15th St.
NYC 10009	Mon.-Sat.10-8, Sun. 11-6
Lower East Side	**212-533-8608**
94 Delancey Street	bet. Ludlow/Orchard
NYC 10002	Mon.-Sun. 10-7
NoHo	**212-995-0381**
734 Broadway	at 8th St.
NYC 10003	Mon.-Sat. 9-9, Sun. 12-6
Lower Manhattan	**212-608-3640**
89 South Street Seaport	Pier 17
NYC 10038	Mon.-Sat. 10-9, Sun. 10-8

Forman's   M/W

Shop here for designer sportswear, separates and outerwear at terrific discounted prices. Labels include Jones New York, Evan Picone, Ralph Lauren, Kasper and Liz Claiborne. To top it off, Forman's also offers an extensive petite and plus-size department. The merchandise changes all the time, so if you're in the neighborhood, it's well worth a visit. End-of-season sale an additional 40% off.

Midtown East	**212-681-9800**
145 East 42nd Street	bet. Lex./Third Ave.
NYC 10017	Mon.-Thurs. 8-9, Fri. 8-4:30, Sat. closed, Sun. 10-6
Lower East Side	**212-228-2500**
82 Orchard Street	bet. Broome/Grand
NYC 10002	Mon.-Wed. 9-6, Thurs. 9-8, Fri. 9-2, Sat. closed, Sun. 9-7
Fifth Avenue	**212-719-1000**
560 Fifth Avenue	at 46th St.
NYC 10017	Mon.-Thurs. 8-9, Fri. 8-2, Sat. closed, Sun. 10-6
Lower Manhattan	**212-791-4100**
59 John Street	at Williams St.
NYC 10039	Mon.-Wed.7:30-7,Thurs.7:30-8, Fri. 7:30-2, Sat. closed Sun. 11:30-5:30

Forreal   W

While Forreal Basics targets gen-xers, Forreal appeals to contemporary women in search of fashion forward, dressier looks. Find a selection of slim-fitted pants by Vertigo and Fred Sun; also jackets, sweaters, and T-shirts perfect for mixing and matching.

Upper East Side	**212-396-0563**
1369 Third Avenue	bet. 78/79th St.
NYC 10021	Mon.-Sat. 11-7, Sun. 12-6

Forreal Basics   W

While mothers bring their teenage daughters to Forreal for the hip assortment of jeans and casual basics, they invariably can't resist purchasing a thing or two for themselves. Shop a coveted jean selection of labels like Diesel, Miss

Sixty, Mavi, Diab'less and more. There's an abundance of fitted tees and T-shirts from makers like Michael Stars, 3 Dot, Petit Bateau and more. Alas, it's too bad that the sales assistants aren't much help.

Upper East Side	212-734-2105
1335 Third Avenue	bet. 76/77th St.
NYC 10021	Mon.-Sat. 11-7, Sun. 12-5

Upper East Side	212-717-0493
1200 Lexington Avenue	bet. 81/82nd St.
NYC 10028	Mon.-Sat. 11-7, Sun. 12-6

Fortuna Valentino   W

This is the place to shop for those hard-to-find zebra or leopard striped stiletto pumps, gold rhinestone elastic sandals, or dark blue python booties. If you're in the market for a pair of too-hot-to-handle exotic shoes, at over the top prices, a visit to Fortuna is a must!

SoHo	212-941-5811
422 West Broadway	bet. Prince/Spring
NYC 10012	Mon.-Wed. 11-7, Thurs.-Sat. 11-8, Sun. 12-7

Fragile   W

The survival of this shop stems solely from its trendy merchandise, and not its seedy interior, blaring music and dreary atmosphere. Find a great mix of styles by Parisian-based designers and young undiscovered New York talent. Choose from sexy tops, filmy shirts, see-through dresses, and sweaters. These are edgy looks heavily influenced by the music and fashion industry.

Lower East Side	212-982-5437
189 Orchard Street	bet. Houston/Stanton
NYC 10002	Mon.-Sun. 12-8

Franceska   W

There's certainly a lot going on at Franceska—maybe too much! Find a cornucopia of women's clothing and lingerie, as well as men's and boy's swimwear by Vilebrequin. Lingerie labels include Gossamer, Anti-Flirt, Faust and Lilli Ros, while snug-fitting tops, dresses, pants and sweaters complete the assortment. Handbags and jewelry are worth a second look.

Upper East Side	212-744-5400
1070 Madison Avenue	at 81st St.
NYC 10028	Mon.-Fri. 11-6, Sat. 11-7, Sun. 12-6

Frank Shattuck   M

Frank Shattuck has taken over where his mentor Henry Stewart, one of New York's most distinguished old-world tailors, left off. Each suit is hand-made from start to finish, from construction and drafting to the final five hour pressing process. Pay $3,500 for one of these luxurious suits and expect it to wear for a lifetime.

Frank Stella

Midtown East   212-371-5805
18 East 53rd Street, Room 8W   bet. 5th/Madison
NYC 10022   by appointment

Frank Stella   M/W

The husband and wife team of Frank and Stella deliver a no-nonsense menswear collection with tailored looks. Find classic suits by Jack Victor, dress shirts by Ike Behar, as well as sportscoats, sweaters, ties and outerwear. A minimal selection for women.

Upper West Side   212-877-5566
440 Columbus Avenue   at 81st St.
NYC 10024   Mon.-Fri. 11-8, Sat. 11-6, Sun. 12-6

Midtown West   212-957-1600
921 Seventh Avenue   at 58th St.
NYC 10019   Mon.-Fri. 10-7, Sat. 10-6, Sun. 12-5

Fratelli Rossetti   M/W

This fine Italian manufacturer began making shoes for cyclists and skaters in the 1950's, and later introduced the first brown loafer to the fashion world. Welcome to Rossetti's world of superbly crafted, classic loafers and lace-ups. Their design watchwords: quality, elegance, comfort and practicality. Styles are best suited for daytime wear.

Midtown East   212-888-5107
625 Madison Avenue   at 58th St.
NYC 10022   Mon.-Fri. 10-6:30, Thurs. 10- 7,
    Sat. 10-6, Sun. 12-5

Frederic Fekkai   W

We all recognize the Frederic Fekkai name (a) because it's one of New York's exclusive beauty salons and (b) a haircut by Frederic himself is worth its weight in gold, literally ($300+). However, if you've experienced neither, you always have his chic Madison Avenue boutique to fall back on. Find Frederic's complete product lines that range from hair care, fragrances and cosmetics to sunglasses, great looking handbags, hair accessories and scarves.

Upper East Side   212-583-3300
874 Madison Avenue   bet. 71/72nd St.
NYC 10021   Mon.-Sat. 10-6, Thurs. 10-7

Freed of London   M/W/C

This respected English establishment supplies the world's top dancers with their selection of ballet, jazz, ballroom and flamenco attire, as well as rehearsal garments. (You can even get the Royal Ballet's regulation apparel.) Footwear runs (no pun intended) from tap, jazz and ballroom to ballet, Flamenco and theatrical. Freed's most sought-after item: hand-crafted, peach satin pointe shoes that can be made to any dancer's specifications.

Midtown West   212-489-1055
922 Seventh Avenue   at 58th St.
NYC 10019   Mon.-Sat. 10-6

French Connection M/W
A British company featuring a contemporary line of sportswear geared toward an under 30 crowd. It's street-wise, chic clothing at affordable prices. Find suits to please the young professional, shirts, sweaters, T-shirts in abundance, pants, outerwear and underwear, all with a touch of international flavor. www.frenchconnection.com

Upper West Side	**212-496-1470**
304 Columbus Avenue	bet. 74/75th St.
NYC 10023	Mon.-Sat. 11-9, Sun. 10-7
Midtown West	**212-262-6623**
1270 Sixth Avenue	at 51st St.
NYC 10020	Mon.-Fri. 9-9, Sat. 10-8, Sun. 12-7
West Village	**212-473-4699**
700 Broadway	bet. Astor Pl./4th St.
NYC 10003	Mon.-Sat. 11-9, Sun. 12-8
SoHo	**212-219-1197**
435 West Broadway	bet. Prince/Spring
NYC 10012	Mon.-Sat. 11-9, Sun. 11-7

French Sole W
French Sole has the city's best selection of ballet flats in every color under the sun. They come quilted or plain, in leather or suede, and feature an adjustable lace to ensure a comfortable fit. If you're looking for a dressier style, select from their "Frankie & Baby" collection featuring Chinese slippers and beaded mules.

Upper East Side	**212-737-2859**
985 Lexington Avenue	bet. 71/72nd St.
NYC 10021	Mon.-Fri. 10-7, Sat. 11-6

Fuchsia W
Fuchsia is a bargain seeker's delight packed with factory samples and vintage pieces by coveted designer names. Find a mix of discounted merchandise by labels like Daryl K, Missoni, Tahari, St. John, Azzedine Alaia, Cynthia Rowley, Michael Kors, Fendi, Joseph, and Prada. Watch out for the blaze of pink shag carpeting as you enter.

NoLiTa	**(pager) 917-990-9895**
126 Baxter Street	bet. Hester/Canal
NYC 10013	Mon.-12-5, Tues.-Sun. 12-8

Furla W
Great looking Italian handbags with up-to-date styling. Crisp, structured lines with minimal hardware account for Furla's enduring designs. Their belt selection offers fashionable accoutrements that do a lot more than just hold up your pants. Also find key chains, coin purses and wallets that make amusing gifts or stocking stuffers. Furla gets top marks for quality, originality and prices.
888-FURLA-US www.furla.it

Upper East Side	**212-755-8986**
727 Madison Avenue	bet. 63/64th St.
NYC 10021	Mon.-Sat. 10-6, Thurs. 10-6:30

Gabbriel Ichak

Upper West Side   212-874-6119
Domo 159A Columbus Avenue   at 67th St.
NYC 10023   Mon.-Sat. 11-7, Sun. 12-6

SoHo   212-343-0048
430 West Broadway   bet. Spring/Prince
NYC 10012   Mon.-Sat. 11-7, Sun. 12-6

Gabbriel Ichak   W

Gabbriel Ichak makes one-of-a-kind handbags from recycled materials. Magazine covers, CD jackets and product packaging (like Goya Rice and El Paso Taco boxes) serve as amusing fronts and backs to these clear plastic, functional handbags. Prices $25 and up.

East Village   212-673-0673
430 East 9th Street   bet. 1st/Ave. A
NYC 10009   Mon.-Sat. 12-8

Gallery of Wearable Art   W

As the name suggests, this shop features clothing items that are one-of-a-kind works of art. From unusual day wear and limited edition evening gowns to non-traditional bridal wear, furs and accessories, Gallery of Wearable Art is your source for non-conformist fashions.

Upper East Side   212-425-5379
34 East 67th Street   bet. Madison/Park Ave.
NYC 10021   Tues.-Sat. 10-6

Galo   W/C

A veteran of Madison Avenue shoe retailing, Galo offers a collection of loafers, flats, pumps, sandals and boots. For children, find styles from casual and contemporary basics to dress up. From toddler to size 5. Prices range from moderate to expensive. Handbag selection includes leather clutches, straw totes and shoulder bags.

Upper East Side   212-832-3922
825 Lexington Avenue   at 63rd St.
NYC 10021   Mon.-Sat. 10-7, Sun. 12:30-5:30

Upper East Side   212-688-6276
692 Madison Avenue   bet. 62/63rd St.
NYC 10021   Mon.-Sat. 10-7, Sun. 12:30-5:30

☆ Gamine   W

Walk into this jewel box boutique and be dazzled by its unique selection of clothing and accessories. Shop an ultra-feminine collection, sprinkled with a dash of ethnic trendiness, from flirty daytime dresses to informal eveningwear made up of sari prints, beading and embroidery. Gamine has an exotic selection of girlie designs that you won't find anywhere else. Fabulous handbags and colored stone jewelry round out the assortment.

Upper East Side   212-472-6918
1322 Third Avenue   bet. 75/76th St.
NYC 10021   Mon.-Sat. 11-8, Sun. 12-6

Gant M/B

Gant specializes in men's and boy's sportswear and accessories. Find three floors of casual basics devoted to jeans, khakis, fleece outfits, rugby shirts, sweatpants, knits and outerwear. Fleece outerwear is their best bet.

Fifth Avenue 212-813-9170
645 Fifth Avenue bet. 51/52nd St.
NYC 10022 Mon.-Sat. 10-7, Sun. 12-6

☆ Gap M/W

Gap caters to just about everyone, and there's no better place to buy affordable wardrobe staples. The Gap is casual weekend wear for the professional, an essential wardrobe for the college student and a uniform for teenagers. Choose from racks of jeans, khakis, shirts, sweaters, T-shirts, belts and accessories. The Gap is a consistent, dependable source for comfortable clothing for all ages at the best prices in town. Unbelievable sales. New this year: the Gap Body Collection featuring intimates, sleepwear and bath & body products. 800-427-7895 www.gap.com

Upper East Side 212-517-5763
1164 Madison at 86th St.
NYC 10028 Mon.-Fri. 10-7, Sat. 10-7, Sun. 11-7

Upper East Side 212-794-5781
1511 Third Avenue at 85th St.
NYC 10028 Mon.- Fri. 9-9, Sat. 10-9, Sun. 11-7

Upper East Side 212-879-9144
1066 Lexington Avenue at 75th St.
NYC 10021 Mon.-Fri. 10-8, Sat. 10-7:30, Sun. 11-6

Upper East Side 212-472-4555
1131-49 Third Avenue at 66th St.
NYC 10021 Mon.-Fri. 9-8, Sat. 10-8, Sun. 11-7

Upper West Side 212-864-3600
2551 Broadway at 96th St.
NYC 10025 Mon.-Sat. 10-9, Sun. 11-8

Upper West Side 212-873-1244
2373 Broadway at 86th St.
NYC 10024 Mon.-Sat. 10-9, Sun. 11-8

Upper West Side (W) 212-873-9272
335 Columbus Avenue at 76th St.
NYC 10023 Mon.-Sat. 11-9, Sun. 10-6:30

Upper West Side 212-787-6698
2109 Broadway at 73rd St.
NYC 10023 Mon.-Sat. 10-9, Sun. 11-8

Upper West Side 212-721-5304
1988 Broadway at 67th St.
NYC 10023 Mon.-Sat. 10-9, Sun. 11-9

Midtown East 212-751-1543
734 Lexington Avenue bet. 58/59th St.
NYC 10022 Mon.-Fri. 9-9, Sat. 9-8, Sun. 10-8

Midtown East 212-980-2570
545 Madison Avenue at 55th St.
NYC 10022 Mon.-Fri. 9-8, Sat. 9-8, Sun. 10-8

Gap Kid and Baby Gap

Midtown East   212-223-5140
757 Third Avenue   at 47th St.
NYC 10017   Mon.-Fri. 8-8, Sat. 10-8, Sun. 11-6

Midtown East   212-697-3590
657-659 Third Avenue   at 42nd St.
NYC 10017   Mon.-Fri. 9-8:30, Sat.11-7, Sun. 11-6

Midtown East   212-754-2290
900 Third Avenue   at 54th St.
NYC 10022   Mon.-Fri. 9-8, Sat. 10-6, Sun. 11-5

Midtown East   212-213-6007
549 Third Avenue   bet. 36/37th St.
NYC 10016   Mon.-Fri. 9-8:30, Sat. 10-8:30, Sun. 11-7

Midtown West   212-956-3142
250 West 57th Street   bet. B'way/8th Ave.
NYC 10019   Mon.-Fri. 10-9, Sat. 9-9, Sun. 11-6

Midtown West   212-764-0285
1212 Sixth Avenue   bet. 47/48th St.
NYC 10036   Mon.-Fri. 9-9, Sat. 9-8, Sun. 11-7

Midtown West   212-768-2987
1466 Broadway   at 42nd St.
NYC 10036   Mon.-Sat. 9-10, Sun. 9-9

Midtown West   212-643-8960
60 West 34th Street   at Broadway
NYC 10001   Mon.-Sat. 9-9, Sun. 10-8

Fifth Avenue   212-977-7023
680 Fifth Avenue   at 54th St.
NYC 10019   Mon.-Sat. 10-8, Sun. 11-7

Flatiron   212-989-0550
122 Fifth Avenue   bet. 17/18th St.
NYC 10011   Mon.-Fri. 10-9, Sat. 10-8, Sun. 11-7

East Village   212-353-2090
133 Second Avenue   at St. Marks Place
NYC 10003   Mon.-Thurs. 10-9, Fri. Sat. 11-9, Sun. 12-8

East Village (M)   212-674-1877
750 Broadway   at 8th St.
NYC 10003   Mon.-Sat. 10-9, Sun. 11-8

West Village   212-727-2210
345 Sixth Avenue   at 4th St.
NYC 10014   Mon.-Sat. 10-9, Sun 10-8

Lower Manhattan   212-374-1051
89 South Street   South Street Seaport Pier 17
NYC 10038   Mon.-Sat. 10-9, Sun. 11-8

Lower Manhattan   212-432-7086
157 World Trade Center   bet. Church/Vesey
NYC 10046   Mon.-Fri. 7:30-8, Sat. & Sun.12-7

Gap Kid and Baby Gap   B/G

Gap sets the trends for moderately priced children's clothing. Find jeans, T-shirts, overalls, shirts, pants, sweatshirts, sweaters, dresses, pajamas, shoes and accessories. From outdoor weekend wear to back-to-school basics, Gap has it all at the best prices in town. From newborn to 13 years.
www.babygap.com

Gap Kid and Baby Gap

Upper East Side 212-423-0033
1535 Third Avenue bet. 86/87th St.
NYC 10028 Mon.-Fri. 9-9, Sat. 9-9, Sun. 10-7

Upper East Side 212-517-5763
1164 Madison Avenue at 86th St.
NYC 10028 Mon.-Fri. 10-8, Sat. 10-7, Sun. 11-7

Upper East Side 212-327-2614
1037 Lexington Avenue at 74th St.
NYC 10021 Mon.-Fri. 10-8, Sat. 10-7:30, Sun. 11-6

Upper East Side 212-472-4555
1131-49 Third Avenue at 66th St.
NYC 10021 Mon.-Fri. 9:30-8, Sat. 10-8, Sun. 11-7

Upper West Side 212-873-2044
2300 Broadway at 83rd St.
NYC 10024 Mon.-Sat. 10-9, Sun. 11-8

Upper West Side 212-721-5119
1988 Broadway at 67th St.
NYC 10023 Mon.-Sat. 10-9, Sun. 11-9

Upper West Side 212-875-9196
341 Columbus Avenue bet. 76/77th St.
NYC 10023 Mon.-Sat. 10-8, Sun. 11-7

Midtown East 212-980-2570
545 Madison Avenue at 55th St.
NYC 10022 Mon.-Fri. 9-8, Sat. 10-7, Sun. 11-6

Midtown East 212-223-5140
757 Third Avenue at 47th St.
NYC 10017 Mon.-Fri. 8-8, Sat. 10-7, Sun. 12-5

Midtown East 212-697-3590
657-659 Third Avenue at 42nd St.
NYC 10017 Mon.-Fri. 9-8:30, Sat. 11-7, Sun. 11-6

Midtown East 212-213-6007
549 Third Avenue bet. 36/37th St.
NYC 10016 Mon.-Sat. 9-8:30, Sun. 11-7

Midtown West 212-315-2250
250 West 57th Street bet. B'way/8th Ave.
NYC 10019 Mon.-Fri. 9-9, Sat. 10-8, Sun. 11-6

Midtown West 212-302-1266
1466 Broadway at 42nd St.
NYC 10036 Mon.-Sat. 9-10, Sun. 9-9

Midtown West 212-764-0285
1212 Sixth Avenue bet 47/48th St.
NYC 10036 Mon.-Fri. 9-9, Sat. 9-8, Sun. 11-7

Midtown West 212-643-8995
60 West 34th Street at B'way
NYC 10001 Mon.-Sat. 9-9, Sun. 10-8

Fifth Avenue 212-977-7023
680 Fifth Avenue at 54th St.
NYC 10019 Mon.-Sat. 10-8, Sun. 11-7

Flatiron 212-989-0550
122 Fifth Avenue bet. 17/18th St.
NYC 10011 Mon.-Fri. 10-9, Sat. 10-8, Sun. 11-7

Geiger

West Village   **212-777-2420**
354 Sixth Avenue   at Washington Pl.
NYC 10011   Mon.-Sat. 10-9, Sun. 11-8

Lower Manhattan   **212-786-1707**
89 South Street,   South Street Seaport Pier 17
NYC 10038   Mon.-Sat. 10-9, Sun. 11-8

Lower Manhattan   **212-945-4090**
225 World Financial Center   at Liberty St.
NYC 10281   Mon.-Fri. 9:30-7, Sat. 11-5, Sun. 12-5

Geiger   W

This Austrian manufacturer is famous for its "boiled wool" outerwear. Find jackets and coats in traditional Alpine colors with embossed silver buttons, as well as a traditional sportswear collection. No Austrian burgher's wardrobe is complete without a Geiger jacket.

Midtown East   **212-644-3435**
505 Park Avenue   at 59th St.
NYC 10022   Mon.-Sat. 10-6, Thurs. 10-8, Sun. 1-5

Genny   W

Newly appointed designer Josephus Thimister is now at the design helm of this Italian sportswear company. Shop a 2,200-sq. ft. store that runs the gamut from $80 T-shirts to $5,000 evening gowns. Find a collection of smart, wearable clothes that include chiffon tops and dresses, pants, tweed skirts, sweaters, leathers and coats.

Upper East Side   **212- 249-9660**
831 Madison Avenue   bet. 68/69th St.
NYC 10021   Mon.-Sat. 11-7

Geoffrey Beene   W

Shop this designer's small, elegant boutique, known for highly personalized service, showcasing Geoffrey Beene's collection of couture and ready-to-wear. Designs feature unexpected fabric combinations, impeccable workmanship with an emphasis on cut and attention to detail. The end result: a classic, well-tailored look with timeless wearability. While his elegant and feminine suits are perfect for ladies who lunch, Beene is perhaps most admired for his beautiful evening gowns that are soft, feminine and fit like a dream.

Fifth Avenue   **212-935-0470**
783 Fifth Avenue   bet. 59/60th St.
NYC 10022   Mon.-Fri. 10-6, Sat. 11-5

Gerry Cosby & Co.   M/B

A great source for pro sports equipment and apparel for basketball, football, baseball and hockey. Shop here for an NFL, NBA or NHL jersey or souvenir from your favorite team.

Midtown West   **212-563-6464**
3 Penn Plaza   at Madison Square Garden
NYC 10001   Mon.-Fri. 9:30-7:30, Sat. 9:30-6, Sun. 12-5

Ghost　　　　　　　　　　　　　　　　　　　　　　M/W
"Ghost-busters" will no longer have to make do with the very limited selection found in uptown department stores now that designer Tanya Sarne has opened her first free-standing store in super-hip NoHo. Ghost is best known for soft, feminine clothing dyed in vibrant hues and manufactured in special crinkly rayons, which are wrinklefree and machine washable. The assortment includes wash-and-wear dresses (long and short), peasant tops, sweaters, and drawstring pants.

NoHo　　　　　　　　　　　　　　　　**646-602-2891**
28 Bond Street　　　　　　　　　　bet. Bowery/Lafayette
NYC 10012　　　　　　　　　Mon.-Sat. 11-7, Sun. 12-6

Ghurka　　　　　　　　　　　　　　　　　　　　　M/W
Ghurka features classic, expertly hand-crafted handbags, luggage and accessories (that invoke days of the Raj or an African Safari). Their signature leather-trimmed canvas travel bags and handbags are great looking and durable. In addition, find a selection of Trafalgar suspenders exclusive to Ghurka. 800-587-1584 www.ghurka.com

Midtown East　　　　　　　　　　　　　**212-826-8300**
41 East 57th Street　　　　　　　　bet. Madison/Park Ave.
NYC 10022　　　　　　　　　Mon.-Sat. 10-6, Thurs. 10-7

Gianfranco Ferre　　　　　　　　　　　　　　　　M/W
Inside this sleek, futuristic brushed steel interior, find Ferre's romantic and feminine ready-to-wear collection. Ferre's trademark: beautifully detailed blouses in soft silhouettes. For men, find a modern collection of suits and sportswear.

Upper East Side　　　　　　　　　　　**212-717-5430**
845 Madison Avenue　　　　　　　　　bet. 70th/71st St.
NYC 10021　　　　　　　　　Mon.-Sat. 10-6, Sun. 12-5

Gianni Versace　　　　　　　　　　　　　　　　　M/W
Since taking over the helm of this high-energy fashion house, Donatella Versace has successfully stepped into her brother's design shoes and proven her talents to the world. She continues his legacy by fusing together the worlds of fashion and music, earning the sobriquet "rock 'n' roll designer." Like her brother, Donatella's talent lies in energetic, sensational, eye-catching designs. Find ready-to-wear, sportswear, casualwear, shoes and accessories with looks that are adventuresome and aggressive. A Versace design is sexy, and glitzy. According to rockstar Bon Jovi, "Wearing a Versace is like driving a Ferrari with the top down at 70 mph."

Upper East Side　　　　　　　　　　　**212-744-6868**
815 Madison Avenue　　　　　　　　　　bet. 68/69th St.
NYC 10021　　　　　　　　　　　　　　Mon.-Sat. 10-6
Fifth Avenue　　　　　　　　　　　　**212-317-0224**
647 Fifth Avenue　　　　　　　　　　　bet. 51/52nd St.
NYC 10022　　　　Mon.-Sat. 10-6:30, Thurs. 10-6:30

Gilcrest Clothes Company　　　　　　　　　　M
This menswear discount retailer operates from a third floor loft. Choose from a good selection of European styled suits by labels like Jane Barnes, Ungaro, Louis Feraud, Baumler and more. In addition, find sportcoats, blazers, slacks, overcoats, raincoats and tuxedos. It's all 40% less than department store prices. Suit prices run from $339 to $600.

Chelsea　　　　　　　　　　　　　　**212-254-8933**
900 Broadway, 3rd Floor　　　　　　　bet. 19/20th St.
NYC 10003　　　　　Mon.-Fri. 8-5:30, Sat. 9-5, Sun. 9-4

Giordano's　　　　　　　　　　　　　　　　W
Anyone with tiny feet will appreciate Giordano's great selection of casual and dressy shoes in sizes 4 to $5^1/_2$. Labels include Donna Karan, Anne Klein, Stuart Weitzman, Fendi, Via Spiga and more.

Upper East Side　　　　　　　　　　**212-688-7195**
1150 Second Avenue　　　　　　　　　bet. 60/61st St.
NYC 10021　　　　　　　　　　Mon.-Fri. 11-7, Sat. 11-6

Giorgio Armani　　　　　　　　　　　　M/W
Armani continues to make everyone's "best dressed list" with his minimalist approach to fashion. For the past 25 years, men and women have adored his immaculate, well-proportioned clothing that is the epitome of elegance. An Armani design is simple, smart and relaxed; shapes are easy and uncontrived. In his women's collection, Armani applies a masculine cut with a neutral color palette, while never losing sight of his most important ingredient: femininity. From ready-to-wear to eveningwear to accessories, sophistication and wearability are the rule. Don't mistake Armani's minimalism for bland timidity; according to the master himself, "Elegance doesn't mean being noticed; it means being remembered." www.giorgioarmani.com

Upper East Side　　　　　　　　　　**212-988-9191**
760 Madison Avenue　　　　　　　　　　at 65th St.
NYC 10021　　　　　　　　Mon.-Sat., 10-6, Thurs. 10-7

Giraudon　　　　　　　　　　　　　　　M/W
Giraudon's footwear line delivers a utilitarian, unisex look, and lots of chunky rubber soles. Find two lines designed by Alain-Guy Giraudon featuring everything from rugged boots and sporty loafers with lug soles to leather-soled dressy lace-ups and slip-ons.

Chelsea　　　　　　　　　　　　　　**212-633-0999**
152 Eighth Avenue　　　　　　　　　　bet. 17/18th St.
NYC 10011　　　　　　　Mon.-Sat. 11:30-7:30, Sun. 1-6

Giselle　　　　　　　　　　　　　　　　　W
You are now entering a time warp. Giselle caters to a mature, conservative customer in search of no-nonsense work suits, blouses, sportswear and coordinating accessories, all at 20% below retail. Labels include Escada Sport, Miss V (Valentino), Ferre Studio and Baslere.

Lower East Side 212-673-1900
143 Orchard Street bet. Delancey/Rivington
NYC 10002 Sun.-Thurs. 9-6, Fri. 9-4, Sat. closed

Givenchy W

With this year's recent move, the house of Givenchy has finally joined the ranks of other Madison Avenue designer boutiques. The shop's modern interior, combined with designer Alexander McQueen's new fashion direction, aims to attract a younger, hipper customer. Shop a color coordinated pret-a-porter line of form-fitted suits, sensual, tailored skirts and dresses, as well as strong-shouldered jackets. Clean, simple lines, feminine styling and McQueen's modern interpretation of classic mixed with sexy looks define a Givenchy design. Handbags and shoes also available.

Upper East Side 212-688-4338
710 Madison Avenue at 63rd St.
NYC 10021 Mon.-Sat. 10-6, Sun. 11-5

Goffredo Fantini M/W

Goffredo Fantini is a fresco painter turned cobbler (no, we didn't make this up) and he has invented the "Fressura," a space-age shoe with a permanent (read: indestructible) sole and changeable, elastic tops. You need to see it to believe it. Also, a small collection of urban, chunky heeled shoes.

NoLiTa 212-219-1501
248 Elizabeth Street bet. Prince/Houston
NYC 10012 Tues.-Fri. 12-7, Sat. 12-6, Sun. 12-7

Gorsart M

It's worth the trek to Gorsart's inconvenient location for its well-priced menswear collection. Find suits by Joseph Abboud, Hickey-Freeman, Burberrys and Gieves & Hawkes. Prices range from $450 to $975 with free custom alterations. Sportswear, shirts, ties and outerwear are all private label. Find shoes by Aldon and Cole Haan. The Gorsart look is classic American with an easy-to-wear feel.

Lower Manhattan 212-962-0024
9 Murray Street bet. B'way/Church
NYC 10007 Mon.-Fri. 9-6, Sat. 9-5:30

Granny-Made W/B/G

This shop specializes in unique hand-knits from Italy, England and the U.S. Mothers can shop an adorable collection of children's novelty sweaters, featuring appliques, sweet embroideries, cute animals and floral motifs. For adults, a similar selection by labels like Christine Foley, Ronie Rapl and Carol Horn. Accessories include socks and novelty pillows.

Upper West Side 212-496-1222
381 Amsterdam Avenue bet. 78/79th St.
NYC 10024 Mon.-Fri. 11-7:30, Sat. 10-6, Sun. 12-5

Great Feet B/G

Simply the best children's footwear selection in New York. If you can't find it here, you won't find it anywhere. Brand names include Stride-Rite, Keds, Nike, Hilfiger, Sam & Libby and Dr. Martens. Styles range from casual weekend wear to back-to-school classics and party shoes. They also carry the very latest in skateboard shoes. Socks, tights and slippers available.

Upper East Side   212-249-0551
1241 Lexington Avenue   at 84th St.
NYC 10028   Mon.-Sat. 9:30-5:30, Fri. 9:30-7:30

Greenstones & Cie B/G

For the past 19 years, Greenstones & Cie has been dressing kids in a variety of looks, from intricate European clothing to practical American-made togs. Find brand names such as Marese, Kenzo (girls), Naf Naf, Portofino, Mini Man and Catamini. Whether it's school-time, play-time or party-time you'll always be pleased with the selection. Greenstones' hats are an absolute must. Sizes from newborn to 12 years.

Upper East Side   212-427-1665
1184 Madison Avenue   bet. 86/87th St.
NYC 10028   Mon.-Sat. 10:30-6:30

Upper West Side   212-580-4322
442 Columbus Avenue   bet. 81/82nd St.
NYC 10024   Mon-Sat 10-7, Sun. 12-6

Gucci M/W

Can we all agree that Gucci designer Tom Ford is a genius? Ford has revived this 93-year-old Italian leathergoods company and turned it into the world's most glamorous fashion house. Welcome to the world of Gucci where the look is strictly avant-garde, the color palette predominately black and the testosterone level dangerously high. Ford is the master at creating sexy glamour. Shop a ready-to-wear collection that features clothing that's slick, seductive and has a surprisingly classic fit. Gucci is also one of the trendiest places to shop for cutting edge shoes. Leathergoods and handbags incorporate classic Italian styling with a contemporary flair. Suggestive, slinky and oh-so-Hollywood defines Gucci today. **New 35,000-sq. ft. flagship store.** 800-234-8224

Fifth Avenue   212-826-2600
685 Fifth Avenue   at 54th Street
NYC 10022   Mon.-Wed., Fri. 10-6:30,
    Thurs. & Sat. 10-7, Sun. 12-6

Guess? M/W

Guess? is back and better than ever with their collection of apparel and accessories that combine "sexy collegiate looks" with European flair. Shop for casual wear in simple styles with cool attitude. Basics include fashion jeans, khakis, shirts, T-shirts, outerwear and shoes that are always in keeping with the latest trends. Accessories include wallets, watches and sunglasses trademarked with the visible Guess logo. Some dressier styles for women.

SoHo   212-226-9545
537 Broadway   bet. Prince/Spring
NYC 10012   Mon.-Sat. 11-9, Sun. 11-7

Lower Manhattan   212-385-0533
23-25 Water Street   at South Street Seaport
NYC 10038   Mon.-Sat. 10-9, Sun. 11-8

Gymboree   B/G

A children's shop featuring casual clothing. Find four lines of coordinating play clothes that are fun, colorful and easy-to-wear. Styles are popular with kids and prices will please Mom and Dad. From newborn to size 7/8. 800-222-7758

Upper East Side   212-717-6702
1120 Madison Avenue   bet. 83/84th St.
NYC 10028   Mon.-Fri. 10-7, Sat. 11-6, Sun. 12-5

Upper East Side   212-517-5548
1332 Third Avenue   at 76th St.
NYC 10021   Mon.-Sat. 10-7, Sun. 12-6

Upper East Side   212-688-4044
1049 Third Avenue   at 62nd St.
NYC 10021   Mon.-Sat. 10-7, Sun. 12-6

Upper West Side   212-595-9071
2271 Broadway   at 82nd St.
NYC 10024   Mon.-Fri. 10-9, Sat. 10-8, Sun. 11-6

Upper West Side   212- 595-7662
2015 Broadway   bet. 68/69th St.
NYC 10023   Mon.-Fri. 10-8, Sat. 10-7, Sun. 12-6

H. Herzfeld   M

Traditionally styled menswear is the name of the game at H. Herzfeld, especially in their outstanding haberdashery department that carries shirts, neckwear, sweaters, sportswear, underwear, pajamas and accessories, as well as shoes by Alden. Although suits are generally custom-made, you will find a selection of Hickey-Freeman and private label. Off-the-rack suits start at $1,200, while custom will run you $2,200. Herzfeld delivers tailored looks with classic English styling.

Midtown East   212-753-6756
507 Madison Avenue   at 52/53rd St.
NYC 10022   Mon.-Fri. 9-6, Sat. 9-5:30

Hanae Mori   W

A Japanese designer who favors "old-world couture rather than flights of fancy." Mori's distinctive trademark is her use of luxurious fabrics, often featuring floral motifs and oriental themes. A mature customer shops here for formal suits, cocktail dresses, knits and eveningwear. The look is feminine, refined and Japanese classic.

Upper East Side   212-472-2352
27 East 79th Street   bet. 5th/Madison
NYC 10021   Mon.-Sat. 10-6

Hans Koch W

This shop specializes in handcrafted, one-of-a-kind belts, handbags and jewelry. Koch's passion for color drives all his designs. Belts are simple and easy-to-wear, while handbag styles range from soft to constructed and incorporate bold color combinations.

SoHo   **212-226-5385**
174 Prince Street   bet. Sullivan/Thompson
NYC 10012   Mon.-Thurs. 12-8, Fri. & Sat. 12-9, Sun. 1-8

Harriet Love W

Formerly a vintage shop, Harriet Love now sells "retro" look casual wear that can be dressed up or down. This small boutique is a leader in antique-inspired clothing.

SoHo   **212-966-2280**
126 Prince Street   bet. Wooster/Greene
NYC 10012   Tues.-Sun. 11-7

Harry Rothman's M

A good source for well-priced men's clothing, Rothman's offers discounts of up to 40% on brand names like Hickey-Freeman, Canali, Joseph Abboud, Gieves and Hawkes, and Hugo Boss. Also find a selection of shirts, ties, underwear, sport jackets, outerwear and shoes in a full range of sizes.

Flatiron   **212-777-7400**
200 Park Avenue South   at 17th St.
NYC 10003   Mon.-Fri. 10-7, Thurs. 10-8,
   Sat. 9:30-6, Sun. 12-5:30

The Hat Shop W

This whimsical world of toppers guarantees the perfect fit for every head. Choose a selection of hats from over 40 talented New York designers. Labels include Deborah Harper, Abigail Aldridge, Brenda Lynn, Eric Javits and Jacqueline Lamont. Styles range from a classic straw boater to a wide-brimmed show-stopper. Every Thursday is open house for milliners, an ideal time to stop in for custom fittings.

SoHo   **212-219-1445**
120 Thompson Street   bet. Prince/Spring
NYC 10012   Mon.-Sat. 12-7, Sun. 1-6,

Hatitude W

It's always fun to browse in this eclectic hat boutique. Despite the store's name, hats take a back seat to the selection of dolls and vintage jewelry. When you do finally spot the hats, you'll find them in all shapes, sizes and fabrics with an emphasis on vintage. Look for Wendy Carrington to increase her collection this fall when she adds several new designers. www.wendycarrington.com

TriBeCa   **212-571-4558**
93 Reade Street   bet. W. B'way/Church
NYC 10013   Mon.-Fri. 12-7, Sat. 12-5

Hedra Prue W

Owners Anna Kim and Tracy Mayer are known for culling the hottest items from each season's new designers. You'll find clothes in interesting silks, colors and fabrics, from younger undiscovered designers. Find a collection of basics, as well as unusual one-of-a-kind pieces. Choose from form-fitted sundresses, skirts, suits, pants and accessories that are a perfect crossover between evening and daywear. Labels include Martin, Trosman & Churba, Barney Cheng and more.

NoLiTa 212-343-9205
281 Mott Street bet. Houston/Prince
NYC 10012 Mon.-Sat. 11:30-7:30, Sun. 12-6:30

Helene Arpels W

Helene Arpels opened her Park Avenue shoe salon 38 years ago, and over time it has changed very little. Her clientele includes royalty and socialites from all over the world. Arpels features pumps, loafers, slippers, ornate evening shoes, custom jewelry and caftans. Prices are over-the-top—a pair of loafers sells for $575.

Midtown East 212-755-1623
470 Park Avenue bet. 57/58th St.
NYC 10022 Mon.-Sat. 10-6:30

Hello Sari W

Hello Sari is strictly devoted to authentic Indian merchandise. This matchbox interior is home to beaded and embroidered dresses, shawls, scarves, saris and amusing sandals and shoes. It's a perfect place to shop for an unusual ethnic piece to spice up your wardrobe.

NoLiTa 212-274-0791
261 Broome Street bet. Allen/Orchard
NYC 10002 Sat. & Sun. 12-7
  weekdays call for hours

Helmut Lang M/W

Lang's seductive vision of urban dressing keeps the crowds coming back for more. Staying true to form, he continues to turn out edgy-looking clothes defined by sensual shapes and artistic detailing. Each collection is based on three elements: luxury fabrics, sober color palettes, and clean looks. Find a ready-to-wear line that boasts trouser suits, shirts, cardigans, tops, shearlings and beautifully cut coats, all in the natural luxe of wools, cashmeres, thick silks and leathers. Modern, relaxed chic defines the Lang label. Check out his "hipper-than-thou" jeans assortment packed with lots of attitude. New this year: shoes and handbags.
www.helmutlang.com

SoHo 212-925-7214
80 Greene Street bet. Spring/Broome
NYC 10012 Mon.-Sat. 11-7, Sun. 12-6

★ H & M (Hennes & Mauritz) M/W

The Swedish have landed and taken New York by storm. H & M, short for Hennes & Mauritz, is a Scandinavian version of Club Monaco delivering high fashion, designer looks (straight off the runways) at incredibly low prices. Think Gap, Old Navy and Club Monaco all rolled into one. Shop a 35,000-sq. ft. store featuring 20 lines of trendy clothing that include sexy leather pants at $95, jeans trimmed in sequins at $35, embroidered tank tops for as little as $5.50, accessories and cosmetics, as well as plus sizes. Fashion forward looks at very affordable prices. These clothes aren't built to last, but at these unbelievable prices do we really care? www.hm.com

Fifth Avenue   212-489-0390
640 Fifth Avenue   at 51st St.
NYC 10019   Mon.-Sat. 10-8, Sun. 11-7

Midtown West
34th Street   bet. Fifth/Sixth Ave.
NYC 10001   Mon.-Sat. 10-8, Sun. 11-7

Henri Bendel W

Once considered the place to shop for eclectic fashions and accessories, Bendel's, now owned by The Limited, has become more mainstream. One of the nicest things about Bendel's is its relatively small size — you can be in and out in a flash. Cosmetics and accessories areas are compact and easy to shop, while clothing departments are small, well-organized and well-staffed. Bendel's continues to showcase some of the brightest new designers like Dirk Bikkembergs, Gharani Strok and Nanette Lepore, along with favorites like Kors, Vivienne Tam, Gaultier, Susan Lazar, Anna Molinari and Nicole Miller. Sweaters, hats, hosiery, casual wear and outerwear departments round out Bendel's assortment. Find a Garren hair salon and a Salon de The on upper levels. 800-423-6335

Fifth Avenue   212-247-1100
712 Fifth Avenue   bet. 55/56th St.
NYC 10019   Mon.-Sat. 10-7, Sun. 12-6

Henry Lehr W

Henry Lehr's offers a collection of brand labels for those in search of comfortable casual wear. Find jeans by Levi's, Helmut Lang, A. Gold E. and Earl. Shirts, knits and T-shirts round out the assortment.

NoLiTa   212-274-9921
232 Elizabeth Street   bet. Prince/Houston
NYC 10012   Mon.-Sun. 11-7

Henry Lehr W

Henry Lehr's second SoHo shop showcases T-shirts in an abundance of styles. Find labels by Juicy Couture, Jet, 3 Dot, Michael Stars, Skimpiez and more. In addition, choose from large totes, sarongs for the summer months and clogs by Gretel Clogs. A good source for basic, casual tops at reasonable prices.

Holland & Holland

NoLiTa   212-343-0567
268 Elizabeth Street   bet. Prince/Houston
NYC 10012   Mon.-Sun. 11-7

Hermès   M/W

Although Hermès does, in fact, sell ready-to-wear, nearly everyone comes here for their distinctive neckties, scarves and handbags. Discreetly colorful ties (at $120) feature amusing prints. Collecting Hermès scarves is a religion for some women—even at $275 per scarf—while their Kelly bag is coveted by the ultra chic. In clothing, rich, refined and "sporty posh" define a collection of beautifully tailored basics, including pleated pants, shirts, cashmeres, jackets and outerwear. These are classic fashions, free from the trendiness of other luxury houses. **New 20,000-sq. ft. flagship store.** 800-441-4488

Upper East Side   212-751-3181
691 Madison Avenue   bet. 62/63rd Street
NYC 10022   Mon.-Sat. 10-6, Thurs. 10-7

Heun   W

Owned by the same folks who brought you Juno shoes, Heun is a good destination for trendy merchandise, including filmy shirts, hip pants, dresses, jackets, cashmere sets and T-shirts. In the back, find a large selection of shoes to go with your outfit. Labels include Heun, Ensemble and Loretta Di Lorenzo.

SoHo   212-625-2560
543 Broadway   bet. Prince/Spring
NYC 10012   Mon.-Sat. 10:30-8, Sun. 11-8

Himaya   W

The design team of Gig Ferrante and Cezar Lim are the talents behind Himaya, which means "sublime" in the Far East. Find a sophisticated ready-to-wear collection manufactured in advanced wools, silks, and leathers with stretch capability for comfort and wrinkle resistance. Himaya's customer layers her looks with tailored, and deconstructed jackets, dresses, suits, and separates, and couture evening gowns. It's European chic with American ease.
www.himaya.com

Fifth Avenue   212-973-9107
551 Fifth Avenue, Suite 1620   at 45th Street
NYC 10176   Mon.-Sat. 10-6

Holland & Holland   M/W

What Hermès is to the equestrian world, Holland & Holland is to the hunting world. Originally a purveyor of hunting rifles, this shop now specializes in refined, luxurious sportswear perfect for both city and country living. Find jackets in tweeds and suedes, shirts, pants, sweaters, outerwear and accessories with bucolic looks. A note of caution: even the mega-rich have been known to blink twice at the price tags. Their impressive gun room and fine art and book department are worth a look.

Hotel Venus

Midtown East	**212-752-7755**
50 East 57th Street	bet. Madison/Park
NYC 10022	Mon.-Fri. 10-6:30, Sat. 10-6

Hotel Venus   M/W

Owned by Patricia Field, Hotel Venus takes the same familiar fashion approach as her other downtown shop (Patricia Field's). We're talking faddish clothes where rough biker meets diva. Shop a daring and colorful selection of vinyl bustiers, sheer fitted shirts, leather halter tops, micro-minis, hard-core rubberized patent leather outfits, funky clubwear, boas, lingerie, shoes and accessories. Labels include Clutch, Lip Service and Hysteric Glamour. It's worth a trip just to experience the shopping environment and amusing sales staff. For the fearless and campy.

SoHo	**212-966-4066**
382 West Broadway	bet. Broome/Spring
NYC 10012	Mon.-Sun. 12-8

House of Dormeuil   M/W

This French clothier specializes in custom, made-to-measure and off-the-rack suits. Available in fabulous fabrics, custom suits and shirts start at $2,850 and $135, respectively. Also find ties, bench-made shoes by Edward Green and luxurious accessories. Dormeuil's tailor even makes office visits.

Upper East Side	**212-396-4444**
21 East 67th Street	bet. Madison/Fifth Ave.
NYC 10021	Mon.-Sat. 10-6

Hunting World   M/W

If you're headed to Africa for a safari, a stop at Hunting World is a must. Outfit yourself in the latest bush gear of safari jackets, pants, vests, silk scarves, hats and shoes, then pack it all in their signature travel bags. Fishing gear and apparel for the complete angler also available.
800-833-1251

Midtown East	**212-755-3400**
16 East 53rd Street	bet. Madison/Fifth Ave.
NYC 10022	Mon.-Sat. 10-6

Iceberg   M/W

An Italian retailer appealing to those who want to keep up with today's fashions without being too trendy. Iceberg features a ready-to-wear collection in high-tech fabrics, modern designs and form-fitted shapes. Find dresses, blouses, skirts, jackets and knits, all color coordinated. It's sophisticated clothing with an edge. A small sportswear selection for men.

Upper East Side	**212-249-5412**
772 Madison	at 66th St.
NYC 10021	Mon.-Sat. 10-6, Thurs. 10-7

If   W

A SoHo purveyor of avant-garde clothing and accessories. Find a collection of ready-to-wear from designers such as

Commes des Garcons, Ivan Grundahl, Marc Le Bihan and Vivienne Westwood. Shoes, hats, handbags and accessories also available.

SoHo	**212-334-4964**
94 Grand Street	bet. Mercer/Greene
NYC 10013	Mon.-Sat. 11-7, Sun. 11-6:30

Il Bisonte   M/W

Durable, handcrafted leather goods, embossed with a bison logo and perfect for weekends. Find a complete line of handbags, small leathergoods, briefcases and luggage. Undyed leather and brass hardware define a Bisonte design. Styles are functional and good for travel.

Upper East Side	**212-717-4771**
22 East 65th Street	bet. Fifth/Madison Ave.
NYC 10021	Mon.-Sat. 11-6
SoHo	**212-966-8773**
72 Thompson Street	bet. Broome/Spring
NYC 10012	Tues.-Sat. 12-6:30, Sun. & Mon. 12-6

Ina   M/W

Ina's self-described mission: " To select only what's in fashion from those who are in fashion, for those who want to be in fashion." Welcome to this consignment shop where the fashion cognoscenti part with their designer clothes. Find the hottest designer names like Prada, Gucci, Kors, Marni, Armani, Calvin Klein and Versace. Handbags, scarves and shoes by Blahnik, Gucci, Chanel and Hermès round out the assortment. Ina's secret recipe: her wares are in pristine condition, but her prices can't be beat.

SoHo	**212-941-4757**
101 Thompson Street	bet. Spring/Prince
NYC 10012	Mon.-Sun 12-7
NoLiTa	**212-334-9048**
21 Prince Street	bet. Mott/Elizabeth
NYC 10012	Sun.-Thurs. 12-7, Fri. & Sat. 12-8
NoLiTa (M)	**212-334-2210**
262 Mott Street	bet. Houston/Prince
NYC 10012	Sun.-Thurs. 12-7, Fri. & Sat. 12-8

Infinity   B/G

Infinity is your answer for those "hard-to-shop-for" preteens. Find activewear, sportswear and dressy suits from London. Labels include Rocky T, Ikkes, Sermonetta and David Charles. Looks run from basic to borderline funky.

Upper East Side	**212-517-4232**
1116 Madison Avenue	at 83rd St.
NYC 10028	Mon.-Sat. 10-6

Inside Story   W

A tiny boutique stocked with the latest in sexy underpinnings. Whether it's a saucy bra or a fetching teddy, it's all by

Institut

top-of-the-line European brand names like Aubade, Lise Charmel and La Perla. Find looks guaranteed to flatter.

Upper West Side   212-874-2773
198 Columbus Avenue   bet. 68/69th St.
NYC 10023   Mon.-Sat. 11-8, Sun. 12-7

Institut   W

Institut's party-like ambience, colorful interior design and trendy selection of European and American designers draws young New Yorkers. Find a contemporary collection of urban street fashions. Choose from stretch pants by Tark, flowy dresses, leathers, jackets, body-hugging knits, tight tops, skirts and accessories, and fun jewelry. Remember that this is trendy fashion, not high fashion. Best for the under 40 crowd. Fun jewelry.

SoHo   212-431-5521
97 Spring Street   bet. Mercer/B'way
NYC 10012   Mon.-Sun. 11-8

SoHo   212-431-1970
99 Spring Street   bet. Mercer/B'way
NYC 10012   Mon.-Sun. 11-8

Intermix   W

The Intermix's buyers do a bang-up job of bringing you the hottest designers and the latest looks. Find up-to-the-minute fashions by Tracy Feith, Helmut Lang, Paul & Joe, Rebecca Taylor, Vivienne Tam, Anna Sui, Theory, Sigerson Morrison shoes and more. Although this shop reeks of trend, you won't look like you're trying too hard.

Upper East Side   212-249-7858
1003 Madison Avenue   bet. 77/78th St.
NYC 10021   Mon.-Sat. 10-7, Sun. 12-6

Flatiron   212-533-9720
125 Fifth Avenue   bet. 19/20th St.
NYC 10003   Mon.-Sat. 11-8, Sun. 12-6

In the Black   W

A SoHo boutique whose focus is basic black eveningwear (cocktail dresses, suits and formal wear). Labels include Vertigo, Transit, Artwork and more. Moderate prices.

SoHo   212-420-7800
130 Thompson Street   bet. Houston/Prince
NYC 10012   Tues.-Sat. 12-7, Sun. 12-6

Iramo   M/W

Here's an innovative concept in retailing: When you want to open another hip-hop shoe store in the same neighborhood with exactly the same merchandise, but want to stay "original," what should you do? Spell the name of your first store backwards and, voila, you've created a totally "new" store. If this makes no sense to you, go to Omari and read all about Iramo!!!

SoHo   212-334-9159
89 Spring Street   bet. Mercer/W. B'way
NYC 10012   Mon.-Sat. 11-8, Sun. 11-7:30

Issey Miyake   M/W
Home to Miyake's signature women's and men's collections, the shop is a magnet for artsy, avant-garde types seeking extreme, head-turning fashions. Unusually shaped, sculpture-like designs, synthetic materials and lots of color are Miyake's trademarks. Many of the looks are sheer and revealing and might not be for everyone.

Upper East Side   212-439-7822
992 Madison Avenue   at 77th St.
NYC 10021   Mon.-Fri. 10-6, Sat. 11-5

J. Crew   M/W
J. Crew is where you shop for work-week basics and weekend staples. It's classic, dependable clothing that's easy to wear year round. J. Crew covers all its bases by offering three dressing options: casual Friday clothes, dressy looks with classic styling and weekend wear. Shop for chinos, dress pants, cashmere, button-down shirts, relaxed jeans, T-shirts, dresses, swimsuits, sleepwear and underwear, accessories and shoes. The J. Crew image epitomizes an active "all American" lifestyle. Great bang for the buck. 800-562-0258
www.jcrew.com

Fifth Avenue   212-765-4227
30 Rockefeller Center at 50th St.   bet. 5th/6th Ave.
NYC 10022   Mon.-Sat. 10-7, Sun. 11-7

Flatiron   212-255-4848
91 Fifth Avenue   bet. 16/17th St.
NYC 10003   Mon.-Fri. 10-8, Sat. 11-6, Sun. 11-6

SoHo   212-966-2739
99 Prince Street   at Mercer
NYC 10012   Mon.-Sat. 10-8, Sun. 12-6

Lower Manhattan   212-385-3500
203 Front Street   at South Street Seaport
NYC 10038   Mon.-Sat. 10-9, Sun. 11-8

J. McLaughlin   M/W
Preppy, conservative clothing is the name of the game at McLaughlins'. Women can choose from a collection of career and sportswear that runs the gamut from dress suits and blazers to sweaters and jackets. For men, find sportswear perfect for urban weekend living.

Upper East Side   212-369-4830
1311 Madison Avenue   bet. 92/93rd St.
NYC 10028   Mon. & Fri. 10-6, Tues.-Thurs. 10-7,
                                     Sat. 11-6, Sun. 12-6

Upper East Side   212-879-9565
1343 Third Avenue   at 77th St.
NYC 10021   Mon. & Fri. 11-8, Tues.-Thurs. 11-9,
                                    Sat. 10:30-6, Sun. 12-6

J. Mendel   W
A luxury fur shop selling both contemporary and traditional coats, running from sporty chic to glam evening. Shop

the finest quality furs that include mink, chinchilla, sable, fisher and fox, as well as cashmere overcoats and rainwear lined or trimmed in one of these coveted pelts. Mendel's delivers European styling with simple elegance and just the right degree of fashion edge. Expect to pay top dollar; however, at the end of the season, prices are negotiable.

Upper East Side   212-832-5830
723 Madison Avenue   bet. 63/64th St.
NYC 10021   Mon.-Sat. 9:30-6

J.M. Weston   M/W

An expensive French footwear retailer renowned for handmade, classic shoes. Find conservative styles for loafers, lace-ups and boots, all hand-stitched to endure a lifetime of wear. For a slice of this luxury, you'll have to pay anywhere from $400 to $600. 877-4-Weston

Upper East Side   212-535-2100
812 Madison Avenue   at 68th St.
NYC 10021   Mon.-Sat. 10-6

J. Press   M

One of the oldest menswear shops in New York, J. Press prides itself on its selection of traditional suits, furnishings, sportswear, formalwear, outerwear and accessories—all in good taste at reasonable prices. A great shop for young career men. Suit prices start at $285.

Midtown East   212-687-7642
7 East 44th Street   bet. Fifth/Madison
NYC 10017   Mon.-Sat. 9-6

J.S. Suarez   W

The Suarez family has been selling copies of famous maker handbags for nearly 50 years. Find brand name knock-offs of Gucci, Hermès, Chanel and more. Quality workmanship and styling go into each one of these handbags. Prices generally run 30% to 50% below retail. Belts, scarves and small leathergoods also available.

Midtown East   212-753-3758
450 Park Avenue   bet. 56/57th St.
NYC 10022   Mon.-Fri. 10-6, Sat. 10-5

Jacadi   B/G

A successful French company that makes shopping for your children a pleasure. Clothing is neatly displayed according to size, color and style. Find back-to-school basics and casual play clothes, as well as shoes and accessories. Looks range from adorable smocked dresses to embroidered and appliqued overalls. A great sweater and blouse selection. A layette department selling everything from bumpers to towels. Newborn to age 12. Good sales.

Upper East Side   212-369-1616
1281 Madison Avenue   bet. 91/92nd St.
NYC 10128   Mon.-Wed, Fri., Sat., 10-6,
   Thurs. 10-7, Sun. 12-5

Upper East Side 212-535-3200
787 Madison Avenue bet. 66/67th St.
NYC 10021 Mon.-Wed., Fri., Sat. 10-6,
Thurs. 10-7, Sun. 12-5

Jack Silver Formal Wear M

Looking for a tuxedo for your wedding or a gala event? Rent or buy at Jack Silver. Choose from labels like Oscar de la Renta, Pierre Cardin, After Six and Ralph Lauren. Tuxedos for purchase must be ordered; rentals are in stock. Shirts, bow ties, cummerbunds, suspenders and shoes also available.

Midtown West 212-582-0202
1780 Broadway, 3rd Fl. bet. 57/58th St.
NYC 10019 Mon. & Thurs. 9-7

Jack Spade M

For the past five years, fashionistas of the female persuasion have trumpeted handbags by Kate Spade. Good news, gentlemen, it's your turn now with husband Andy Spade's collection of snappy, efficient bags. Find travel bags, day bags, informal briefcases, totes, messenger bags, banker's envelopes, wallets and more, all under the semi-eponymous Jack Spade label. They come in three fabrications: canvas, nylon and water-repellent, waxed cotton canvas. Lots of extra amenities like pockets for cell phones and pens. Bags start at $200. Shooting coats and Mackintosh rainwear also available.

SoHo 212-625-1820
56 Greene Street bet. Spring/Broome
NYC 10012 Mon.-Sat. 11-7, Sun. 12-6

Jaeger W

A British purveyor of conservative sportswear and career wear that rolls along year after year. Jaeger caters to the executive-type seeking secure, tailored business attire for the office and casual wear for weekends. Find mix and match separates pants, skirts and sweaters in traditional English fabrics.

Upper East Side 212-628-3350
818 Madison Avenue bet. 68/69th St.
NYC 10021 Mon.-Sat. 10-6

☆ Jamin Puech W

A sophisticated handbag shop from the owner of Calypso St. Barths. Find vintage-inspired handbags that are refreshingly modern, chic and stylish. Each bag is hand-made in France and detailed to perfection. Style fabrications range from crocheted and sequined to beaded, leather and straw. Shoes also available.

NoLiTa 212-334-9730
252 Mott Street bet. Houston/Prince
NYC 10012 Mon.-Sat. 11-7, Sun. 12-7

Janet Russo W

Janet Russo's passion has always been for collecting unusual fabrics. Every year she travels far and wide in search of beautiful cloths that come from all over the world, from Indian saris and Chinese silks to Liberty of London prints. These materials are then turned into her very own collection of feminine frocks. Find lots of dresses, tops, sweater sets and eveningwear, as well as cardigans and camisoles by Mary Beth's design. Accessories include antique purses, earrings and everyday bags. Styles are best suited for the curvaceous woman seeking looks with a romantic edge.

NoLiTa   212-625-3297
262 Mott Street   bet. Houston/Prince
NYC 10012   Sun.-Wed. 11-6, Thurs.-Sat. 11-7

☆ Jay Kos   M

Shopping at Jay Kos is like shopping at your own personal club. An intimate atmosphere of beautifully displayed merchandise makes you want to buy it all. Shop a luxurious collection of classic Italian suits (ready-made or custom), tweed shooting jackets, all-weather coats (including Macintosh jackets and Austrian Loden coats), Scottish silk-lined cashmere sweaters, hand-cut shirts from one of the oldest workshops in Switzerland, neckwear and English corduroys. In addition, find furnishings and accessories that include fabulous English cufflinks, Swain Adney & Brigg umbrellas and Borsalino and Lock hats. Kos' appeal is based on traditional styling, luxury fabrics and pure elegance. Expensive.

Upper East Side   212-327-2382
986 Lexington Avenue   bet. 71/72nd St.
NYC 10021   Mon.-Thurs. 10-7, Fri. & Sat. 10-6

Jeffrey New York   M/W

If you want your fashion fresh and cutting edge, head for the meat-packing district where Jeffrey Kalinsky is in charge of his 18,000-sq. ft. multi-designer emporium. Kalinsky's unique ability to cull the highlights from each designer's collection sets this mini-department store apart from the rest. Outfit yourself in sophisticated and hip labels like Jil Sanders, Helmut Lang, Alexander McQueen, Narciso Rodriguez, Marc Jacobs and Saint Laurent Hommes. The real prize at Jeffrey's may well be his fabulous shoe selection. Treat your feet to a pair of shoes by Gucci, Robert Clergerie, Manolo Blahnik, Ferragamo and Weitzman. New this year: Order a pair of shoes over the phone and have it delivered the same day.

Chelsea   212-206-1272
449 West 14th Street   bet. 9/10th Ave.
NYC 10014   Mon.-Sun. 11-8, Thurs. 11-9

Jennifer Tyler   M/W

A designer line of cashmere furnishings from Italy and Scotland. Find multiple sweater styles, coats, pants, shawls, capes, blankets and accessories, all available in a range of weights and colors.

Upper East Side   212-772-8350
854 Madison Avenue   at 70th St.
NYC 10021   Mon.-Fri. 10-8, Sat. 10-7 Sun. 12-6

Jennifer Tyler, Two W
A bridge line of cashmeres imported from Hong Kong, designed exclusively by Jennifer Tyler. Find sweaters, pants, dresses, twin sets and cardigans in single-ply weights. Lower prices attract a younger clientele.

Midtown East 212-644-9175
705 Lexington Avenue at 57th St.
NYC 10022 Mon.-Sat. 10-7, Sun. 12-6

Jenny B. M/W
Jenny B.'s ever-changing selection of merchandise keeps her customers coming back for more. Find feminine ballet flats, hipster boots and sexy in-your-face stilettos under the Jenny B. and Varda labels. For men, styles run from classic and dressy to hip and funky.

SoHo 212-343-9575
118 Spring Street bet. Mercer/Greene
NYC 10012 Mon.-Sun. 11-7

Jill Anderson W
Jill Anderson has created a following for her subtly modern, feminine clothing. For Anderson, design is a kind of yoga "where the space of her calm contentment feeds her imagination." This shop's tranquil atmosphere is a perfect backdrop for her collection of dresses, skirts, jackets, tops and outerwear which are cut in clean, unusual lines to accentuate the female form. Jillanderson@mindspring.com

East Village 212-253-1747
331 East 9th Street bet. 1st/2nd Avenue
NYC 10003 Mon.-Sun 12-8

Jill Stuart W
The winning formula for Stuart's collection is the combination of tasteful and approachable clothes with a feel-good dose of feminine light-heartedness. Simple, unfussy lines, easy-to-wear practicality and just the right amount of punch infuse her designs. Find dresses, skirts, jackets, cashmeres and tops in pared-down shapes. Shoes and handbags also available.

SoHo 212-343-2300
100 Greene Street bet. Prince/Spring
NYC 10012 Mon.-Sat. 11-7, Sun. 12-6

Jimin Lee / Translatio W
The flagship store for this hot new designer carries a collection of Asian-influenced separates. The line's core features silk organza jackets, printed tulles, hand-woven silks, leathers, evening gowns, and cashmeres from the Loro Piana mills. Lee's hallmark: designing reversible clothes with a double personality. For example, a dress with the Aramaic alphabet on one side reverses to reveal a snakeskin pattern. Couture-like attention to detail and fabrics, which have an ageless softness, define the sophisticated aesthetic of her clothes.

Jimmy Choo

TriBeCa	**212-219-9146**
13 White Street	bet. 6th Ave./W. B'way
NYC 10013	Tues.-Sat. 11-7, Sun. 12-5

☆ Jimmy Choo   W

Princess Diana (who knew a thing or two about shoes) helped make Jimmy Choo a success on the other side of the pond; now he has hit New York. This three-story shoe emporium will cause women to throw logic to the winds and pay from $225 to $865 for a Choo original. His design philosophy emulates that of Blahnik's: styles feature narrow toes, high heels and decorative detailing. Find day shoes, evening shoes and boots offered in a range of heel heights.

Fifth Avenue	**212-593-0800**
645 Fifth Avenue	at 51st St.
NYC 10022	Mon.-Sat. 10-6

Joan & David   W

Joan & David draws customers for a variety of reasons. One customer is the professional in search of classic career clothing, while another is here to shop for a pair of Joan & David shoes. Find a collection of casual and sporty styles, as well as evening and business dress shoes. Traditional designs are the rule here.

Upper East Side	**212-772-3970**
816 Madison Avenue	bet. 68/69th St.
NYC 10021	Mon.-Sat. 10-6

John Anthony   W

Strictly couture! For grand occasions that require an elegant ballgown or dressy suit, John Anthony is at your service. Choose from his ready-made collection or custom order your own. Cosmically high prices; expect to pay $10,000 for a ballgown.

Midtown East	**212-888-4070**
153 East 61st Street (penthouse)	bet. Lex./Third Ave.
NYC 10021	by appointment

John Fluevog Shoes   M/W

Welcome to a shoe store for the youth of the next millennium! With their 6" platform heels, Fluevog claims that they will "keep you above the urban trash." You have to be young and gutsy to wear these towering clodhoppers and, frankly, young and confused to pay these prices. 800-381-3338
www.fluevog.com

SoHo	**212-431-4484**
104 Prince Street	bet. Greene/Mercer
NYC 10012 Mon.-Wed. 11-7, Thurs.-Sat. 11-8, Sun. 12-7	

John Lobb   M

Since 1850, John Lobb's handmade shoes have been caressing the feet of distinguished gentlemen and reassuring them with their motto, "Some things are forever." Now Britain's venerable shoemaker opens his new, freestanding boutique. Find straight cap oxfords, loafers, buckle shoes, jodhpur boots, evening slip-ons and classic moccasins. Beautiful craftsmanship and traditional styling define the Lobb label. Shoes start at $750, while custom-made start at $3,000.

Upper East Side   **212-888-9797**
680 Madison Avenue   bet. 61/62nd St.
NYC 10021   Mon.-Sat. 10-6, Sun. 12-6

Johnston & Murphy   M

Since 1850 this men's footwear retailer has satisfied their customers. Find a full range of shoe styles, from dress and formal shoes to casual basics and weekend wear. Prices range from $90 to $325. 800-424-2854.
www.johnstonandmurphy.com

Midtown East   **212-527-2343**
520 Madison Avenue   at 54th St.
NYC 10022   Mon.-Sat. 9-7, Sun. 12-6

Midtown East   **212-697-9375**
345 Madison Avenue   bet. 44/45th St.
NYC 10017   Mon.-Fri. 9-7, Sat. 10-6, Sun. 12-5

Lower Manhattan   **212-321-3909**
1 World Trade Ctr.   bet. Liberty/Vesey
NYC 10048   Mon.-Fri. 8-7:30, Sat. 11-6

Joovay   W

A small lingerie boutique stocked with top-of-the-line American and European labels. Looks run from dainty and sweet to sexy and hot. Find bras, panties, teddies, nightwear, camisoles and slips. Labels include Lise Charmel, Marvel, LeJaby and La Perla. Hosiery by Oroblu also available.

SoHo   **212-431-6386**
436 West Broadway   at Prince
NYC 10012   Mon.-Sun. 12-7

Joseph   W

This London retailer keeps its customers coming back for more by sticking to what it knows best: keeping the same basic styles running every season, but updating them with the fabric, color and texture of the moment. Fashionistas shop here for contemporary fashions with a classic edge. Find trousers, shirts, jackets, modern separates in easy-to-wear shapes, leathers and shearlings, as well as that one drop-dead, high-end piece that's introduced into each collection. Although prices run high, the Joseph label will have you looking urban chic year after year. Check out his very happening pants shop down the block.

Upper East Side   **212-570-0077**
804 Madison Avenue   bet. 67/68th St.
NYC 10021   Mon.-Sat. 10-6:30, Thurs. 10-7

Joseph

The concept of "just pants" is one of Joseph's claims to fame (in New York and elsewhere). Find edgy styles designed in chino, cotton sateen, denim in heavy colors and gabardine. If you're feeling adventuresome, go for a brushed urethane or a PVC number. Ask for their hottest seller, "The Joker," a straight leg pant that retails for $245, or the "Cinno," a low-waisted chino-like pant with a comfort fit in every fabric imaginable. A Joseph pant is sexy, form-fitted and urban chic. Sizes run from XS to XL.

Upper East Side (pants only)	**212-327-1773**
796 Madison Avenue	bet. 67/68th St.
NYC 10021	Mon.-Sat. 10-6:30, Thurs. 10-7
SoHo (pants only)	**212-343-7071**
115 Greene Street	bet. Prince/Spring
NYC 10012	Mon.-Sat. 11-7:30, Sun. 12-6

Joseph A. Banks M

A Boston retailer featuring tailored career clothing for the conservative dresser. In keeping with its solid New England origins, Banks offers a comforting shopping environment. Find a complete selection of suits, sportswear, shirts, ties and underwear, as well as a Cole-Haan shoe department. Every fall, Banks invites you to trade in an old suit and get $100 credit towards a new one. 800-285-2265

Midtown East	**212-370-0600**
366 Madison Avenue	bet. 46/47th St.
NYC 10017	Mon.-Sat. 9-7, Thurs. 9-8, Sun. 12-5

Judith Leiber W

Judith Leiber features over 500 bags for evening and daytime wear. Choose a classic alligator style or an elaborately detailed design for fancy nights out. True Leiber aficionados, however, shop here for Leiber's rhinestone evening bags and jewel-encrusted minaudières. These bags are often seen in the clutches of society types, including Nancy Reagan.

Upper East Side	**212-327-4003**
987 Madison Avenue	bet. 76/77th St.
NYC 10021	Mon.-Sat 10-6

Julian and Sara B/G

A shop stocked with children's clothing lines from France and Italy. Find back-to-school basics, play clothes and accessories hand-picked from top labels like Charabia, Lili Gaufrette, Petit Boy, Jean Bourget, Arthur, Confetti and Elsy. Newborn through age 12.

SoHo	**212-226-1989**
103 Mercer Street	bet. Prince/Spring
NYC 10012	Tues.-Fri. 11:30-7, Sat. & Sun. 12-6

Julie Artisan's Gallery W

Open since 1973, this shop is an artisan's gallery showcasing techniques like weaving, hand painting, stitching, quilting and knitting. Each piece is a lovingly handcrafted work of art, either one-of-a-kind or sold in limited editions. Women shop here for intricate evening kimonos, loomed knitted jackets, colorful sweaters, hand-dyed shirts and more. Labels include Tim Harding and Linda Mendelson. For a mature customer who values an artistic approach to dressing.

Upper East Side	212-717-5959
762 Madison Avenue	bet. 65/66th Street
NYC 10021	Mon.-Sat. 11-6

Jungle Planet W

Find a "jungle" of merchandise from all parts of the planet, from Nepal to little ol' Gotham. Choose from a selection of Mandarin dresses, shirts, jeans, T-shirts, sarongs, scarves, beaded handbags and jewelry, as well as a few vintage pieces.

West Village	212-989-5447
175 West 4th Street	bet. 6th/7th Avenue
NYC 10014	Sun.-Thurs. 12-8, Fri. & Sat. 12-9

Juno M/W

For the fashion crazed who absolutely must have the very latest in footwear. Find boots, casual day shoes and lace-ups, all in black and boasting thick rubber soles. If you look carefully, you may find something suitable for a toned down affair.

Flatiron	212-647-9064
170 Fifth Avenue	at 22nd Street
NYC 10010	Mon.-Sat. 10:30-8, Sun. 12-7
SoHo	212-925-6415
550 Broadway	bet. Prince/Spring
NYC 10012	Mon.-Sat. 10:30-8, Sun. 11-8

Jutta Neumann M/W

For a one-of-a-kind, handcrafted sandal, Jutta Neumann is your weumann! Enter this closet-size shop and add a little beauty and a lot of color to your wardrobe. Although she carries a variety of other styles and sizes, her forté is handmade sandals and handbags. Choose from a variety of leathers and a surfeit of colors (turquoise, bright yellow and orange, as well as traditional browns and blacks). Have a pair of sandals or a handbag designed in basic leather or an exotic skin like stingray or snake. From simple one-straps to slip-on thongs to thick-heeled slides that fit like a dream. Custom sandals range from $140 to $300 with a three-week delivery. Accessories include leather jewelry and wallets.

East Village	212-982-7048
317 East 9th Street	bet. 1st/2nd Ave.
NYC 10003	Tues.-Sat. 12-8

Katayone Adeli W

Nominated for the Perry Ellis Award for new design talent, Katayone Adeli has taken New York by storm with "her savvy take on urban hip without pretension." Anyone can always shop for the Katayone Adeli label in department stores; however, true fashionistas shop an exclusive collection available only in the NoHo store. This 3,500-sq. ft. minimalist space is the backdrop for an everyday wardrobe of great looking mix and match pieces, including dresses, pants, skirts, sweaters and coats. For example, toss a pair of

Kate Spade

Adeli's super fitted pants with a stretch top or cashmere sweater. These are contemporary fashions with sculpted looks, perfect for cutting-edge urbanites.

NoHo 212-260-3500
35 Bond Street bet. Lafayette/Bowery
NYC 10012 Mon.-Sat. 11-7, Sun. 12-6

Kate Spade   W

Everyone is talking about Kate Spade and her bags. Each season she reinvents traditional bags through her fabric and color combinations such as bright leathers, textured burlap, nylon, canvas, corduroy and seersucker. Find a selection of bags in a variety of looks, from practical shoulder and tote bags to sleek and stylish shapes. Spade's signature square silhouettes are simple, functional and chic. Raincoats, shirts and pajamas also available. New this year: great looking, girlie shoe styles that include mules, slingbacks and slides.

SoHo 212-274-1991
454 Broome Street at Mercer
NYC 10012 Mon.-Sat. 11-7, Sun. 12-6

Kavanagh's Designer Resale Shop   W

Owner Mary Kavanagh (formerly director of personal shopping at Bergdorf Goodman) sells pre-owned, but pristine, high-end designer clothing. Her specialty is Chanel suits priced at $900. In addition, find clothing by Armani, Ungaro, Bill Blass, Jil Sanders, Prada and more. Choose shoes from labels like Manolo Blahnik, Tod's, Gucci, Prada and Hermès. Hermès ties for $85, as well as accessories.

Midtown East 212-702-0152
146 East 49th Street bet. Lex./Third
NYC 10017 Tues.-Fri. 11-6, Sat. 11-4

Kazuyo Nakano   W

At the age of ten, designer Kazuyo began to acquire her skills by apprenticing in her father's handbag company. Fashion thrill seekers come here for fresh, new looks in handbags. Find constructed leather styles, multi-colored python baguettes, evening bags covered in pastel paillettes, leather bags trimmed in feathers and Indian beading, and printed pony bags. These innovative, pretty handcrafted pieces will add color and life to any outfit.
www.kazuyonakano.com

NoLiTa 212-941-7093
223 Mott Street bet. Spring/Prince
NYC 10012 Wed.-Mon. 12:30-7

Keiko   M/W

Have you ever wondered where a sizzling swimsuit featured in a fashion magazine comes from? Have you always dreamed of owning a swimsuit with that perfect fit? Well then, a trip to Keiko's is a must! Find a collection of bathing attire in mouthwatering colors. Prices start at $120 and include alterations. Keiko's tour de force, however, is a custom designed suit that will minimize the negatives and maximize the positives. Custom prices start at $250 with a four to six week delivery.

SoHo   212-226-6051
62 Greene Street   bet. Spring/Broome
NYC 10012   Mon.-Fri. 11-6, Sat. 12-6, Sun. 1-6

Kelly Christy   M/W

Kelly Christy now has her own hat boutique, after selling her chic toppers in Barneys for many years. Christy describes her styles as "classic with a twist," and her designs highlight her unique use of trim. Find fedoras, boleros, cloches, berets and boaters. Choose from off-the-rack or indulge in a made-to-measure.

NoLiTa   212-965-0686
235 Elizabeth Street   bet. Houston/Prince
NYC 10012   Tues.-Sat. 12-7, Sun. 12-6

☆ Keni Valenti   W

Located in the heart of the garment district is this four-room showroom that specializes in vintage couture. At Keni Valenti it's all about retro, one-of-a-kind pieces featuring looks that run from designer dresses and eveningwear to shoes and accessories. You may just come across a beautiful Chanel couture suit, an Yves Saint Laurent or Halston outfit from the 70's, a Dior ensemble from the early 50's all the way up to a current John Galliano, a Paco Rabanne leather dress, a Pucci gown, a Courreges frock and more. Expect to pay high couture designer prices for a little slice of vintage luxury.

Midtown West   212-967-7147
247 West 30th Street, 5th Floor   bet. 7th/8th Ave.
NYC 10001   by appointment only

Kenneth Cole   M/W

Kenneth Cole once hawked his wares from a broken down trailer, but now he commands a $300 million fashion empire built on his edgy advertisements and prolific shoe designs. "Kenneth Cole New York" and his secondary line "Reaction" feature a broad range of styles, from career and dress shoes to trendy and casual basics. Find loafers, updated ankle boots, pumps, boots, traditional oxfords, sneakers and bridal shoes. In short, find high fashion shoes at affordable prices. Briefcases, outerwear, handbags, scarves and sunglasses round out the assortment. New this year: men's and women's sportswear. 800-487-4389 www.kencole.com

Upper West Side   212-873-2061
353 Columbus Avenue   at 77th St.
NYC 10024   Mon.-Sat. 10-8, Sun. 11-7

Flatiron   212-675-2550
95 Fifth Avenue   at 17th St.
NYC 10003   Mon.-Sat. 10-8, Sun. 11-7

SoHo   212-965-0283
597 Broadway   bet. Prince/Houston
NYC 10012   Mon.-Sat. 10-8, Sun. 12-7

Kenzo

M/W

Now that Kenzo's founding designer, Takada, has retired, it's time for a new team of designers to take charge. The first step was signing on ready-to-wear director Alexander Keller. The second step is to preserve the Kenzo spirit—an ethnic flavor inspired by every corner of the world from Africa to Asia. Find suits and separates, their bridge line, "Jungle," offering fun, functional sportswear; and "Kenzo Jeans," a selection of denim, T-shirts and casualwear. Kenzo designs are colorful, versatile and ideal for mixing and matching. Looks run from classic and tailored to loose and relaxed.

Upper East Side 212-717-0101
805 Madison Avenue bet. 67/68th St.
NYC 10021 Mon.-Sat. 10-6

SoHo **Opening 2001**
80 Wooster Street bet. Spring/Broome
NYC 10012 Mon.-Sat 10-6, Sun. 12-6

Kerquelen

M/W

Named after the Kerquelen Islands in the southern Indian Ocean, this shop carries over 700 pairs of men's and women's shoes for hipsters seeking avant-garde footwear. Enter a gallery-like space and choose from styles by up-and-coming designers from Germany, Spain, and Italy. On a raised platform is a parade of high-fashion heels, flats, and casual shoes (like multi-colored sneakers, fringed sandals, modern shaped clogs, slip-ons, mules, boots, and espadrilles). Labels include Callaghan, Farrutx, Graye, Joop!, Shu Think, and Jamie Mascaro. www.kerquelen.com

SoHo 212-431-1771
44 Greene Street bet. Grand/Broome
NYC 10013 Mon.-Sat. 10:30-8, Sun. 11-6

SoHo 212-226-8313
430 West Broadway bet. Spring/Prince
NYC 10012 Mon.-Sat. 10:30-8, Sun. 11-6

Kids Are Magic

B/G

A good selection of clothing at competitive prices. Find casual basics, back-to-school and trendy fashion pieces. Girls and boys will rejoice in hip labels like Wrangler, Dollhouse, French Toast, Bonnie Jean and Calvin Klein, while newborns and infants will look adorable in Baby Dior. Newborn to size 16 girls and 20 boys.

Upper West Side 212-875-9240
2293 Broadway bet. 82/83rd St.
NYC 10024 Mon.-Wed. 10-8,
Thurs.-Sat. 10-9, Sun. 12-6:45

Kids Foot Locker

B/G

Kids Foot Locker has a large selection of children's athletic wear, from baseball jerseys and tennis outfits to top-of-the-line sneakers. Brand names include Adidas, Nike and Reebok. From infants to size 6.

Upper East Side   212-396-4567
1504 Second Avenue   bet. 78/79th St.
NYC 10021   Mon.-Sat. 10-8, Sun. 11-6

Kinnu   W

Enter Kinnu and experience a world of Indian color, fabric, and design. Hand-woven, iridescent silks and cross-dyed cottons (made up in kurta-styled tunics, dresses, asymmetrical wraps, and drawstring pants) define the collection. Gold brocade trim on hems and cuffs, intricate embroidery, mirror-work, and hand-dying reflect the elaborate workmanship that goes into each design. Decorative items like quilted bedspreads, wall-hangings, and art work also available.

NoLiTa   212-334-4775
43 Spring Street   bet. Mott/Mulberry
NYC 10012   Mon.-Sun. 11:30-7

☆ Kirna Zabête   W

Owners Sarah Hailes (nicknamed Kirna) and Beth Shepherd (nicknamed Zabête) have started a new wave in retailing with their trendy 5,000-sq. ft. fashion emporium. This mini fashion department store is enlivened with little slices of amusement like a pet section and a candy section. Kirna Zabête's main draw is still its clothing. Fashionistas will relish browsing the racks of frocks in 60 hard-to-find designer names like Olivier Theyskens, Balenciaga, Wink, Martine Sitbon, Bruce, Clements Ribeiro, Alice Roi, and A.S. Vandevorst. The Kirna Zabête concept: mixing and matching labels rather than dressing from head to toe in one designer. Accessories include handbags, hats, lingerie, shoes, and lotions and potions.

SoHo   212-941-9656
96 Greene Street   bet. Spring/Prince
NYC 10012   Mon.-Sat. 11-7, Sun. 12-6

Kleinfeld and Son   W

The barons of bridal wear! It may be a trek to Kleinfeld's, but the savings alone make it worth the trip. Find over 1,000 gowns in stock at all times. Designer labels include Carolina Herrera, Scassi and Dior.

Brooklyn   718-765-8500
8202 Fifth Avenue   Tues., Thurs. 11-9,
Brooklyn 11209   Wed., Fri., Sat. 11-6 by appt.

Klein's of Monticello   W

An Orchard Street institution for over 20 years, Klein's of Monticello is where savvy shoppers go for luxury European clothing. Best of all, their prices are 25% less than anywhere else. Find suits, jackets, trousers, cashmere sweaters, blouses and outerwear from designers such as Luciano Barbera, Max Mara, Les Copains, Malo, Agnona, Rene Lezard, Gunext, Antonio Fusco, Clara Cottman and more. Accessories include belts, hats and scarves. A small selection of men's sportcoats.

Koh's Kids

Lower East Side   212-966-1453
105 Orchard Street   at Delancey
NYC 10002   Sun.-Fri. 10-5, closed Sat.

Koh's Kids   B/G
A tribe's children's shop selling a unique clothing selection, particularly their hand-knit sweaters. Find European and American labels like Naf Naf, Flapdoodles, Cherry Tree, Zutano and Le Petit Bateau, as well as shoes by Elephanten. Toys and accessories also available. Newborn to size 8.

TriBeCa   212-791-6915
311 Greenwich Street   bet. Chambers/Reade
NYC 10013   Mon.-Fri. 11-7, Sat. 10-6, Sun. 11-5

Krizia   M/W
Krizia creator Mariuccia Mandelli believes that clothing is our second skin; hence her ready-to-wear designs are body-conscious and comfortable. Shop a collection that runs the gamut from an $8,000 glam dress to a simple T-shirt, and includes sculpted black crepe suits, pants, stretch cashmere twinsets, separates and coats. Her best items are luxury knitwear designed in lean shapes, from cling-to-the-body dresses to form-fitted sweaters. Eveningwear includes glamorous beaded chiffon gowns and slinky, black jersey dresses. Felinistas will purr with delight when they see her signature "cat" sweaters. Men's fashions border on avant-garde.

Upper East Side   212-879-1211
769 Madison Avenue   bet. 65/66th St.
NYC 10021   Mon.-Fri. 10-7,
    Thurs. 10-8, Sat. 10-6

La Galleria La Rue   W
Personalized, attentive service is the watchword at La Galleria La Rue, a boutique that celebrates the beauty of all ages. Find a collection of lifestyle-friendly separates in tactile, techno fabrics that are appropriate for work, cocktails, or dinner.

Flatiron   212-807-1708
12 West 23rd Street   bet. 5th/6th Ave.
NYC 10010   Mon.-Fri. 12-8, Sat. & Sun. 12-6

West Village   212-352-0961
385 Bleecker Street   at Perry Street
NYC 10014   Mon.-Thurs. 12-8, Fri. 12-9,
    Sat. 11-7, Sun. 12-6

La Layette   B/G
Attention, doting grandmothers! La Layette will meet all your exacting standards with their line of luxury, European clothing. From hand-embroidered outfits and beautiful christening gowns to linens and hand-painted furniture, each item is prettier than the next. Expensive. Newborn to size 2.

Upper East Side   212-688-7072
170 East 61st Street   bet. Third/Lex.
NYC 10021   Mon.-Fri. 11-6, Sat. 11-5

Lady Foot Locker

La Perla W
Totally in, fiendishly expensive. A designer's showcase of feminine intimates under the expensive La Perla label. Find a collection of lingerie that runs from tasteful and elegant to seductive and sexy. La Perla also features a fashion line of bustiers and bodysuits with built-in bra cups. Swimwear and sleepwear also available. Be prepared to pay up to a few hundred dollars for a single item, but remember, La Perla is the caviar of lingerie.

Upper East Side 212-570-0050
777 Madison Avenue bet. 66/67th St.
NYC 10021 Mon.-Sat. 10-6

☆ La Petite Coquette W
In business for twenty years La Petite Coquette is still the in-place to shop for high-end sexy lingerie. Just ask regulars like model Cindy Crawford and actress Sarah Jessica Parker. Once you've seen the storefront windows, it's impossible to resist stopping in. Enter what feels more like a boudoir than a shop and find an incredible selection of silk intimates in a multitude of colors. Looks run from alluring corsets and garters to flirty nighties and feminine basics. Labels include La Perla, Ravage, Elle of Italy, Andre Sarda, Natori, Cosabella and Aubade. One of the best lingerie shops in the city.

NoHo 212-473-2478
51 University Place bet. 9/10th St.
NYC 10003 Mon.-Sat. 11-7, Sun. 12-6

☆ La Petite Etoile B/G
Mothers shop here for designer children's wear labels. Find casual play clothes, back-to-school basics, and dressy ensembles, all with European labels like Tartine et Chocolat, Cacharel, Les Copains, Florianne, Lui et Lei, I Pinco Pallino, Petit Bateau, Simonetta and La Perla. Newborn to 14 years.

Upper East Side 212-744-0975
746 Madison Avenue bet. 64/65th St.
NYC 10021 Mon.- Sat. 10-6, Thurs. 10-7, Sun. 12-5

Lacoste M/W
The originator of the pique polo shirt, Lacoste is in full swing again with their crocodiles. Find a sportswear collection suitable for golf, tennis and weekend relaxation. Accessories include golf bags, belts, hats, socks and sunglasses. 800-4-LACOSTE www.lacoste.com

Midtown East 212-750-8115
543 Madison Avenue bet. 54/55th St.
NYC 10022 Mon.-Sat. 10-5, Thurs. 10-8, Sun. 12-5

Lady Foot Locker W
Lady Foot Locker features athletic wear and footwear strictly for women. Find workout clothes for fitness and basketball. Choose from a range of footwear lines suitable for run-

ning, tennis, basketball or cross training. Brand names include Nike, Reebok, Adidas, Fila and New Balance.
800-877-5239 www.ladyfootlocker.com

Upper East Side 212-396-4567
1504 Second Avenue bet. 78/79th St.
NYC 10021 Mon.-Sat. 10-8:30, Sun. 11-6:30

Midtown West 212-967-1239
901 Sixth Avenue bet. B'way/33rd St.
NYC 10001 Mon.-Sat. 10-8, Sun. 11-6

Lower Manhattan 212-732-7240
89 South Street at South Street Seaport
NYC 10038 Mon.-Sat. 10-9, Sun. 11-8

Lana Marks W

Handbag aficionados shop here for those coveted Lana Marks' exotic skins. We're talking alligator, ostrich and lizard. Designs are classic and fashionable, and the color assortment runs from black to vivid pink. Trying one on your shoulder is almost impossible, as a tangle of chains and locks secures each bag to the display.

Midtown East 212-355-6135
645 Madison Avenue bet. 59/60th St.
NYC 10022 Mon.-Fri. 10-7, Thurs. 10-8, Sat. 10-6

☆ Language W

There's always something wonderful here to whet your appetite and tickle your fancy. The buyers at Language are endlessly discovering new talent from South America, Europe, and the Far East. Shop a contemporary showroom that combines art with fashion, featuring products for the body, mind and home. Find everything from hand-embroidered evening dresses by Jemima Khan and sheer lace clothing by Clarissa Hulse to a Tufi Duek tight-fitting leather suit. Looks run from hip and contemporary to soft and feminine. Accessories include handbags, pashminas and unique jewelry. Interspersed are works of art, "objets" and furniture for the home. New this year: The "Patuche," a 100% pure pashmina shawl that makes the old, blended pashmina feel run of the mill.

NoLiTa 212-431-5566
238 Mulberry Street bet. Prince/Spring
NYC 10012 Mon.-Sat. 11-7, Thurs. 11-8, Sun. 12-6

Laundry, by Shelli Segal W

Although she continues to supply major department stores, Shelli Segal also has her own shop. Find a sportswear collection that features everyday essentials, from cashmere tops to drawstring pants. Mix and match separates, and wear them with confidence. Clothes are nicely styled, softly shaped and reasonably priced. A Segal design is feminine, elegantly understated and easy-to-wear.

SoHo 212-334-9433
97 Wooster Street bet. Prince/Spring
NYC 10012 Mon.-Sat. 11-7, Sun. 12-6

Laundry Industry M/W
A sleek shop featuring designer clothing from Amsterdam. Designed by two women, Laundry is about fad-free functional fashions with a hip, European edge. Find a collection of sportswear in simple, modern designs, a minimal color palette and a tight fit. Laundry's design mix: a little techno, a little sexy and a lot of basics.

SoHo 212-343-2225
122 Spring Street at Greene
NYC 10012 Mon.-Sun. 11-7

Laura Ashley W/G
Renowned for their home furnishings and their trademark floral fabrics, Laura Ashley also features clothing for women and girls. Customers with a traditional sensibility shop here for dress-down work attire and weekend wear. Find long dresses, man-tailored shirts, slacks, knits, T-shirts and accessories, all color coordinated. In addition, mothers can dress their daughters in a cheerful selection of smocked dresses, knits, sweaters and more. From size 2 to 9.

Upper West Side 212-496-5110
398 Columbus Avenue at 79th St.
NYC 10024 Mon.-Wed., Sat. 10-7,
Thurs. & Fri. 10-8, Sun. 12-6

Laura Beth's Baby Collection B/G
Previously a buyer for Barneys' baby department, Laura Beth decided to go solo and open her own showroom. This is one-stop-shopping for expectant mothers in search of perfect nursery accoutrements to add the finishing touches to their baby's room. Find crib linens, pillows, bumpers, bedskirts and decorative accessories like bookends, mirrors, mobiles and lamps. It all comes at 20% below retail. She even does birth announcements.

Upper East Side 212-717-2559
300 East 75th Street, Suite 24E at Second Ave.
NYC 10021 by appointment only

Laura Biagiotti W
Biagiotti's claim to fame is luxurious, featherweight knitwear. Find a sportswear collection of suits, dresses, pants, separates and coats in cashmere, silk and linen fabrications. A Biagiotti design is versatile, functional and comfortable. Although Biagiotti may not be for the hip and trendy, she does have a loyal following that includes royalty.

Midtown West 212-399-2533
4 West 57th Street bet. 5th/6th Ave.
NYC 10019 Mon.-Sat. 10-6

The Leather and Suede Workshop W
Owner Ron Shahar's moniker is "The Leather Man." On sabbatical from his tailoring days, he's happiest when talking leather. Choose from a variety of skins like suede,

Leather Corner

cowhide, leather and snakeskin, all in a multitude of colors. Shop for pants, jackets, skirts (long and short), dresses, shirts, coats and even hats. Pants start at $350, while jackets start at $450. Shahar will custom tailor a micro mini or a pair of black leather pants to fit like a glove.

Midtown East   **212-688-1946**
107 East 59th Street   bet. Lex./Park Ave
NYC 10022   Mon.-Fri. 10-7, Sat.11-7, Sun. 11:30-6:30

Leather Corner   M/W

Find good value in leather outerwear in this decidedly unglam ambience. Men and women can choose from a variety of styles, such as short and long leather coats, biker and bomber jackets, and casual weekend wear. Labels include Kenneth Cole, Nine West, Andrew Marc and Tibor. Expect to pay $120 for plain leather and up to $800 for a full-length coat trimmed in fur.

Lower East Side   **212-475-7231**
144 Orchard Street   at Rivington
NYC 10002   Mon.-Sun. 9-6:30

Leather Rose   M/W

Head to Leather Rose for custom-made pants by South African-born Aldo Kleyn. He'll make you any style in any skin or color. Pick from swatches of lambskin, alligator, deer hide, black mamba snake skin or plain buttery leather. Expect a two-month wait for delivery, but his creations will last a lifetime. Prices start at $800.

East Village   **212-529-6790**
412 East 9th Street   bet. 1st/Ave. A
NYC 10009   Tues.-Sun. 2-8

Le Corset   W

Owner Selima Salaun is a master at spotting new trends in lingerie and pleasing her customers. Entering Le Corset, you immediately feel the allure of its fabulous selection of new and vintage lingerie that runs from flirty to unabashedly sexy. Find satin and silk bustiers, feminine camisoles, demi-cup bras to accentuate cleavage, bodysuits, lacey panties, chemises, garter belts and more. Labels include Dr. Boudoir, Le Corset, Leigh Bantivoglio, Colette Dinnigan, Aubade and Lise Charmel.

SoHo   **212-334-4936**
80 Thompson Street   bet. Spring/Broome
NYC 10012   Mon.-Sat. 11-7, Sun. 12-7

Lederer   M/W

Lederer is best known for their classically styled, private label handbags; however, they are also an excellent source for reproductions from the houses of Gucci, Hermès and Channel. Also find briefcases, small leathergoods, hunting clothes, Wellington boots and Barbour outerwear.

Midtown East   **212-355-5515**
457 Madison Avenue   at 51st St.
NYC 10022   Mon.-Sat. 9:30-6, Thurs. 9:30-6:30

Lee Anderson W

For 17 years Lee Anderson has been dressing New York matrons with her couture collection, as well as offering custom tailoring. Find classic suits, pants, blouses, jackets and coats, as well as after-five and special occasion dress. Choose from off-the-rack or order custom down to the very last button. An Anderson design is lady-like and uptown traditional.

Upper East Side   212-772-2463
23 East 67th Street   bet. 5th/Madison
NYC 10021   Mon.-Sat. 11-6 or by appt.

Legacy W

A boutique that sells "vintage inspired" clothing. You get a vintage look, but without the musty smell or tattered wear and tear. Find dresses, skirts, blouses, pants and more with a retro feel and a distinctive look.

SoHo   212-966-4827
109 Thompson Street   bet. Prince/Spring
NYC 10012   Mon.-Sun. 12-7

Leggiadro W

Leggiadro features resort wear that will travel almost anywhere. Find clothing and swimwear by Sugar, Lilly Pulitzer and Leggiadro. It's all in lots of preppy prints and bright colors, perfect for Palm Beach or the Nantucket seaside. Accessorize with a wrap, skirt, sarong or shirt. Sweaters and Jackie Roger sandals also available.

Upper East Side   212-753-5050
700 Madison Avenue   bet. 62/63rd St.
NYC 10021   Mon.-Sat. 10:30-6

Legs Beautiful W

Mostly legwear. Find a fabulous selection of hosiery with brand names like DKNY, CK, Hue, Hanes and Dim, but also sexy lingerie, Danskin apparel, amusing socks and tights. If only legs beautiful was on every street corner!

Upper East Side   212-750-3730
1025 Third Avenue   bet. 60/61st St.
NYC 10022   Mon.-Fri. 10-8, Sat. 9:30-7, Sun. 12-7

Midtown East   212-688-9599
CitiCorp Center, 153 East 53rd St.   at Lexington Ave.
NYC 10022   Mon.-Fri. 8-8, Sat. 11-6, Sun. 12-5

Midtown East   212-949-2270
Metlife Bldg., 200 Park Ave.   bet. 44/45th St.
NYC 10166   Mon.-Fri. 7:30-8

Lower Manhattan   212-945-2858
225 Liberty St.   World Financial Ctr.
NYC 10281   Mon.-Fri. 8-7, Sat. 11-6, Sun. 12-5

Leonard Logsdail M

Once a Saville Row tailor, Leonard Logsdail now provides New York bankers, diplomats and high-powered lawyers with his bespoke tailoring. He takes your measurements,

Les Copains

cuts his paper pattern and then ships your order to London to be hand-stitched. Conservative suits of the best pedigree start at $2,200, while pricier suits will run you $3,800. Expect to wait 2 1/2 months for delivery.

Midtown East   212-752-5030
9 East 53rd Street, 4th Fl.   bet. 5th/Madison Ave.
NYC 10022   by appointment

Les Copains   W

Les Copains is restructuring its business in order to modernize its image. The first step was the appointment of two new designers, Stefano Guerriero and Antonio Marras. The classic "Les Copains" line features clean and lean silhouettes that include tailored suits, wool jackets, tweed pieces, knitwear and coats. The look is classic chic with an avant garde edge. The Trend label is fashion forward and meant for the young and unabashedly trendy. If you're after a casual, sporty appearance, look for the "Blue Eagle" label.

Upper East Side   212-327-3014
807 Madison Avenue   bet. 67/68th St.
NYC 10021   Mon.-Sat. 10-6

LeSportSac   M/W

LeSportSac features a wide range of functional bags perfect for traveling. They're manufactured in 100% nylon, double stitched on the insides and, best of all, machine washable. Find travel totes, weekend duffels, cosmetic clutches, handbags and more. Color assortment includes metallics, solids, pastels and brights. New for the year: LeSportSac's new Kiki bag, similar to the Fendi baguette, is heating up the competition, especially when it only retails for a mere $68.
800-486-BAGS www.lesportsac.com

SoHo   212-625-2626
176 Spring Street   bet. W. B'way/Thompson
NYC 10012   Mon.-Sat. 10-7, Sun. 12-6

Lester's   B/G

A nondescript shop that features a good selection of back-to-school basics, casual play clothes and trendy sportswear for hard-to-please juniors. Brand names include Juicy, Hard Tail and Quicksilver. Find a full service layette and shoe department. Accessories also available. From newborn to size 16.

Upper East Side   212-734-9292
1522 Second Avenue   at 79th St.
NYC 10021   Mon.-Fri. 10-7, Thurs. 10-8,
    Sat. 10-6, Sun. 12-5

Levi Strauss   M/W

Faced with stiff competition in the jeanswear market, Levi Strauss, an American institution, has launched a highly publicized, radical "Engineered Jeans" line retailing for $75 in this floor-to-ceiling denim emporium. Their international size chart makes shopping for tourists a breeze. There's a jean and fit for everyone here at an average cost of $54. Ladies can even custom fit a pair of "512's" if they're willing to wait two weeks for delivery. Casual basics and accessories also available. New this year: Levi's Lot 53 and Levi's Red collection of jeans and jackets modeled after vintage designs. 800-872-5384 www.levi.com

Midtown East 212-826-5957
750 Lexington Avenue bet. 59/60th St.
NYC 10021 Mon.-Sat. 10-8, Sun. 12-6

Midtown East 212-838-2188
3 East 57th Street bet. 5th/Madison Ave.
NYC 10022 Mon.-Sat. 10-8, Sun. 12-6

Lexington Formalwear M

For 50 years this Midtown men's formalwear shop has satisfied demanding New Yorkers. Located in a 3,000-sq. ft. converted library, the store offers an enormous selection of tuxedos, dinner jackets, white tie and tails, as well as morning suits. Tailoring is included in the price. Shirts, shoes and accessories also available. Tuxedo rentals by Perry Ellis, Givenchy and Chaps run from $100 to $149.

Midtown East 212-867-4420
12 East 46th Street, 2nd Fl. bet. 5th/Madison Ave.
NYC 10017 Mon.-Wed. 9-5:30,
Thurs. & Fri. 9-6:30, Sat. 10-4

Lilliput/SoHo Kids B/G

Inspired by the Lilliputians in *Gulliver's Travels*, this store carries a soup-to-nuts collection of children's clothing, ideal for play, school, and dress-up. For boys, mothers can choose from jeans, khakis, dress shirts, sweaters, T-shirts, and windbreakers. For girls, find a wide range of looks, running from adorable print dresses and Madeline T-shirts to cool, fashionable leather jeans paired with a hip top. And for babies, they've got it all, from onezies in washable silks and cashmeres to a basic Petit Bateau undershirt. Labels include Lili Gaufrette, Honore, Baby Go-Go, I Golfini della Nonna, Baby Gordon, Diesel, and Maxon Kids. Shoes, hats, pajamas, bags, and toys round out the assortment. From newborn to 18 years old. www.lilliputsoho.com

SoHo 212-965-9567
265 Lafayette Street bet. Spring/Prince
NYC 10012 Tues.-Sat. 11-7, Sun. 12-6

SoHo 212-965-9201
240 Lafayette Street bet. Spring/Prince
NYC 10012 Tues.-Sat. 11-7, Sun. 12-6

The Limited W

A huge success with the younger set, The Limited features functional, casual and sporty clothing with a fashion edge. Designs are contemporary, color and size availability terrific and price points moderate. 800-307-5984

Lina Tsai

Lower Manhattan   212-488-9790
503 World Trade Center   bet. Church/Vesey
NYC 10048   Mon.-Fri. 10-7, Thurs. 10-8,
Sat. 10-6, Sun. 12-5

Lina Tsai   W

In a town obsessed with basic black, it's refreshing to find a boutique packed with vivid shades of pink, green, purple and orange. The owner adores sweets, and thinks of her clothing in terms of candy colors. Find dresses, skirts, tops, slim pants and three-quarter-length coats with sexy, yet sweet looks.

East Village   212-529-8231
436 East 9th Street   bet. 1st/Ave. A
NYC 10003   Mon.-Fri. 1:30-7, Sat. 1-8, Sun 1-6

Linda Dresner   W

Tired of the hustle and bustle atmosphere of high-end department store shopping? Let Linda Dresner come to your rescue with her top-of-the-line collection of cutting-edge designers like Ann Demeulemeester, Marni, Martin Margiela, Wink, Dries Van Noten, John Galliano, Helmut Lang, Chloe and Jil Sanders. Choose from classic and timeless pieces or indulge in hip and trendy designs. Whether it's a lavish gown or a stylish suit, Dresner carries the best of the best with prices to match. Limited selection of shoes and accessories.

Midtown East   212-308-3177
484 Park Avenue   bet. 58/59th St.
NYC 10022   Mon.-Sat. 10-6

Lingerie on Lex   W

An intimate apparel shop that features European brand labels. Find lingerie, sleepwear, loungewear, hosiery and children's robes. Brand names include Hanro, Lise Charmel, La Perla, Le Jaby and Ritratti.

Upper East Side   212-755-3312
831 Lexington Avenue   bet. 63/64th St.
NYC 10021   Mon.-Fri. 10-6, Sat. 11-6

Lisa Shaub   M/W/C

A relative newcomer to Mulberry Street, Lisa Shaub features a collection of classic toppers. Emphasis is on comfort and fit with designs that feature subtle color combinations. The selection includes fedoras, cloches, boaters, wide-brimmed Panama's, berets, and newborn cotton baby hats. Custom also available.

NoLiTa   212-965-9176
232 Mulberry Street   bet. Prince/Spring
NYC 10012   Wed. 12-5, Thurs.-Sat. 12-7, Sun. 1-6

Little Eric Shoes   B/G

A shop that boasts Italian footwear made exclusively for Little Eric. The sales staff claims these shoes will outwear your child. At Little Eric's, it's all about the fit. Find casual basics, back-to-school essentials, formal dress shoes and trendy must-haves. Mothers shop here for those high fashion styles that teenagers covet. A good source for all ages, especially for your baby's first walking shoes. Expensive. From infants to size $8^1/_2$.

Upper East Side   212-717-1513
1118 Madison Avenue   bet. 83/84th St.
NYC 10028   Mon.-Sat. 10-6, Sun. 12-5

Upper East Side   212-288-8987
1331 Third Avenue   at 76th St.
NYC 10021   Mon.-Fri. 10-7, Sat. 10-6, Sun. 12-6

Liza Bruce   W

Liza Bruce, one of Barneys' most popular swimwear labels, has opened her doors to New Yorkers with a new teensy-weensy SoHo shop. Find a brightly colored collection of swimwear that includes one-pieces, bikinis, tankinis, and bandeaus, with looks that run from classic to sexy. Top quality Lycras, comfortable linings and sophisticated styling define the Liza Bruce label. Pay anywhere from $130 to $300, with sizes that run from S, M, and L and she's happy to make any necessary alterations. In addition, check out her ready-to-wear line that includes Lycra dresses, tank tops, sarongs, T-shirts and more.

SoHo   212-966-3853
80 Thompson Street   bet. Spring/Broome
NYC 10012   Mon.-Sun. 11-6

Liz Claiborne   W

Liz Claiborne, a brand synonymous with traditional styling and dependable comfort, continues to be a mainstay for career women. This spacious Fifth Avenue flagship store carries the various Claiborne lines, from relaxed sportswear and casual basics to career wear. A Liz Claiborne design is practical, office-friendly and affordable. An extensive petite section, shoes and accessories also available.
www.lizclaiborne.com

Fifth Avenue   212-956-6505
650 Fifth Avenue   at 52nd St.
NYC 10019   Mon.-Fri. 10-8, Sat. 10-7, Sun. 12-6

☆ Liz Lange Maternity   W

A former *Vogue* magazine editor, Liz Lange continues to apply her chic style to the maternity world. With her new, ground floor location on Madison Avenue, mothers-to-be can shop an upscale collection of fashionable clothing. Find clean and modern styles without the cutesy bows and patterns, from capri pants to a spaghetti strap evening dress. Lange's design philosophy: fitted shapes that accentuate the beauty of a pregnant woman's body without compromising style and elegance. Ask celebrities like Cindy Crawford and Elle MacPherson who have compared Lange's designs to Michael Kors and Calvin Klein. 888-616-5777

Loehman's

Upper East Side	**212-879-2191**
958 Madison	bet. 75/76th St.
NYC 10021	Mon.-Sat. 10-7, Sun. 12-5

Loehman's M/W

Wise shoppers make Loehman's their first stop when looking for top brand names at value prices. Find men's and women's apparel, a petites' section, accessories and shoes. Loehman's main attraction, however, is without doubt the "Back Room," a department stocked with designer labels like Calvin Klein, Donna Karan, Armani and more. And by the way, if you're not satisfied, Loehman's has a 14 day, get-your-money-back return policy.

Chelsea	**212-352-0856**
101 Seventh Avenue	bet. 16/17th St.
NYC 10011	Mon.-Sat. 9-9, Sun. 11-7

☆ Longchamp W/M

This venerable French leathergoods manufacturer returns to Madison Avenue with its classic collection of handbags, briefcases, luggage and small leathergoods. Find structured handbag styles in leather, suede and nylon that are in keeping with Longchamp's tradition of understated elegance and modern chic. Not to be missed is their Pliages collection of nylon fold-up travel totes in a rainbow of colors. Belts, scarves and gloves also available.

Upper East Side	**212-223-1500**
713 Madison Avenue	bet. 63/64th St.
NYC 10021	Mon.-Sat. 10-7

Lord & Taylor M/W/C

While most New York department stores have undergone major changes over the years, Lord & Taylor has remained true to its original mission of merchandising the "American Look": conservative and affordable clothing for sensible people. Lord & Taylor has devoted much of its floor space to extensive petite, career and sportswear collections, as well as dresses by American designers. Other departments include cosmetics, accessories, children's, men's, lingerie, outerwear and large sizes. 800-223-7440

Fifth Avenue	**212-391-3344**
424 Fifth Avenue	bet. 38/39th St.
NYC 10018	Mon. & Tues. 10-7,
	Wed.-Fri. 10-8:30, Sat. 10-7, Sun. 11-7

Lord of the Fleas W

This shop wins top prize for the wittiest store name, and carries trendy, tight-fitting, hip clothing for juniors and pre-teens. Find T-shirts galore, tops, pants, jackets, knits and accessories.

Upper West Side	**212-875-8815**
2142 Broadway	bet. 75/76th St.
NYC 10023	Mon.-Sun. 11-8:30
East Village	**212-260-9130**
305 East 9th Street	bet. 1st/2nd Ave.
NYC 10009	Mon.-Sun. 12-8:30

Louis Vuitton

Loro Piana M/W
With cashmere, it's all about altitude, not attitude. Apparently the higher a goat climbs, the finer its cashmere. If this theory is correct, then Loro Piana's goats must have reached the highest peaks. Recently settled in their fancy Madison Avenue digs, Loro Piana is better than ever, although the sales staff could use a minor attitude adjustment. Find a ready-to-wear collection featuring elegant knitwear, outerwear, pants, shirts and jackets in sumptuous fabrics like cashmere, silk and super-fine wool. In addition, choose from a luxurious assortment of cashmere shawls, scarves, stoles and capes in mouthwatering shades. Prices are sky high, but remember, so were those goats!

Upper East Side 212-980-7961
821 Madison Avenue bet. 68/69th St.
NYC 10021 Mon.-Sat. 10-6, Thurs. 10-7

Louie W
Owner Laura Pedone says, "Remember when women came down to shop in SoHo (about ten years ago) to find something special? Well, that's what my boutique is all about—preserving those one-of-a-kind looks that you won't find anywhere else." Find undiscovered design talents like Julien Segura, Lauren Moffatt and Booty Wear by Judy B. whose styles reflect New York chic. Choose from skirts, pants, dresses, separates and accessories. The look is refreshingly feminine without being girly. Great looking handbags.

SoHo 212-274-1599
68 Thompson Street bet. Spring/Broome
NYC 10012 Tues.-Sat. 12-7, Sun. 12-6

Louis Féraud W
Because Louis Feraud's five-member design team sticks to tradition rather than pursuing the latest fashion trends, you'll find a feminine collection where classic designs are the rule. Find a pret-a-porter line that caters to the corporate woman who wants desk-to-dinner versatility, from a ladylike luncheon dress to a suit paired with a skirt or pants. You can expect a full-bodied cut, tailored looks and sizing that runs from 4 to 16. Feraud's sportswear collection, "Contraire," hopes to draw a younger shopper in search of versatile basics that are all designed to be mixed and matched. Accessories also available.

Midtown West 212-956-7010
3 West 56th Street bet. 5th /6th Ave.
NYC 10019 Mon.-Sat. 10-6

Louis Vuitton M/W
Is it possible that two prestigious initials, "LV," can make your travels more luxurious? Find Vuitton's collection of luggage, handbags, travel accessories, as well as a ready-to-wear line by designer Marc Jacobs. A Vuitton design is

defined by craftsmanship, refinement and elegance. So if you crave initials other than your own (and, let's be honest, need a status boost), march down to Vuitton and drop a bundle for one of these monogrammed classics. They're truly vintage chic. 800-847-2956 www.vuitton.com

Midtown East — 212-371-6111
49 East 57th Street — bet. Madison/Park Ave.
NYC 10022 — Mon.-Fri. 10-6, Thurs. 10-7, Sat. 10-5:30, Sun. 12-5

SoHo — 212-274-9090
116 Greene Street — bet. Spring/Prince
NYC 10012 — Mon.-Sat. 11-7, Sun. 12-5

Luca Luca — W

Luca Luca thrives on color, from bold brights to soft pastels. Find dress suits, pants, dresses and eveningwear in feminine designs. Luca Luca is for women who want to look perfectly matched and completely color coordinated.

Upper East Side — 212-288-9285
1011 Madison Avenue — at 78th St.
NYC 10021 — Mon.-Sat. 10-6:30, Thurs. 10-8, Sun. 12-5

Upper East Side — 212-755-2444
690 Madison Avenue — at 62nd St.
NYC 10021 — Mon.-Sat. 10-6:30, Thurs. 10-8, Sun. 12-5

Lucky Brand Dungarees — W/M

In the beginning there was Levi's; now there's Lucky Brand, a California-based company that features a floor-to-ceiling selection of jeans, loungewear and everything in between. Pay an average of $70 for a pair of jeans. "Lucky You" and a four-leaf clover logo mark the lining of each pair. Will they bring you good luck? Only time spent in a pair of Lucky Brands will tell. www.luckybrandjeans.com

SoHo — 212-625-0707
38 Greene Street — at Grand
NYC 10013 — Mon.-Sun. 11-7

Lucy Barnes — W

Located in the center of the meat-packing district, Lucy Barnes brings New Yorkers her collection of detail oriented designs in which she likes to put strange combinations together. Her trademark: the extensive use of handwork where items are lovingly made by the art of crocheting, beading, patchwork and knitting. Shop a collection of taffeta bustiers, bustle skirts in iridescent silks, tops with intricate stitching, beaded leather pieces, accessories and more. These are edgy, feminine fashions with a touch of sexiness. Maternity and bridal by special order, as well as a menswear line to follow.

Chelsea — 212-255-9502
422 West 15th Street — bet. 9/10th Ave.
NYC 10011 — Tues.-Sat. 11-7, Sun. & Mon. by appointment only

Luichiny W
This Eighth Street footwear retailer is for the fearless and funky. Luichiny only does platforms, manufactured in Spain in bold colors. Find sandals, maryjanes, wedges and even stilettos mounted on the highest of platforms.

West Village   212-477-3445
21 West 8th Street   bet. 5/6th Ave.
NYC 10011   Mon.-Sat. 11-9, Sun. 12-8

Macy's M/W/C
Macy's has just about everything under the sun. There are extensive men's, women's and children's departments, home furnishings and cosmetics, as well as places to grab a bite to eat. The end result: the world's largest department store, packed with aggressive shoppers in search of the ultimate bargain. While designer labels are scarce, you'll find an ample selection of labels like Jones New York, Evan Picone and Tommy Hilfiger. Extensive shoe departments for men, women and children have everything from sneakers to dress-up shoes. Another bonus is the vast array of services Macy's provides, such as hair salons, restaurants, post office, theater tickets and jewelry appraising. 800-431-9644

Midtown West   212-695-4400
Broadway at Herald Square   bet. B'way/34th St.
NYC 10001   Mon., Thurs., Fri. 10-8:30,
    Tues., Wed., Sat. 10-7, Sun. 11-6

Madison Ave. Maternity & Baby W
Pregnant movie stars, models and socialites come to this shop for sophisticated, chic maternity clothes without a hint of dowdiness. Find casual, career and eveningwear designs that come direct from Milan and Paris, all exclusive to Madison Avenue Maternity. Choose from dresses, slacks, separates and dressy suits. Prices run from $89 to $1,400.

Upper East Side   212-988-8686
1043 Madison Avenue, 2nd Fl.   bet. 79/80th St.
NYC 10021   Mon.-Fri. 10-7, Sat. 10-6, Sun. 12-5

M-A-G W
M-A-G, a Chinese cashmere company, features a bridge line collection of cashmeres and sportswear. Find an abundance of sweater styles, from twin sets to chunky turtlenecks with an average price of $170. In addition, choose from separates, capri pants, beaded skirts, cargo pants, silk tops and more. Check out their exclusive line of cultured pearls, as well as their fashionable cashmere pieces for babies and children. 888-MAG-0494 www.m-a-g.com

SoHo   212-965-1898
120 Wooster   bet. Prince/Spring
NYC 10012   Mon.-Sat. 11-7, Sun. 12-7

Magic Windows B/G
A full-service children's shop. Find back-to-school essentials, basics, party clothes, as well as special occasion

dress wear, perfect for a bar mitzvah, wedding or christening. A good source for personalized blankets, sweaters, pillows and robes. Newborns to pre-teen.

Upper East Side   212-289-0028
1186 Madison Avenue   bet. 86/87th St.
NYC 10028   Mon.-Sat. 10-6, Sun. 12-5

Make 10   M/W

Make 10 features a collection of footwear packed with fashion attitude, from conservative to downright funky. Brand names include Enzo, Dakota, Steve Madden, Nine West, Franco Sarte and more.

Upper East Side   212-472-2775
1227 Third Avenue   bet. 70/71st St.
NYC 10021   Mon.-Fri. 11-7:30, Sat. & Sun. 12-6

NoHo   212-460-8144
680 Broadway   bet. Bond/W. 3rd St.
NYC 10012   Mon.-Sat. 11-8, Sun. 12-6

Midtown West   212-956-4739
1386 Sixth Avenue   bet. 56/57th St.
NYC 10019   Mon.-Fri. 10-7, Sat. 11-6, Sun. 12-6

Fifth Avenue   212-868-1202
366 Fifth Avenue   bet. 34/35th St.
NYC 10001   Mon.-Fri. 10-7, Sat. 11-7, Sun. 12-6

Makie   M/W/C

Looking for a great pair of pajamas? Well here's a tiny SoHo shop packed with them. At Makie, find classic-styled pajamas, nightshirts and unisex bathrobes manufactured in France by Bains-Plus. Men and women can choose from a selection of solids with contrasting piping, jacquards, checks, stripes and florals in top quality cottons with comfy, elasticized waists. Prices start at $140. Buy kiddie pj's (from 4 to 12 yrs for $70), as well as rompers and adorable handmade dresses. Canvas totes, vintage buttons and other goodies complete their assortment.

SoHo   212-625-3930
109 Thompson Street   bet. Prince/Spring
NYC 10012   Mon.-Sat. 12-7, Sun. 11-6

Makola   W

Venetian designer Ilaria Makola brings New Yorkers a collection of day and evening dresses that are ultra-feminine and lively in color. Choose from luxurious silks and whimsical, cotton print dresses styled with dainty waistlines and full petticoat skirts. The end result: romantic looks reminiscent of the 50's. Coordinating accessories include shoes, handbags, jackets and hats.

Upper East Side   212-772-2272
1045 Madison Avenue   bet. 79/80th St.
NYC 10021   Mon.-Sat. 10-6, Sun. 12-5

Malia Mills   W

Does the idea of shopping for a swimsuit provoke panic? Well, fear not, Malia Mills has come to the rescue. Her talent lies in creating bathing suits that fit like lingerie. Choose from a variety of looks with amusing names like "Bust-A-Move," "D-Mure," "It's A Cinch" and "Skinny Dipper." Find a line of hip, functional swimwear designed to be mixed and matched by size, color and fabric. Styles range from daring bikinis to reassuring maillots. So if you want an itsy bitsy top paired with a fuller bottom, Mills has just that. Sizes run from AA to DD cup. Bags, slippers, skirts and hair ornaments also available. www.maliamills.com

NoLiTa   212-625-2311
199 Mulberry Street   bet. Spring/Kenmare
NYC 10012   Mon.-Sun. 12-7

Malo M/W

There's cashmere, and then there's Malo's cashmere! Malo's comes from frigid Mongolia, and the colder the weather, the better the cashmere. New Yorkers flock here for luxury knitwear in traditional and non-traditional styles. A Malo sweater is recognized for quality, cut and shape. Find crewnecks, cardigans, v-necks, turtlenecks, twin sets, cablestitch pullovers and more. Malo's home collection includes pajamas, robes, slippers, pillows and blankets. New this year: ready-to-wear that complements their knitwear.

Upper East Side   212-396-4721
814 Madison Avenue   at 68th St.
NYC 10021   Mon.-Sat. 10-6, Thurs. 10-7

SoHo   212-941-7444
125 Wooster Street   bet. Prince/Spring
NYC 10012   Mon.-Sat. 11-7, Sun. 12-6

☆ Manolo Blahnik W

Forced to choose between their jewelry or their Blahnik's, many women might well choose the latter. So for sexy footwear that sets off all fashion trends, arm yourself with a pair of Blahnik's. A Manolo design is feminine, seductive (but never vulgar) and fabulously comfortable. Find stilettos, elegant pumps, classic loafers and strappy sandals to match any mood or dress. Your walk down the aisle won't be complete without a pair of Blahnik bridal shoes. Manolo loyalists include Faye Dunaway, Madonna and Diane von Furstenberg.

Midtown West   212-582-3007
31 West 54th Street   bet. 5th/6th Ave.
NYC 10019   Mon.-Fri. 10:30-6, Sat. 10:30-5:30

Manrico M/W

Manrico's sweaters are deliciously pure, soft and warm. Styles include polos, zip fronts, cardigans, twin sets, crews, 16-ply cable stitch pullovers and vests in 100% cashmere or silk and cashmere blends. Don't leave town during their winter and summer sales when prices are 30% to 50% off.

Upper East Side   212-794-4200
802 Madison Avenue   bet. 67/68th St.
NYC 10021   Mon.-Sat. 10-6, Sun. 12-5

Maraolo M/W

An Italian company that manufactures its own shoes, as well as those for Giorgio Armani. Find a collection of loafers, lace-ups, pumps, boots, sandals and casual weekend shoes, manufactured in quality leathers and suedes. Best to shop during their sales when prices can be as low as cost.

Upper East Side 212-535-6225
1321 Third Avenue bet. 75/76th St.
NYC 10021 Mon.-Sat. 11-8, Sun. 1-6

Upper East Side 212-628-5080
835 Madison Avenue bet. 69/70th St.
NYC 10021 Mon.-Sat. 9:30-7, Sun. 12:30-5:30

Upper East Side 212-832-8182
782 Lexington Avenue bet. 60/61st St.
NYC 10021 Mon.-Sat. 10-8, Sun. 12:30-6

Upper West Side (Maraolo Outlet) 212-787-6550
131 West 72nd Street bet. Amsterdam/Columbus Ave.
NYC 10023 Mon.-Fri. 10:30-8, Sat. 10-7, Sun. 12-6

Midtown East 212-308-8793
551 Madison Avenue at 55th St.
NYC 10022 Mon.-Fri. 9:30-7, Sat. 11-7, Sun. 12-6

Marc Jacobs W

From the designer who brought you the "grunge" look, comes a collection of clothes that is a mixture of cut-to-the-chase urbanity and hushed indulgence. Find a ready-to-wear line of coordinating separates in luxury fabrics and classic designs that can be mixed and matched in all sorts of combinations. His most coveted commodity, however, is his knitwear, particularly his beautiful, hand-knit cashmere sweaters. Accessories include scarves, belts, hats and jewelry, as well as a selection of shoes. Prices are sky high. New this year: handbags and leathergoods ranging from $85 for a pencil case to $5,700 for an alligator duffel.

SoHo 212-343-1490
163 Mercer Street bet. Houston/Prince
NYC 10012 Mon.-Sat. 11-7, Sun. 12-6

Marc Jacobs M

Marc Jacobs' second store, exclusively for men, offers a full range of ready-to-wear. Enter a pure and clean interior, and find suits and sportswear imbued with classic modernism and elegance. Complement your suit with a selection of men's furnishings that includes ties, scarves, hats, small leathergoods, bags, underwear and shoes. Outerwear designs run from P-coats and fitted parkas to military-styled coats. The Marc Jacobs label is defined by luxury fabrics, clean cuts and understated looks. For men who don't want to look like they're wearing designer.

West Village 646-638-1185
403 Bleecker Street bet. West 11th/Hudson
NYC 10012 Mon.-Sat. 11-7, Sun. 12-6

MarcoArt
M/W

Best known for designing and painting watch faces for Swatch, Marco also has designed a collection of hand-printed T-shirts, halter tops, dresses and bags. A typical Marco design is a brightly colored T-shirt with an amusing slogan.

Lower East Side   212-253-1070
186 Orchard Street   bet. Houston/Stanton
NYC 10002   Mon.-Sat. 10-6

Mare
M/W

This uncluttered, neat shop carries sleek Italian shoes under the Mare label. Looks run from classic to trendy. Good price points.

SoHo   212-343-1110
426 West Broadway   bet. Prince/Spring
NYC 10012   Mon.-Fri. 11-8, Sat. 11-7, Sun. 12-7

Margie Tsai
W

After apprenticing with Donna Karan and Vivienne Tam, Tsai has struck out on her own with a collection that combines industrial and feminine fabrics. Styles range from gossamer-thin butterfly lace dresses and heavy rubber coats to hand-painted organdy shirts paired with acetate skirts. This multi-cultural designer says her clothing is "functional art," that tells a story with fabric. For those of you with fond memories of the 60's, Margie Tsai stocks white, sheath style paper dresses that are disposable!   www.margietsai.com

NoLiTa   212-334-2540
4 Prince Street   bet. Elizabeth/Bowery
NYC 10012   Mon.-Sun. 12-7

Marianne Novobatzky
W

Can't stand basic black one minute longer? Craving a little color and "pizzazz" in your evening wardrobe? Check out Marianne Novobatzky's SoHo showroom. It's packed with designs perfect for evening and special occasion dress. Find raw silk taffeta ballgown skirts, bustiers, fancy-dress suits, taffeta gowns, dresses and jackets. You can mix and match from the collection or simply have Madame Novobatzky design your very own.

SoHo   212-431-4120
65 Mercer Street   bet. Spring/Broome
NYC 10012   Mon.-Fri. 12-7, Sat. 12-5

Marina Rinaldi
W

Marina Rinaldi, a division of Max Mara, is a luxury boutique for the plus-sized woman. Find dresses, suits, pants, blouses, sweaters and outerwear, perfect for all times of day, manufactured in Italy under the Marina Rinaldi label. It's about sumptuous fabrics, classic designs and expert tailoring guaranteed to flatter even the fullest figure. Sizes range from 10 to 22. Customer service is exceptional. A limited selection of shoes.

Mark Christopher

Upper East Side	212-734-4333
800 Madison Avenue	bet. 67/68th St.
NYC 10021	Mon.-Sat. 10-6, Thurs. 10-7

Mark Christopher   M

This downtown custom tailor is convenient for the Wall Street crowd. Get measured for a suit, shirt or tie and expect delivery in approximately three weeks. Suit prices start at $500 and expect to pay $145 for a shirt. Of course, prices depend on fabric selection.

Lower Manhattan	212-509-2355
80 Wall Street	bet. Water/Beaver
NYC 10005	Mon.-Fri. 9-5, Sat. by appointment

Mark Montano   W

This well-established downtown designer creates "dress-me-up" clothing with Barbie Doll flair. Find dresses, tops, skirts, jackets and pants in vibrant colors and lively patterns. Accessories include handbags and jewelry. Best for evening.

East Village	212-505-0325
434 East 9th Street	bet. 1st/Ave. A
NYC 10009	Tues.-Fri. 1-7, Sat. 12-8, Sun. 1-6

☆ Mark Schwartz   W

Welcome to this charming shop featuring fabulous shoe styles where unusual heel shapes and bursts of color are the rule. Not surprisingly, designer Mark Schwartz believes "a woman should begin (her wardrobe) with her shoes and build from there." Find pony-skin mules, creamy suede flats, python pumps, sexy, strappy, evening shoes, wooden-bottom sandals, and other styles in printed fabrics and silk plaids. These shoe designs are guaranteed to make any leg look fun and sexy. www.markschwartzshoes.com

NoLiTa	212-343-9292
45 Spring Street	bet. Mott/Mulberry
NYC 10012	Mon.-Sat. 11-7, Sun. 12-6

Marsha D.D.   G

Perhaps the hottest ticket in town for cool, trendy pre-teen clothes. Don't let the disorganized interior deter you; Marsha D.D. will satisfy even the ficklest kids. Find jeans and pants galore, shirts, sweatshirts, minis and accessories under fashion forward labels like Paris Blues, Hollywood, Hard Tail, Juicy Couture, Roxy, Betsey Johnson Kids, Le Petit Bateau (up to size 18), Profetto and more. The look is hip and happening. From 7 years to 16.

Upper East Side	212-534-8700
1324 Lexington Avenue	bet. 88/89th St.
NYC 10028	Mon.-Sat. 10-6

Marsha D.D.   B

Boys from 5 to 13 years old will gives thumbs up to Marsha D.D.'s cool selection of merchandise. Find looks where surf meets streets with sought-after labels like Quiksilver, Rusty,

Metropolitan Prairie, and Diesel. Casual wear includes cargo pants, collared shirts, lots of flannel, T-shirts, swim suits, jeans, sweats, underwear by Calvin Klein, as well as great accessories including a terrific selection of G-Shock watches. It's cool duds for cool dudes. Size 8 to 20.

Upper East Side   212-876-9922
1324 Lexington Avenue   bet. 88/89th St
NYC 10028   Mon.-Sat. 10-6

Martier   W

You get two shops rolled into one: upstairs is filled with fashion forward collections for trend seekers, while downstairs holds a superabundance of sexy lingerie (plus some swimwear). You'll find just about every popular label worn by New York's young fashionistas, including William B, Exte, Rebecca Taylor, Gili, Mandalay and Ferre. Looks run from slim, fitted pants and printed body-hugging tops to long flowing skirts and satin corsets. And downstairs, discover colorful selection of daring intimates by La Perla, NA, Malizia, Valery, Ritratti, Aubade and others. Sales staff is friendly and helpful.

Upper East Side   212-758-5370
1010 Third Avenue   at 60th St.
NYC 10022   Mon.-Sat. 10-8, Sun. 12-6:30

Martinez Valero   W

A convenient neighborhood shoe shop featuring fashion forward styles at attractive prices. Shop a varied selection of footwear, from classic to trendy. Find looks that will complement any outfit whether it's satin evening pumps, boots, summer sandals, or more. Prices run from $125 to $265.

Upper East Side   212-753-1822
1029 Third Avenue   at 61st St.
NYC 10021   Mon.-Fri. 10-8, Sat. 11-7, Sun. 12-6

Mary Efron   W

Mary Efron sells eclectic vintage pieces from the turn of the century to the 1950s. Find a collection of silk and embroidered Chinese jackets, dresses from the 1920s, evening and special occasion wear, as well as antique handbags that come beaded, jeweled or painted. Go back in time and experience Ms. Efron's mini-museum of antique clothing.

SoHo   212-219-3099
68 Thompson Street   bet. Broome/Spring
NYC 10012   Tues.-Sun. 1-7

Mason's Tennis Mart   M/W/C

Mason's is the oldest and most respected tennis retailer in the city. Find tennis gear and apparel for both the professional and novice player. Equipment brand names include Dunlop, Wilson, Volkl, Head and Prince, while labels Ellesse, Polo, Fila, Nike and Lacoste make up their apparel collection. Great children's department. Same day stringing for rackets.

Maternity Work

Midtown East   212-755-5805
56 East 53rd Street   bet. Madison/Park Ave.
NYC 10022   Mon.-Fri. 10-7, Sat. 10-5

Maternity Work   W

This is the outlet store for Mimi Maternity, Pea in the Pod and Motherhood. Shop here for on-sale items from all three lines, whether it's for career wear or casual basics.

Midtown West   212-399-9840
16 West 57th Street, 3rd Fl.   bet. 5th/6th Ave.
NYC 10019   Mon.-Wed. 10-7, Thurs. 10-8,
Fri. & Sat. 10-6, Sun. 12-6

Mavi   M/W/C

Mavi is getting hotter by the minute. Celebrities are slipping into this Turkish jeans manufacturer's sexy, low-rise styles, and now Mavi is wardrobing the stars of the television hit show "Sabrina the Teenage Witch." Choose from a huge selection of low-waisted, form-fitted and light-weight jeans that retail from $52 to $58. Find them in every size and length, making Mavi a good source for models with itsy bitsy waists and long legs.

SoHo   212-625-9458
510 Broome   bet. Thompson/W. B'way
NYC 10013   Mon.-Sun. 11-8

Max Fiorentino   W

A good neighborhood shop for knock-off designer handbags. Find familiar shapes and styles that include the Fendi baguette, an Hermès classic or even a Gucci. Prices run from $250 to $900 depending on your selection. Also, shop an enormous selection of pashmina shawls retailing at $155.

Upper East Side   212-751-5553
1024 Third Avenue   bet. 60/61st St.
NYC 10021   Mon.-Fri. 10-8, Sat. & Sun. 11-7

Max Mara   W

Max Mara caters to women who appreciate simplicity and ease over trendiness and fashion drama. Find two floors of luxury basics that include beautifully tailored suits, dresses, shirts, separates and outerwear. Designs are clean, crisp and classic and always incorporate a fresh, feminine appeal. Discover the best selection of overcoats, perfect over the simple chic of a Max Mara skirt and separate. Shoes and accessories also available.

Upper East Side   212-879-6100
813 Madison Avenue   at 68th St.
NYC 10021   Mon.-Sat. 10-6, Thurs. 10-7

Max Studio   W

Designer Leon Max carries a line of modern and up-to-date clothing that includes knitwear, dresses, pants, skirts—but sorry, no shoes. In short, find contemporary sportswear at contemporary prices. www.maxstudio.com

Men's Warehouse

SoHo   212-941-1141
415 West Broadway   bet. Prince/Spring
NYC 10012   Mon.-Thurs. 11-7,
Fri. & Sat. 11-8, Sun. 12-6

Mayle   W

Designer/owner Jane Mayle sells ultra-feminine, vintage inspired designs. Shop four clothing racks, grouped by color, and featuring looks that go from day to evening. Find sexy, backless ultra-suede dresses, pinstriped pants, lace and crochet pieces, "cowgirl" tops in pink leopard prints, army inspired sweaters, and coats. A Mayle design fuses sleek shapes with a gypsy spirit. Accessories include handbags, shawls, and patch purses.

NoLiTa   212-625-0406
252 Elizabeth Street   bet. Prince/Spring
NYC 10012   Mon.-Sat. 12-7, Sun. 12-6

Meghan Kinney Studio   W

If you're tired of paying uptown designer prices, then hustle down to Meghan Kinney's East Village shop. She specializes in polished, multi-purpose sportswear. Separates play a major role in her collection: match a full pant with a double-knit wool jersey and accompany it with a jacket or coat. Each season she introduces a new blend of fabric and texture combinations into her neutral color palette. These are classic fashions with an urban edge. Designs are cut to shape.

East Village   212-260-6329
312 East 9th Street   bet. 1st/2nd Ave.
NYC 10003   Mon.-Fri. 1-8, Sat. 12-8, Sun. 12-6

Ménage À Trois   W

Social engagement coming up fast? Let Ménage À Trois solve your last-minute concerns. Select a style from their collection and have it made in the color, size and fabric of your choice. Looks include cocktail and dinner suits, chiffon slip-dresses, iridescent silk-taffeta ballgowns and even sexy leather pants suitable for downtown party girls. Allow two to three weeks for delivery and expect to pay anywhere from $750 to $2,200 for dressy evening looks.

Upper East Side   212-396-2514
799 Madison Avenue, 2nd Floor   bet. 67/68th Street
NYC 10021   Mon.-Fri. 9-6, Sat. 10-5

Men's Wearhouse   M

Tired of the headaches and hassles of department store shopping? Make your way to Men's Wearhouse—they have the same merchandise, but 25% cheaper on average. Find suits by Hugo Boss, Canali, DKNY, Chaps Ralph Lauren, Gianfranco Ferre and more. Men's furnishings, dress shirts, tuxedos, casual sportswear, outerwear, socks and underwear complete the assortment. A complete shoe department with labels by Cole-Haan, Bostonian, Florsheim and more.
800-776-7848

Midtown East   212-856-9008
380 Madison Avenue   at 46th St.
NYC 10017   Mon.-Fri. 8:30-7:30, Sat. 10-6, Sun. 12-6

Metro Bicycle   M/W/C

With six locations throughout Manhattan, Metro Bicycle delivers service. Bikes come with a three-year warranty that includes gear and brake adjustments, as well as replacement of defective parts. Find mountain, road and suspension bikes from makers such as Specialized, Trek, Raleigh and Gary Fisher at competitive prices. Bicycles are available for rent by the hour or the day.

Upper East Side   212-427-4450
1311 Lexington Avenue   at 88th St.
NYC 10128   Mon.-Sun. 9:30-6:30,
Wed. & Thurs. 9:30-7:30

Midtown West   212-581-4500
360 West 47th Street   at 9th Ave.
NYC 10036   Mon.-Fri. 9-7, Sat. 10-6, Sun. 10-5

Chelsea   212-255-5100
546 Sixth Avenue   at 15th St.
NYC 10011   Mon.-Sun. 9:30-6:30

East Village   212-228-4344
332 East 14th Street   bet. 1st/2nd Ave.
NYC 10003   Mon.-Sun. 9:30-6

TriBeCa   212-334-8000
417 Canal Street   at 6th Ave.
NYC 10013   Mon.-Sun. 9:30-6:30

☆ Michael Kors   W

The long-awaited opening of the Michael Kors store has finally come. Between designing for the French luxury brand Celine and launching his own retail shop, Kors is a busy man. Polished, sophisticated looks combined with feminine chic is his message. Find textured suits, sleek, tailored jackets, shift dresses, blouses, beautiful cashmeres and knits, eveningwear and a healthy dose of fur. It's classic, all-American clothing that goes from sporty to high glam.

Upper East Side   212-452-4685
974 Madison Avenue   at 76th Street
NYC 10021   Mon.-Sat. 10-6

Michael's, The Consignment Shop for Women   W

For 45 years Michael's has set the pace in the consignment industry by featuring the ultimate in pre-owned couture clothing and bridal wear. Brides-to-be can select from magnificent creations by Vera Wang, Arnold Scassi or Dior. So whether you're searching for a designer frock on a limited budget or you simply love the thrill of the hunt, you'll find one of New York's largest selections of previously owned outfits by Prada, Hermès, Armani, Chanel, Gucci and more, at a fraction of the original cost.

Miller's Harness Company

Upper East Side 212-737-7273
1041 Madison Avenue, 2nd Fl. bet. 79/80th St.
NYC 10021 Mon.-Sat. 9:30-6, Thurs. 9:30-8

☆ Michelle Roth & Co. W
Michelle Roth specializes in European couture wedding dresses that reflect the requirements of today's modern bride. Roth's trademarks: a perfect fit, a profuse use of color (from Wedgwood blue and celadon to maize yellow), a dramatic silhouette and, yes, a sexy and high fashion look. Choose from exclusive collections by Elizabeth Emanuel (who designed Princess Diana's wedding dress), Peter Langner, Domo Adami, and Max Chaoul. Prices run from $3,000 to $18,000. And if you're nervous about getting wet from a sudden rain shower or a tipsy guest spilling champagne, ask for designer Emanuel's "Plastic Fantastic" little number: a tight-fitting bodice and bouffant skirt that's entirely waterproof, and a mere $18,000.
www.michelleroth.com

Midtown West 212-245-3390
24 West 57th Street, Suite 203 bet. 5th/6th Ave.
NYC 10019 by appointment only

Mika Inatome W
A TriBeCa shop for the bride in search of a non-traditional wedding dress. Japanese designer Mika Inatome specializes in slim, form-fitted gowns, rather than a romantic, full petticoat dress. Styles include fashionable column dresses, either plain or embroidered with pearls and lace. Best to custom order your own. Prices start at $1,500.

TriBeCa 212-966-7777
11 Worth Street, Suite 4B bet. W. B'way/Hudson
NYC 10013 by appointment only

Milen Shoes M/W
This Eighth Street shoe shop features European brand name footwear. Find styles that range from work shoes and evening to casual and relaxed. Choose from mules, sandals, boots and evening shoes. For men, find leather and suede loafers, boots and sandals. Brand names include Stephane Kelian, Massimo, Enrico Atantoniri and others.

West Village 212-254-5132
23 West 8th Street bet. 5th/6th Ave.
NYC 10011 Mon.-Sat. 11-9, Sun. 12-9

Miller's Harness Company M/W/C
Miller's features world-class riding attire and equipment for dressage, show and hunt. From children's size 4 to adults, find riding boots (fitted and custom), saddles, clothing (casual and show) and training equipment. Miller's also offers brand name saddles, including Colby, Collegiate, Lancer and Hermès. Trot on down and discover the perfect attire for you and your favorite equine.

Mimi Maternity

Flatiron	**212-673-1400**
117 East 24th Street	bet. Park/Lex. Ave.
NYC 10010	Mon.-Sat. 10-6, Thurs. 10-7

Mimi Maternity W

Don't fall into a fashion rut just because you're pregnant. There are sources for stylish maternity wear, and Mimi Maternity is one of them. Find a selection of clothing that delivers fashionable comfort.

Upper East Side	**212-737-3784**
1125 Madison Avenue	at 84th St.
NYC 10028	Mon.-Fri. 10-7, Sat. 10-6, Sun. 12-6

Upper East Side	**212-832-2667**
1021 Third Avenue	bet. 60/61st St
NYC 10021	Mon.-Fri. 10-7, Thurs.10-8,
	Sat. 10-6, Sun. 11-6

Upper West Side	**212-721-1999**
2005 Broadway	bet. 68/69th St.
NYC 10023	Mon.-Thurs. 10-8, Fri. & Sat. 10-7, Sun. 12-5

Missoni M/W

Enter this Madison Avenue boutique and discover Missoni's world of slinky and unusual knitwear. Designer Angela Missoni is mad for wild, geometric textures and sharp-edged graphics in bold color combinations. In short, patterns are her message. She's turned knitwear into a complete line of women's ready-to-wear that includes pants, halter dresses, skirts, sweaters and swimwear. For men, sweaters are your best bet. Attenzione: These zig-zag fashions can make you dizzy.

Upper East Side	**212-517-9339**
1009 Madison Avenue	at 78th St.
NYC 10021	Mon.-Sat. 10-6

Miss Pym G

Miss Pym's line for children rises to the level of couture. Owners Lisa Hall and Julia Roshkow are very particular about what they will and won't create. ("We don't do bright colors, lace, Peter Pan collars, puffy sleeves or smocking.") Expensive, sophisticated clothing for mothers who want their children on the best-dressed list.

Upper East Side	**212-879-9530**
1025 Fifth Avenue	bet. 83/84th St.
NYC 10028	by appointment

Miu Miu W

Miu Miu, Prada's spirited secondary line, showcases its sportswear collection on aluminum fixtures against hot red walls. Billed as Prada's reasonably priced line, but don't be fooled, it's still expensive. The look is downtown trendy, where rough meets pretty. Pants suits, shirts, dresses and jackets make up Miu Miu's avant-garde collection. Also find functional and fashionable handbags, as well as shoes to complement your Miu Miu outfit.

SoHo	**212-334-5156**
100 Prince St.	bet. Greene/Mercer
NYC 10012	Mon.-Sat. 11-7, Sun. 12-6

Mom's Night Out / One Night Out

Modell's M/B
One of America's oldest sporting goods chains, Modell's is the city's largest resource for gear and apparel. Find equipment and clothing for fishing, camping, fitness, baseball, swimming and more. Also a large selection of brand name sneakers at low prices. 800-275-6633 www.modells.com

Upper East Side 212-996-3800
1535 Third Avenue bet. 86/87th St.
NYC 10028 Mon.-Sat. 8:30-9, Sun. 10-6:30

Midtown East 212-661-4242
51 East 42nd Street bet. Vanderbilt/Madison
NYC 10017 Mon.-Fri. 8-8, Sat. & Sun. 9:30-6

Midtown West 212-594-1830
901 Sixth Avenue at 32nd St.
NYC 10001 Mon.-Sat. 10-8, Sun. 11-6

Lower Manhattan 212-964-4007
200 Broadway bet. Fulton/John
NYC 10038 Mon.-Fri. 8:30-6, Sat. 10-5, Sun. 11-4

Moe Ginsburg M
With their recent multimillion-dollar renovation, Moe Ginsburg ushers in the millennium with a spacious and comfortable shopping environment. Find five floors of menswear that runs the spectrum from accessories to formal wear. Men can shop for a full range of casual and business attire under the Ginsburg label, as well as designers like Donna Karan, Hugo Boss, Ralph, Joseph Abboud and Burberry. Their largest departments, however, are formal-wear and shoes. Choose from dress and casual footwear styles by Bally, Bostonian, Church's, and Kenneth Cole. Other departments include men's furnishings, a big and tall division, outerwear and jeans. Find a full range of sizes at good prices. On-site tailoring available.

Flatiron 212-242-3482
162 Fifth Avenue at 21st St.
NYC 10010 Mon.-Fri. 9:30-7, Thurs. 9:30-8,
Sat. & Sun. 9:30-6

Mom's Night Out / One Night Out W
Owner Patricia Shilands has covered all her bases when it comes to pleasing women in search of the perfect evening ensemble. Mom's Night Out and One Night Out are separate stores located across a hall. The former caters to expectant mothers, while the latter is for women—can you guess?—without a baby on the way. In both cases the goal is to offer an intimate shopping environment filled with glamorous eveningwear. Both stores allow you to rent, buy or custom-order. Shop a collection of fancy suits, cocktail dresses and ballgowns with designer labels like Vera Wang, Halston, Prada, Gucci and their own signature line. Looks run from fashion forward to downright sexy! So if you want to buy a gown, design your own or merely rent one, this is a perfect destination.

Upper East Side   212-744-6667
147 East 72nd Street, 3rd Floor   bet. Lex./Third Ave.
NYC 10021   Mon.-Fri. 10:30-6, Thurs. 10:30-8

Montmartre   W

This long-time denizen of Columbus Avenue continues to please its customers with a well-balanced assortment of fashionable clothes that runs from casual and contemporary to career and eveningwear. Find trendy labels by Chaiken, Paul and Joe, Jill Stuart, BCBG and Diane Von Furstenberg.

Upper West Side   212-875-8430
2212 Broadway   bet. 78/79th St.
NYC 10024   Mon.-Sat. 11-8, Sun. 12-7

Upper West Side   212-721-7760
247 Columbus Avenue   bet. 71/72nd St.
NYC 10023   Mon.-Sat. 11-8, Sun. 12-7

Morgane Le Fay   W

Argentinean designer Liliane Casabal expertly translates fantasy into wearable reality. Find feminine, soft and clean designs in fabrics from silk charmeuse to dreamy chiffon and organza. The selection includes elegant slacks, jackets and the creamiest ecru wedding gowns. This is the perfect place to shop for refined romantic clothing.

Upper East Side   212-879-9700
746 Madison Avenue   bet. 64/65th St.
NYC 10021   Mon.-Sat. 10-6

SoHo   212-219-7672
67 Wooster Street   bet. Spring/Broome
NYC 10012   Mon.-Sun. 11-7

Moschino   M/W

Moschino's approach is tongue-in-cheek (we think) for both his store design and clothing. Enter a whimsical interior dominated by a spiral staircase adorned with wrought iron question marks; heart and peace sign logos are scattered throughout; and, yes, finally you discover some actual clothing. "Cheap & Chic" is a complete line of ready-to-wear; "Diffusion" is a jean line; and there's also couture. The merchandise, whether it's jeans or couture, is fun and outrageous, and sends the message: let's not take fashion too seriously!

Upper East Side   212-639-9600
803 Madison Avenue   bet. 67/68th St.
NYC 10021   Mon.-Sat. 10-6

Motherhood Maternity   W

A very affordable alternative to the pricier Manhattan maternity boutiques. Find suits, casual wear, lingerie and underwear for mothers-to-be. Fabrics tend to be synthetic.
800-4-MOM-2-BE

Upper East Side   212-734-5984
1449 Third Avenue   at 82nd St.
NYC 10028   Mon.-Fri. 10-7, Thurs. 10-8,
    Sat. 10-6, Sun. 12-6

Midtown West 212-564-8170
901 Sixth Avenue at 33rd St.
NYC 10001 Mon.-Sat. 10-8, Sun. 11-6

Chelsea 212-741-3488
641 Sixth Avenue at 20th St.
NYC 10011 Mon.-Sat. 10-7, Sun. 11-6

M. Steuer Company W

This discounter is known for its selection of inexpensive hosiery and workout wear. From leotards, unitards and leggings to bra tops, bike shorts and socks, find it all at some of the best prices in town. Choose from two brands of hosiery, Steuer's private label line "Diva" and Givenchy. Prices range from $1.75 to $6.

Midtown West 212-563-0052
31 West 32nd Street bet. 5th/B'way
NYC 10001 Mon.-Fri. 7:45-5:20

MZ Wallace W

At MZ Wallace find a collection of tote and travel bags manufactured in durable materials like leather, Cordura nylon, burlap, and printed laminated cottons. These simply shaped weekend bags come in a range of color combinations like fuschia, orange, green, and light blue. The creators' goal: " to create cool bags that have a chic and groovy look."

SoHo 212-431-8252
93 Crosby Street bet. Prince/Spring
NYC 10012 Tues. 1-5, Wed.-Sat. 11-7, Sun. 12-6

N. Peal M/W

N. Peal is the ultimate purveyor of traditional, luxury cashmere sweaters. This 200-year-old private label company features a handsome selection of Scottish knitwear. Styles include v-necks (plain or cabled), round necks, cardigans, twin sets and turtlenecks, from single-ply to six-ply. In addition, find skirts, robes, gloves and socks.

Midtown West 212-826-3350
5 West 56th Street bet. 5th /6th Ave.
NYC 10019 Mon.-Sat. 10-6

☆ Nancy Geist W

Wonderful colors, unusual heel and shoe silhouettes, and femininity define the Geist label. Find stretch leather boots, mules, denim sandals with appliques, snakeskin pumps, baby doll flats, and evening shoes. Looks run from flirty to urban sophisticated. Prices run from $185 to $600.

SoHo 212-925-7192
107 Spring Street at Mercer
NYC 10012 Mon.-Fri. 11-8, Sat. 11-7, Sun. 12-7

☆ Nanette Lepore W

Lepore's unique pieces have been rumored "to inspire cat fights between rock stars." Due to her inspired collections and new SoHo digs (designed by husband Robert Savage),

Lepore is on her way to the big leagues. Her gypsy lifestyle plays a strong role in her clothes. Subtle detailing, lots of color and feminine silhouettes define a Lepore design. Find dresses, satin blouses (open-necked and ruffled), crocodile jackets, fur-trimmed knit coats, and sweaters (plain or embroidered). Accessories include elongated clutches, mohair fuzzy bags and other fun pieces. It's glamour girl meets gypsy looks. www.nanettelepore.com

SoHo   212-219-8265
423 Broome Street   bet. Lafayette/Crosby
NYC 10012   Mon.-Sat. 12-8, Sun. 12-6

Nautica M/B

Great casual and outdoor wear for men and boys. Find shirts, sweaters, jeans, shorts, khakis, swimwear and windbreakers in Nautica's trademark colors and quality fabrics. "Nautica Competition" features workout apparel that's comfortable and stylish.

Upper West Side   212-496-0933
216 Columbus Avenue   at 70th St.
NYC 10023   Mon.-Sat. 10-8, Sun. 12-6

Nellie M. W

Nellie M. is a fashion oasis of contemporary designer labels. Choose from labels like Nicole Miller, Theory, Vivienne Tam and Chaiken. From eveningwear, sportswear and separates to coats and accessories, find a look that's fashionably hip at competitive price points. Kate Spade handbags and accessories also available.

Upper East Side   212-996-4410
1309 Lexington Avenue   at 88th St.
NYC 10128   Mon.-Fri. 10-8, Sat. & Sun. 11-8

New & Almost New (NAAN) W

A SoHo consignment shop that features designer items that are new and almost new. You may come across a Comme des Garçons jacket, an Armani suit, a pair of Prada shoes, a Chanel handbag or even an Hermès scarf. Remember, it's all in the timing, as merchandise changes frequently.

SoHo   212-226-6677
65 Mercer Street   bet. Spring/Broome
NYC 10012   Mon.-Fri. 12-6:30, Sat. 1-6

New Balance New York M/W

New Balance appeals to a range of athletic types. Their impressive sneaker selection covers running, cross-training, hiking, walking, tennis, golf and basketball. The NB apparel line runs from basic shorts and tank tops to microfiber jackets and pants that offer performance, fit and looks. Men's casual shoes and children's sneakers are also available. www.newbalance.com

Midtown East   212-421-4444
821 Third Avenue   bet. 50/51st Street
NYC 10022   Mon.-Fri. 10-7,
  Thurs. to 8, Sat. & Sun 12-5

The New York Look

Midtown West   212-997-9112
51 West 42nd Street   bet. 5th/6th Ave.
NYC 10036   Mon.-Fri. 10-7, Sat. 10-6, Sun. 12-4:45

New Frontier   W
Great for fashionable wardrobe staples that don't cross the threshold of trendiness. Casual basics and work clothes make up New Frontier's collection. Find suits, separates, jackets, dresses and sweaters designed in good taste. New Frontier is stylishly simple.

Upper West Side   212-873-7444
230 Columbus Avenue   bet. 70/71st St.
NYC 10023   Mon.-Sat. 11:30-7:30, Sun. 12-7

New York City Custom Leather   M/W
For years designer Agate Blouse has dressed rock stars and supermodels in her signature custom leather designs, most famously, her 60's inspired, hip-hugging pants with a flared leg made in the best cowhides ("soft, but not wimpy"). She'll cut any pattern you desire, including vests, jackets, bras and hats. Prices run from $700 to $1,000. Delivery dates vary.

Lower East Side   212-375-9593
168 Ludlow Street   bet. Houston/Stanton
NYC 10002   by appointment

New York Golf Center   M/W/C
New York Golf, the city's largest golf store, carries the best equipment for novices and pros. Find clubs from makers like Callaway, Taylor Made, Links and McGregor, as well as golf apparel for men and women. Rainwear, socks, shoes, golf bags, balls, books and accessories also available. Inquire about on-premise lessons.

Midtown West   212-564-2255
131 West 35th Street   bet. 7th Ave./B'way
NYC 10001   Mon.-Fri. 10-8, Sat. 10-7, Sun. 11-5

The New York Look   W
A chain of stores selling contemporary career, casual and eveningwear from French and Italian designers. They've recently upgraded their image, and if you look carefully you can get some great buys. Sales staff tends to be clueless.

Upper West Side   212-765-4758
30 Lincoln Plaza   bet. 62/63rd St.
NYC 10023   Mon.-Thurs. 10-9, Fri. 10-8,
    Sat. 11-9, Sun. 12-7

Upper West Side   212-362-8650
2030 Broadway   bet. 69th/70th St.
NYC 10023   Mon.-Fri. 10-9, Sat.11-9, Sun. 12-7

Midtown West   212-382-2760
570 Seventh Avenue   at 41st St.
NYC 10018   Mon.-Fri. 9-7, Sat. 10:30-7

Fifth Avenue   212-557-0909
551 Fifth Avenue   at 45th St.
NYC 10176   Mon.-Fri. 9-8, Sat. 10-8, Sun. 10-6

Nicole Farhi

SoHo   212-598-9988
468 West Broadway   bet. Houston/Prince
NYC 10012   Mon.-Sat. 11-8, Thurs. 11-9, Sun. 12-8

Nicole Farhi   M/W

Between this London-based designer's strong ready-to-wear collections and her successful in-house restaurant, it appears that Nicole Farhi has adapted quite nicely to New York's fierce retail market. Enter her 16,000-sq. ft. flagship store and find a three-level emporium of product lines, from men's and women's ready-to-wear to a home collection. Farhi calls her clothes "constant friends" and says simplicity is the rule. Choose from nicely cut trousers, skirts, jackets, knits, coats, accessories, shoes and more. Farhi designs with luxury fabrics, clean cuts and a sophisticated ease. Grab a bite downstairs at Nicole's, her modern and sleek looking restaurant.

Upper East Side   212-223-8811
10 East 60th Street   bet. Madison/5th Ave.
NYC 10022   Mon.-Fri. 10-7, Sat. 10-6, Sun. 12-5

☆ Nicole Miller   W

Nicole Miller offers something for everyone. Women shop here for a variety of looks, from ladylike flirtatious to downtown fun. Each season Nicole turns out a collection of bridalwear, cocktail dresses, sportswear and accessories. Shop for chiffon blouses, embroidered bustiers, sweaters, skirts, denim and eveningwear. A Nicole Miller design is modern, clean and fashion forward—a perfect combination of youthful energy and urban sophistication. Also find an ever-changing line of men's ties, featuring her famously tongue-in-cheek prints. Bridal by appointment.
800-365-4721 www.nicolemiller.com

Upper East Side   212-288-9779
780 Madison Avenue   bet. 66/67th St.
NYC 10021   Mon.-Fri. 10-7, Sat. 10-6, Sun. 12-5

SoHo   212-343-1362
134 Prince Street   bet. Wooster/W. B'way
NYC 10012   Mon.-Sat. 11-7, Sun. 12-6

Nicole Vaughn   W

Like other hip-hop stores, Nicole Vaughn sells casual, stretchy clothes, perfect for the Silicon Alley crowd, which needs outfits that will take them from their internet start-up to a night on the town. Find dresses and skirts with matching jackets, pants, tops and a good selection of accessories.

East Village   212-477-3937
110 East 7th Street   bet. 1st/Ave. A
NYC 10009   Mon. 4-8, Tues-Fri. 1-8,
    Sat. 12-8, Sun. 1-8

Niketown   M/W/C

Niketown's exterior mimics the facade of a New York high school (circa 1950), while its interior is a high-tech atrium. Enter through a set of turnstiles to find yourself in a five-floor, futuristic environment replete with video screens con-

stantly plugging Nike products. While most of the merchandise is readily accessible, sneakers ascend at high speed from the basement via a series of five-story clear plastic air tubes. It's all quite thrilling, but that's the point, isn't it?
www.nike.com

Midtown East   212-891-6453
6 East 57th Street   bet. 5th/Madison
NYC 10022   Mon.-Fri. 10-8, Sat. 10-7, Sun. 11-7

The 1909 Company   W

Neo-vintage and vintage clothing fill this well-stocked SoHo shop. Find dresses, suits and jackets from the 1900s to the 1950s, as well as silk lingerie, Edwardian linens, kimonos, robes, handbags and shawls. You may come across a vintage Hermès scarf, a Pucci dress or even a Gucci handbag.

SoHo   212-343-1658
63 Thompson Street   bet. Broome/Spring
NYC 10012   Mon.-Sun. 12-7

99X   M/W

99X features (predominately) English clothing with a retro feel, ranging from 60's flower-power to 80's skinhead. It's packed with funky brand name footwear by Dr. Martens, Creepers and Vegetarian Shoe Co. Styles run from steel-toed shoes to Puma sneakers. Find shirts by Ben Sherman, Lonsdale and Fred Perry. This is clothing and footwear for the hard core punkster.

East Village   212-460-8599
84 East 10th Street   bet. 3rd/4th Ave.
NYC 10003   Mon.-Sat. 12-8, Sun. 12-7

Nine West   W

This retailing conglomerate dominates the footwear industry and claims to "sell two pair of shoes per second." Nine West features a full range of great looking, moderately priced shoes. Designs run from classic and trendy to hip and "in vogue." From sun up to sun down, Nine West carries it all. Find platforms, pumps, flats, loafers, sandals, boots and everything in between. Accessories include handbags, leathergoods, sunglasses and jewelry, as well as an outerwear collection that includes leather, nylon and shearling. New this year: sportswear collection. 800-260-2227
www.ninewest.com

Upper East Side   212-987-9004
184 East 86th Street   bet. Lex./Third Ave.
NYC 10028   Mon.-Fri. 10-8, Sat. 10-7, Sun. 11-6

Upper East Side   212-472-8750
1195 Third Avenue   bet. 69/70th St.
NYC 10021   Mon.-Wed. & Sat. 10-7,
    Thurs. & Fri. 10-8, Sun. 12-6

Upper West Side   212-799-7610
2305 Broadway   bet. 83/84th St.
NYC 10024   Mon.-Fri. 10-8, Sat. 10-9, Sun. 12-7

Nocturne

Midtown East 212-370-9107
341 Madison Avenue at 44th St.
NYC 10017 Mon.-Fri. 8-8, Sat. 10-6, Sun. 12-5

Midtown East 212-486-8094
750 Lexington Avenue bet. 58/59th St.
NYC 10022 Mon.-Fri. 10-8, Sat. 10-7, Sun. 12-5

Midtown East 212-371-4597
757 Third Avenue bet. 47/48th St.
NYC 10017 Mon.-Fri. 8-8, Sat. 11-6, Sun. 12-5

Midtown West 212-397-0710
1230 Sixth Avenue at 49th St.
NYC 10020 Mon.-Fri. 9-8, Sat. & Sun. 10-5

Midtown West 212-564-0063
901 Sixth Avenue bet. 32/33rd St.
NYC 10001 Mon.-Sat. 10-8, Sun. 11-6

Fifth Avenue 212-319-6893
675 Fifth Avenue at 53rd St.
NYC 10022 Mon.-Sat. 10-7, Sun. 10-6

Flatiron 212-777-1752
115 Fifth Avenue at 19th St.
NYC 10003 Mon.-Sat. 10-8, Sun. 11-7

SoHo 212-941-1597
577 Broadway at Prince
NYC 10012 Mon.-Sat. 10-8, Sun. 11-7

Lower Manhattan 212-488-7665
313 World Trade Center Concourse level
NYC 10048 Mon.-Fri. 7:30-8, Sat. 10-6

Nocturne   W

Pop into this little shop for a lovely selection of feminine, delicate nightgowns and robes, mostly made in Brazil. Also find cute children's slippers.

Upper East Side 212-750-2951
698 Madison Avenue bet. 62/63rd St.
NYC 10021 Mon.-Sat. 10-7

Noriko Maeda   W

Japanese designer Noriko Maeda is an authority in designing ultra-feminine clothing. Her superb tailoring skills and classic styling cater to women in search of refined fashions reminiscent of Audrey Hepburn. Find a ready-to-wear collection of simple, ladylike designs in luxury fabrics. Sizes tend to run small.

Upper East Side 212-717-0330
985 Madison Avenue bet. 76/77th St.
NYC 10021 Mon.-Sat. 10-5:30

Norma Kamali   W

For 20 years, Norma Kamali has had a cult following. Her customers range from the young professional to the hip rock star, and everyone in between. Her secret: designing clothes that are seasonless. Shop this unique interior and find sportswear, eveningwear, swimwear and activewear, all

designed to be mixed and matched. Her best bets continue to be her trademark sleeping bag coats, swimwear, and selected items manufactured in parachute material. Not to be missed is Kamali's poly-jersey collection, a line of wrinkle-free clothes. Wear it for day, evening and even to your yoga class. Check out her new high-tech rubber fabric that changes color with your body temperature.
www.normakamali.com

Midtown West   212-957-9797
11 West 56th Street   bet. 5th/6th Ave.
NYC 10019   Mon.-Sat. 10-6

North Beach Leather   W

North Beach Leather lives again, this time in ultra-hip SoHo. Leather, leather and more leather is the message. Choose from racy body-hugging designs that include halter dresses, mini-skirts with matching jackets, bustiers, pants, car coats and cropped jackets. The collection comes in a multitude of colors, from red and turquoise to black and winter white with sexy and sassy looks. Bootcut leather pants retail for $450, classic long coats for $1,000 and jackets for $695. www.northbeachleather.com

SoHo   212-625-8668
523 Broadway   at Spring St.
NYC 10012   Mon.-Fri. 10-8, Sat. 10-9, Sun. 12-6

Nova USA   M/W

Although Nova is a casual sportswear shop for men, curiously 30% of its customers are women. Cameron Diaz and model Helena Christensen are devoted customers of Nova USA's designer Tony Melillo's athletic-inspired, edgy casual clothing. Choose from their signature Judo pants, chinos, T-shirts, zip-collared sweatshirts, and baseball jackets. Sexy basics at affordable prices. Expect a women's collection for Spring 2000.

Lower East Side   212-228-6844
100 Stanton Street   at Ludlow
NYC 10002   Mon.-Sun. 12-6

Nursery Lines   B/G

Nursery Lines specializes in furnishings for your nursery, whether it's window treatments, custom bumpers, linens, monogrammed quilts or interior design for your child's bedroom. They also carry classic Italian and English clothing, including dresses, rompers and sweaters. Best for pajamas and robes, either off the rack or custom made. Tod's shoes also available up to 8 years. From newborn to size 4.

Upper East Side   212-396-4445
1034 Lexington Avenue   at 74th St.
NYC 10021   Mon.-Sat. 11:30-5

Oasis   W

Oasis carries a good selection of merchandise that will work in most women's wardrobes. Shop for everything from stylish suits from Teenflo to sexy outfits from hip labels such as

Yigal Azrouel, Easel and Theory. Also find a broad selection of T-shirts, knits and sexy little dresses. Good sales.
www.oasissoho.com

SoHo   **212-219-0710**
138 Spring Street   at Wooster
NYC 10012   Mon.-Sat. 11:30-8, Sun. 11:30-7:30

Oilily   B/G
Spice up your child's wardrobe with Oilily's bold approach to fashion. Prints, prints, PRINTS everywhere! Even on their shoes! Find patterned dresses, shirts, pants, sweaters, jackets and accessories. Newborn through size 12/14.
800-556-0585

Upper East Side   **212-628-0100**
870 Madison Avenue   bet. 70/71st St.
NYC 10021   Mon.-Sat. 10-6, Thurs. 10-7, Sun. 12-5

Oilily for Women   W
This is the equivalent of "play clothes" for adults. Prints are ubiquitous—on dresses, pants, overalls, jeans, sweaters and accessories. From beachwear to dressier pieces, you can mix and match from past and present seasons. It's cute clothing with easy wearability. 800-850-9551

Upper East Side   **212-772-8686**
820 Madison Avenue   bet. 68/69th St.
NYC 10021   Mon.-Sat. 10-6, Thurs. 10-7, Sun. 12-5

Old Navy Clothing Company   M/W/C
In only five years Old Navy has become a retail behemoth, and their stores are now weighing in at 100,000 sq. feet per location. Teens and adults alike love shopping Old Navy for hip, trendy affordable basics. Old Navy gives you maximum buying power when it comes to casual clothing. This super store is packed with fun essentials like jeans, T-shirts, swimwear, shorts, sweatshirts, sweaters and jackets. Old Navy offers lots of bang for your buck; however, don't expect the clothes to last a lifetime. 800-653-6289
www.oldnavy.com

Midtown West   **212-594-0049**
150 West 34th Street   bet. 6/7th Ave.
NYC 10001   Mon.-Sat. 9-9:30, Sun. 11-8

Chelsea   **212-645-0663**
610 Sixth Avenue   bet. 17/18th St.
NYC 10011   Mon.-Sat. 9:30-9:30, Sun. 11-8

SoHo   **212-226-0865**
503 Broadway   bet. Spring/Broome
NYC 10012   Mon.-Sat. 10-9, Sun. 11-8

Olive & Bette's   W
A boutique packed with trendy designer labels similar to what you might find in Barney's 7th-floor Co-op. Olive & Bette's features a collection of contemporary sportswear that includes skirts, dresses, T-shirts, pants and sweaters. Labels include Theory, Vivienne Tam, Daryl K, Trina Turk and Juicy. www.oliveandbettes.com

Upper East Side	212-717-9655
1070 Madison Avenue	bet. 80/81st St.
NYC 10028	Mon.-Sat. 11-7, Sun. 11-6
Upper West Side	**212-579-2178**
252 Columbus Avenue	bet. 71/72nd St.
NYC 10023	Mon.-Sat. 11-8, Sun. 11-7

Omari M/W

Just another funky SoHo shoe shop for the young and trendy. Chunky heeled sandals, sneaker boots and two-toned patent leather cowboy boots are a few of their styles.

SoHo	212-219-0619
132 Prince Street	bet. Wooster/W. B'way
NYC 10012	Mon.-Sun. 11-7:30

O.M.G. M/W

Glamorous it's not, but do you really care, when you can buy a pair of Levi 501's for $39.99. Other labels include Calvin Klein, Lee, Polo and Dockers.

Midtown East	212-661-6495
850 Second Avenue	at 45th St.
NYC 10017	Mon.-Sat. 9:30-9, Sun. 10:30-7:30
SoHo	**212-925-9513**
546 Broadway	bet. Spring/Prince
NYC 10012	Mon.-Sat. 9-9:30, Sun. 10-8

Only Hearts W

As the name suggests, hearts play a central role here, beginning with the store's exterior heart-shaped door handle. Shop a sweet and flirty collection of lingerie and underpinnings, including camisoles, teddies, lace tanks, sexy underwear and a selection of sleepwear and robes. In addition, find great gift items perfect for bridal showers, from heart-shaped paperweights and candles to sachets and soaps. Great selection of ethnic beaded bags and jewelry.

Upper West Side	212-724-5608
386 Columbus Avenue	bet. 78/79th St.
NYC 10024	Mon.-Sat. 11-8, Sun. 11-6

The Open Door Gallery W

Painter turned fashion designer, Madani views her work as art and that's what makes her collection so refreshing. Movement, color and freedom of expression play vital roles in her designs. She selects silks, linens, cottons and interesting prints, and mixes them together to create one-of-a-kind creations. Finished with raw, zig-zagged edges, her styles often call for wrapping yourself in sarong-like ways. The look is feminine and flowy, and allows you to add your own personal touch.

East Village	212-777-3552
27 East 3rd Street	bet. 2nd Ave/Bowery
NYC 10003	Mon.-Sun. 2-7

Original Leather　　　　　　　　　　　　　　M/W

Original Leather carries clothing that is innovative in styling, deft in cut and fit, and offered at sensible prices. Find an assortment of funky, functional clothing that meets the need and taste of every customer. Their large selection of coats, jackets, pants (in every color, fit, and style), skirts and accessories in durable leathers will convince you that if Original Leather doesn't have it, no one does.

Upper East Side　　　　　　　　　　　　212-585-4200
1100 Madison Avenue　　　　　　　　bet. 82nd/83rd St.
NYC 10028　　　　　　　　　　　Mon.-Sat. 10-7, Sun. 12-6

Upper West Side　　　　　　　　　　　　212-595-7051
256 Columbus Avenue　　　　　　　　　　　at 72nd St.
NYC 10023　　　　　　　　　　　Mon.-Sat. 11-8, Sun. 11-7

Chelsea　　　　　　　　　　　　　　　　212-989-1120
84 7th Avenue　　　　　　　　　　　bet. 15th/16th St.
NYC 10011　　　　　　　　　　　Mon.-Sat. 11-8, Sun. 12-7

West Village　　　　　　　　　　　　　212-675-2303
171 West 4th St.　　　　　　　　　　bet. 6th/7th Ave.
NYC 10014　　　　　　　　　　　　Mon.-Wed. 11-9,
　　　　　　　　　　　Thurs.-Sat. 11-Midnight, Sun. 12-9

West Village　　　　　　　　　　　　　212-777-4362
552 LaGuardia Place　　　　　　　bet. Bleecker/W.3rd St.
NYC 10012　　　　　　　　　　　Mon.-Sat. 11-8, Sun. 12-7

SoHo　　　　　　　　　　　　　　　　　212-219-8210
176 Spring Street　　　　　　　bet. Thompson/W. B'way
NYC 10012　　　　　　　Mon.-Fri. 11-8, Sat. 10-8, Sun. 12-8

Orva　　　　　　　　　　　　　　　　　　　　W

Orva is a good source for the price-conscious woman in search of everyday accessories. Find hats, handbags, knapsacks, gloves and socks, as well as a shoe department featuring labels by Kenneth Cole, Via Spiga, and Nickels. Hosiery by Berkshire, Hanes, Dior, Danskin and Evan Picone are at terrific prices.

Upper East Side　　　　　　　　　　　　212-369-3448
155 East 86th Street　　　　　　　　bet. Lex./Third Ave.
NYC 10028　　　　　　　　　　　Mon.-Sat. 10-9, Sun. 10-8

Orvis　　　　　　　　　　　　　　　　　　M/W

Orvis carries a terrific assortment of equipment for hunting, fishing and bird watching. Outfit yourself in the appropriate attire for a weekend outing or an African safari. Orvis also offers sporting trips, as well as fishing and shooting lessons. New this year: a complete line of Barbour sportswear and outerwear.

Fifth Avenue　　　　　　　　　　　　　212-697-3133
522 Fifth Avenue　　　　　　　　　　　　　at 44th St.
NYC 10017　　　　　　　Mon.-Fri. 9-6, Wed. 9-7, Sat. 10-5

Oshkosh B'Gosh　　　　　　　　　　　　　　B/G

A huge success with Europeans eager to shop for their bambinos. Find everyday wear that includes jeans, overalls, T-shirts, shoes and accessories, all with the Oshkosh B'Gosh

logo. Newborn to size 16. 800-282-4674
www.oshkoshbgosh.com

Fifth Avenue   212-827-0098
586 Fifth Avenue   bet. 47/48th St.
NYC 10036   Mon.-Fri. 10-7, Sat. 10-6, Sun. 12-5

Out of Our Closet M/W

Regular folks, fashion designers and models all bring "last season's" leftovers here for resale. This consignment shop features the ultimate in trendy and hip labels, in near perfect condition. Shop for great basics and street smart looks by DKNY, CK, Diesel, Scoop, Tracy Feith, Tocca and Banana Republic. It all favors cutting-edge looks and better yet, it's all sold well below retail.

Chelsea   212-633-6965
136 West 18th Street   bet. 6th/7th Ave.
NYC 10011   Mon.-Sat. 12-7, Sun. 12-5

Overland Trading Company M/W

A casual shoe outfitter for the wheat and berry set. Find sturdy outdoor shoes and boots from Timberland, Rockport, Birkenstock and Clarks.

Midtown East   212-906-0180
712 Lexington Avenue   bet. 57/58th St.
NYC 10022   Mon.-Fri. 10-8, Sat. 10-7, Sun. 12-6

Oxxford Clothes M

Oxxford is an American menswear institution that has long pleased its customers. Now they've opened a retail shop that will spare you department store headaches. Find classic off-the-rack suits (or custom order one), navy blazers ($1,450 to $1,650), pants ($395 to $695), dress shirts, neckwear, casual sportswear and accessories—an American cut with conservative styling.

Midtown East   212-593-0205
36 East 57th Street   bet. Park/Madison
NYC 10022   Mon.-Sat. 10-6

Paragon Sporting Goods M/W

This is truly a sporting goods store for the 90's. Over 100,000 sq. ft. of space is devoted to equipment and apparel for every sport imaginable. From racket sports, water sports, skiing and hiking to golf, camping, fitness and fishing, the selection is enormous. This well-organized store makes shopping easy and pleasurable. New this year: an extensive golf department. 800-443-9120 www.paragon.com

Chelsea   212-255-8036
867 Broadway   at 18th St.
NYC 10003   Mon.-Sat. 10-8, Sun. 11-6:30

Parke & Ronen M/W

"Body conscious, but forgiving" describes this design team's streamlined, better sportswear geared toward a younger (or at least very trim) customer. In addition to casual pants and shirts, look for knits, vests, scarves and hats. Find a selection of Frank and Daniel belts and Simon Carter sunglasses.

Patagonia

Chelsea	212-989-4245
176 Ninth Avenue	at 21st St.
NYC 10011	Tues-Sat. 12-5, Sun. 1-6

Patagonia   M/W/C

From their modest roots making mountain climbing gear in a tin shed in Ventura, California, Patagonia has evolved into a company with worldwide distribution. Find outdoor, functional clothing for a variety of activities, from kayaking and surfing to climbing, hiking and skiing. The clothes are innovative, reliable and durable. Their polar fleece is excellent. 800-638-6464 www.patagonia.com

Upper West Side	917-441-0011
426 Columbus Avenue	bet. 80/81st St.
NYC 10024	Mon.-Sat. 10-7, Sun. 11-6

SoHo	212-343-1776
101 Wooster Street	bet. Prince/Spring
NYC 10012	Mon.-Sat. 11-7, Sun. 12-6

Patricia Field   M/W

Some call it funky and extreme, others campy and silly. This shop features downtown trendy looks for the club crowd. Find wild styling, from bright patent leather outfits to wigs from the 60's and 70's. Buy it when you see it, as the merchandise changes frequently.

NoHo	212-254-1699
10 East 8th Street	bet. 5th/University Pl.
NYC 10012	Mon.-Sat. 12-8, Sun. 12-8

Paul & Shark   M/W

Paul & Shark, an Italian retailer of yachting attire for, one suspects, the permanently landlocked, fuses urban and nautical influences. This two-level shop sells men's and women's sporty, chic clothing, perfect for yachting or casual sportswear. From sweaters, shirts and warm-up suits to swimwear, light-weight boating jackets, winter-weight coats and a line of polar fleece, it's all specifically fashioned for outdoor living and, best of all, is water-resistant. Golf apparel and canvas and leather boating shoes for men only.

Upper East Side	212-452-9868
772 Madison Avenue	bet. 66/67th St.
NYC 10021	Mon.-Sat. 10-6, Thurs. 10-7

Paul Smith   M

Shop an intimate environment that stands apart from other cookie cutter retail spaces. Designer Paul Smith pleases customers with a collection of refined English-tailored menswear. Find suits, at an average price of $1,200, dress and casual shirts, sport jackets, coats and men's furnishings. Accessories include watches, cufflinks and eyewear. What distinguishes a Paul Smith design is his bold approach to fabric, pattern and color, with a styling that adheres to Old World elegance.

Pearl River

Flatiron   212-627-9770
108 Fifth Avenue   at 16th St.
NYC 10011   Mon.-Sat. 11-7, Thurs. 11-8, Sun. 12-6

☆ Paul Stuart   M/W

Paul Stuart is renowned for outfitting high-powered bankers, lawyers and stockbrokers. From corporate to casual, find tailored designs for the captains of industry seeking that "no nonsense" polished look. For men there are suits, furnishings, shirts, sportswear and outerwear, as well as English bench-made shoes and accessories. Find the same "no-frills" fashions for the corporate woman. Paul Stuart is a great source for traditional clothing that says you mean business. Be prepared to drop a bundle. 800-678-8278

Midtown East   212-682-0320
Madison Avenue   at 45th Street
NYC 10017   Mon.-Fri. 8-6:30, Thurs. 8-7,
    Sat. 9-6, Sun. 12-5

A Pea in the Pod   W

Fret no more about putting together the perfect pregnancy wardrobe. A Pea in the Pod provides expectant mothers with a line of clothes that move easily from day to evening. The clothes are attractive and comfortable, and will make you feel your best at either work or play. 800-4-Mom-2-Be

Midtown East   212-826-6468
625 Madison Avenue   bet. 58/59th St.
NYC 10022   Mon.-Fri. 10-7, Sat. 10-6, Sun. 12-6

Peanutbutter and Jane   B/G

Those in search of high-tech, hip and trendy children's fashions should make the trek to Peanutbutter and Jane. Kids will love it! Find clothing by Flap Doodle, Monkey Wear, Le Tout Petits, Cache Cache, Cherry Tree, Cozy Toes and more. Shoes and accessories also available. From newborn to size 10/12.

TriBeCa   212-620-7952
617 Hudson Street   bet. Jane/W. 12th St.
NYC 10014   Mon.-Sat. 10:30-7, Sun. 12-6

Pearl River   M/W/C

Pearl River lets you experience shopping Asian style without having to leave the island of Manhattan. It's a Chinese department store packed to the rafters with everything from A to Z—appliances, houseware, video rentals, wonderful teas, soaps, food, and yes, even clothing. Find Mandarin jackets, Cheongsam dresses, silk pajamas, kimonos, straw and embroidered slippers and much more at fabulous bargain prices.

NoLiTa   212-966-1010
200 Grand Street   at Mott St.
NYC 10013   Mon.-Sun. 10-7:30

TriBeCa   212-431-4770
277 Canal Street   at Broadway
NYC 10013   Mon.-Sun. 10-7:30

A Perfect Day In Paradise   M/W
The Palm Beach look is in, just for now, and shop owner Denice Summers is capitalizing on this vogue. If you think "paradise" is a sunny resort or country club, then dive into Summer's collection of brightly colored clothing. Women can shop for Lilly Pulitzer-like print dresses, skirts, tops, pants, silk, corduroys, cashmeres and Mackintosh raincoats. Men can shop for corduroys, polos and oxford shirts in a rainbow of bold and pastel colors. Pay $135 for a pair of cords, $350 for a cashmere sweater and $1,500 for a custom-made evening frock.

Upper East Side 212-639-1414
153 East 70th Street bet. Lex./Third Ave.
NYC 10021 Mon.-Fri. 10-6, Sat. 11-5

Peter Elliot   M
One of New York's classic and most civilized men's stores, Peter Elliot is a good alternative to department store shopping and over-hyped designer boutiques. Find suits by Hickey-Freeman and Kiton, blazers, outerwear, shirts, sweaters and accessories. It's all conservatively styled with a touch of panache.

Upper East Side 212-570-2300
1070 Madison Avenue at 81st St.
NYC 10028 Mon.-Fri. 10:30-7, Sat. 10:30-6, Sun. 1-5

Peter Fox Shoes   W
A full-service shoe store that runs the gamut from day to evening. Find casual and dressy styles in classic designs under the Peter Fox label. Brides-to-be can choose from an extensive selection of bridal shoes.

SoHo 212-431-7426
105 Thompson Street bet. Spring/Prince
NYC 10012 Tues.-Sat. 11-7, Sun. 12-5:45

Peter Hermann   M/W
Peter Hermann carries sleek leather goods by popular European makers. Choose from a great assortment of briefcases, luggage, handbags, knapsacks, totes and wallets from labels like Mandarina Duck, Desmo, Jamin Puesch, Tardini and Strenesse. Also find eyewear by the English company of Cutler & Gross.

SoHo 212-966-9050
118 Thompson Street bet. Spring/Prince
NYC 10012 Mon.-Sat. 12-7, Sun. 1-6

Petit Peton   M/W
This Eighth Street upscale shoe store, nominated by *Vogue* and *Elle* magazine as one of the top three shoe stores in the U.S., is a shoe lover's dream come true. Find a collection of sexy, high fashion footwear styles with top designer labels like Valentino, Gianfranco Ferre, Jean Paul Gaultier, Claudio Merazzi and Casadei.

NoHo   212-677-3730
27 West 8th Street   bet. 5th/6th Ave.
NYC 10011   Mon.-Sat. 11-9, Sun. 12-8:30

Philosophy Di Alberta Ferretti   W

Alberta Ferretti's Philosophy line is youthful, refreshing and dedicated to the modern woman. Find a ready-to-wear collection in luxurious and delicate fabrics with simple silhouettes and subtle detailing. A Ferretti design is feminine, fashion forward and wearable.

SoHo   212-460-5500
452 West Broadway   bet. Houston/Prince
NYC 10012   Mon.-Sat. 11-7, Sun. 12-6

Piccione   M/W

Is Italy the true home of custom tailoring? A visit to Signor Piccione's workshop will most likely convince you that it is. He will graciously make a suit, sportcoat or pair of slacks for men, or a pant and jacket ensemble for women. Choose a fabric from the finest mills such as Zegna, Loro Piana, Holland and Sherry and Scabel. Suits prices start at $3,000 with a five-to-six-week delivery time.

Midtown West   212-956-2102
7 West 56th Street   bet. Fifth/Sixth Ave.
NYC 10019   Mon.-Fri. 10-5, Sat. by appointment

Pierre Garroudi   W

Do you need an evening gown, wedding dress or suit created in the next 24 hours? If so, Pierre Garroudi is your man. This designer will re-create any gown from the latest fashion magazines. Garroudi also sells off-the-rack designs that are long, clingy and sheer. A Garroudi original starts at $700 while a custom-made designer wedding dress will run you $1,100 and up. www.pierregarroudi.com

SoHo   212-475-2333
139 Thompson Street   bet. Prince/Houston
NYC 10012   Mon.-Sun. 10-8

Pilar Rossi   W

A Spanish designer known for her collection of bridalwear, evening gowns and dressy suits for special occasions. Choose from off-the-rack styles or custom order your own. A Rossi gown will run you at least $3,000, but you will be smartly, if a little ornately decked out.

Upper East Side   212-288-2469
790 Madison Avenue   bet. 66/67th St.
NYC 10021   Mon.-Sat. 10-6:30

Pleats Please, Issey Miyake   W

You could safely say that Miyake's trademark is his colorful, pressed pleats—he's even named his store and mid-priced clothing collection "Pleats Please." Featherweight, wrinkle-proof and 100% pleated, his ready-to-wear line is form-fitted, non-traditional, rainbow bright and versatile. His

167

Plein Sud

unorthodox style is a hybrid of Eastern and Western influences. While the look isn't for everyone, Miyake devotees swear by the pleats of their pants. www.pleatsplease.com

SoHo 212-226-3600
128 Wooster Street at Prince
NYC 10012 Mon.-Sat. 11-7, Sun. 11-6

☆ Plein Sud W

For ten years French designer Faycal Amor has created wonderfully feminine designs with just the right amount of sex appeal. Find everything from knits and leathers to eye-catching eveningwear. Choose from long dresses cut on the bias, square-shouldered jackets, form-fitted pants, skirts, knits, accessories and shoes, and don't miss his trademark sumptuous leathers and suedes. Sensuous, form-fitted shapes and cutting-edge looks define the Plein Sud label.

SoHo 212-431-6500
70 Greene Street bet. Spring/Broome
NYC 10012 Mon.-Sat. 11-7, Sun. 12-6

Plus Nine Fine Footwear for Women W

For the sophisticated woman in search of designer footwear in larger sizes. Shop in a relaxed atmosphere, aided by a knowledgeable, eager to please sales staff. Choose from brand labels like Stuart Weitzman, Via Spiga, Nichols and Donald Pliner. Sizes run from 9AA to 12AA and 10B to 13B.

Midtown East 212-593-3030
11 East 57th Street, 3rd Fl. bet. Madison/Fifth Ave.
NYC 10022 Mon.-Sat. 10:30-6

Polo Ralph Lauren M/W/B

For the past twenty years, Ralph Lauren has been the industry leader in "lifestyle" retailing. Lauren's collection embraces a number of familiar lifestyle images—the rugged outdoorsy type, the Newport yachtsman, urbane Brit and the waspy, sporty American. Enter Ralph Lauren's anglophile world of instant "Old World" style where you'll find everything from ready-to-wear and "Oscar" caliber eveningwear to sportswear and casual wear that offer timeless wearability. Highlights include blazers, sport jackets, cashmere sweaters and antique jewelry. Lauren has created an "American look," redolent with class and style, and his little polo player has taken over the world.

Upper East Side 212-606-2100
867 Madison Avenue at 72nd St.
NYC 10021 Mon.-Sat. 10-6, Thurs. 10-8

Polo Sport M/W

At Polo Sport, men and women will find the look for just about any lifestyle. The RLX label is a sport's line devoted to the worlds of running, cycling, aquatics and skiwear. "Polo Golf" features the ultimate in classic golfing attire, while "Polo Tennis" caters to both player and spectator with its selection of chic tennis duds. Interspersed, find Ralph's collection of sportswear that includes cashmere sweaters, shirts, jackets, chinos, resort and vintage pieces. It's all under one roof with looks that run from high-tech sporty to classic American.

Upper East Side 212-434-8000
888 Madison Avenue at 72nd St.
NYC 10021 Mon.-Sat. 10-6, Thurs. 10-8

SoHo 212-625-1660
381 West Broadway bet. Broome/Spring
NYC 10012 Mon.-Wed. 12-8,
Thurs.-Sat. 11-8, Sun. 12-6

Portantina   W

A mature customer shops at Portantina to add that unusual, one-of-a-kind piece to her wardrobe. Find an eclectic mix of merchandise, heavily Baroque and Renaissance in feel. Choose from uniquely styled handbags (like hand-painted suede totes and sari print bags), versatile velvet hats, knotted crushed-silk shawls from India and velvet gondolier slippers in rich colors. As for clothing, it's mostly Fortuny-inspired raw silk painted dresses and separates. Pillows, Venetian glassware, throws and more make up their home collection. Lush fabrics, rich colors and an Italian Old World feel define Portantina.

Upper East Side 212-472-0636
895 Madison Avenue at 72nd Street
NYC 10021 Mon.-Sat. 10:30-6

Powers Court Tennis Outlet   M/W/C

Powers Court sells tennis merchandise at some of the lowest prices in town. Find clothing, footwear, racquets and accessories that will meet all your tennis needs. Brand names include Prince, Wilson, Head and K-Swiss.

Chelsea 212-691-3888
132 1/2 West 24th Street bet. 6th /7th Ave.
NYC 10011 Mon.-Fri. 10-6, Thurs. 10-7:15, Sat. 10-4

Prada   M/W

Sleek, versatile and modern are the watchwords for a Prada design. This generations-old Milanese design house continues to be ground zero for celebrity glamour. Find ready-to-wear, sportswear, eveningwear, shoes and accessories. The look is cutting edge, based on simple, form-fitted cuts and a basic color palette. Prada's footwear is also in vogue. Designs are modern, stylized and just this side of funk. Colors, as one might expect, are black and brown. When it comes to handbags, Prada has made nylon a chic respectable fabric and knapsacks an alternative to handbags. Attenzione: Sizing is ridiculously small. New this year: Prada's newest "Bowling Bag" handbag retailing for $700. Also plans to launch a revolutionary new skin care line presented in single dose packaging. www.prada.com

Prada Sport

Upper East Side	**212-327-4200**
841 Madison Avenue	at 70th St.
NYC 10021	Mon.-Sat. 10-6, Thurs. 10-7
Midtown East (Shoes only)	**212-308-2332**
45 East 57th Street	bet. Park/Madison Ave.
NYC 10022	Mon.-Sat. 10-6, Thurs. 10-7
Fifth Avenue	**212-664-0010**
724 Fifth Avenue	bet. 56/57th St.
NYC 10019	Mon.-Sat. 10-6, Thurs. 10-7, Sun. 12-6

Prada Sport M/W

Don't walk into Prada Sport expecting to see work-out or exercise clothing. You won't! Die-hard "Pradanistas," however, won't care; they're happy as pie to discover another outlet for Prada's tight, sexy spandex clothing that looks too good to wear to the gym. Find skirts, tops, jackets, biking shorts, Lycra pants and outerwear in the latest high-tech fabrics at those predictable Prada prices. www.prada.com.

SoHo	**212-925-2221**
116 Wooster Street	bet. Prince/Spring
NYC 10012	Mon.-Sat. 11-7, Sun. 12-6

Precision W

A neighborhood boutique packed with trendy American and European labels. Create the look you're after, whether it's hip contemporary or downtown funky, with their large collection of Tark pants, as well as labels like Earl, Melinda Zoller, Jules, Ticci Tonetto, Mambo and Juicy Couture. Accessories include hats and girly handbags. Best bet: a large pashmina shawl for $149.

Upper East Side	**212-879-4272**
1310 Third Avenue	at 75th St.
NYC 10021	Mon.-Sat. 11-8, Sun. 12-6;30
Midtown East	**212-683-8812**
522 Third Avenue	at 35th St.
NYC 10016	Mon.-Fri. 11:30-8, Sat. 11-7, Sun. 12-6:30

Princeton Ski Shop M/W/C

Avid skiers, snowboarders and skaters will find equipment and apparel. Clothing labels include Bogner, Columbia, Obermayer and Burton, while ski and snowboard equipment is from top-of-the-line manufacturers. www.allskis.com

Flatiron	**212-228-4400**
21 East 22nd Street	bet. B'way/Park Ave. South
NYC 10010	Mon.-Fri. 10-10,
	Sat. 10-7, Sun. 12-6

Product W

Product's design philosophy is simple: give women the basics, but with a twist. The result is women's sportswear (under the Product and By-Product labels) based on quality fabric and creative designs, from stretch denim pants and skirts, simply styled dresses, shirts, jackets and knits. These are functional, sporty fashions with a hint of trendiness. Sizing cut small.

SoHo 212-274-1494
71 Mercer Street bet. Spring/Broome
NYC 10012 Mon.-Sat. 11-7, Sun. 12-6

NoLiTa 212-219-2224
219 Mott Street bet. Prince/Spring
NYC 10012 Mon.-Sat. 11-7, Sun. 12-6

Purdey M

Since 1814 Purdey has been the leading gun manufacturer in the world. Today their business includes hunting apparel and sportswear. Browse a collection of shooting jackets, hunting vests, breeches, shirts, cashmeres, waterproof field jackets, corduroy slacks, ties and accessories. Find them in luxurious tweeds, lodens and lambswools, suitable for hunting in the fields or relaxing in the city. Expensive.
www.purdey.com

Upper East Side 212-639-1500
844 Madison Avenue bet. 69/70th Street
NYC 10021 Mon.-Sat. 10-6

Quiksilver M/W/C

Surf's up! Catch the best waves at Quiksilver, the hottest Boardrider's Club in town. A concept shop where the beach meets the street, where surf and fashion meet to reflect California's active lifestyle. Adults and juniors can shop for the latest in board equipment and fashion trends for surfing, snowboarding or just hanging out. Find surfwear, swimwear, casual wear (including high-tech nylon pants), logo T-shirts, fleece, shirts, sweatshirts, as well as a line of sneakers and accessories. 877-246-7257 www.quiksilver.com

SoHo 212-334-4500
109 Spring Street bet. Mercer/Greene
NYC 10012 Mon.-Sat. 11-7, Sun. 12-7

Rampage Clothing Co. W

A great shop for the perfect mix of hip and fashion forward clothing for the under 30 crowd. Shop a constantly changing selection of merchandise like asymmetrical skirts, dresses, tight tops, pants, jeans and T-shirts, as well as lacy lingerie. Coordinating accessories include handbags, scarves, feather chokers, hats and sunglasses. Find it at affordable prices, but remember this clothing is for one season only.

SoHo 212-995-9569
127 Prince Street at Wooster
NYC 10012 Mon.-Sat. 10-8:0, Sun. 11-7

Rapax W

A good neighborhood shoe store that carries a large selection of fashionable classics. Find simply styled flats, mules, sandals and evening pumps by labels like Pancaldi, Rapax, Claudio Merazzi and Roberto Rinaldi. Prices run from $99 to $300.

Upper East Side 212-734-5171
1100 Madison Avenue bet. 82/83rd Street
NYC 10028 Mon.-Sat. 10-7, Sun. 11-5

Red Tape by Rebecca Dannenberg   W
Uptown and downtown girls alike go out of their way to check out Dannenberg's edgy urban fashions. Her clothes are dedicated to the lean and body-conscious. Her forte is her trouser collection with styles that range from a snug-fitting cigarette pant to a low-waisted bootleg cut. Other duds include sexy knits, skirts, sweaters and jackets.

East Village   **212-529-8483**
333 East Ninth Street   bet. 1st/2nd Ave.
NYC 10003   Mon.-Sun. 12-8

Reebok   M/W/C
A large, futuristic showplace for Reebok's line of fitness, tennis, running and cycling gear. The clothes are practical, good looking and well priced. Reebok's sneaker selection is outstanding, even for kids. www.reebok.com

Upper West Side   **212-595-1480**
160 Columbus Avenue   bet. 67/68th St.
NYC 10023   Mon.-Sat. 10-8, Sun. 12-6

Reebok Golf Shop   M/W
Although not conveniently located (unless you're hitting balls at the Chelsea Pier practice range), the Reebok name nonetheless seems to draw a crowd. Find men's apparel by Reebok and Greg Norman and golf equipment from makers like Wilson, Cobra, Titleist and Callaway. Golf shoes run from $50 to $150 and are available for both men and women.

Chelsea   **212-627-1206**
Chelsea Pier #59   at 23rd Street
NYC 10011   Mon.-Fri. 11-7, Sat. 11-6, Sun. 12-6

Reminiscence   M/W
This shop is a big draw for juniors who want a bit of retro grooviness in their wardrobe. Find fun and affordable Hawaiian T-shirts, baggy tie-string overalls, tube tops, halter tops, bike jackets, wrap skirts, vintage lingerie and boas, as well as military-styled clothing. Accessories include handbags, body glitter, bikini headbands and more.

Chelsea   **212-243-2292**
50 West 23rd Street   bet. 5th/6th Ave.
NYC 10010   Mon.-Fri. 11-7:30, Sat. 11-7:30, Sun. 12-7

René Collections   W
Top signature handbags get knocked off here in style. From Hermès' Kelly bag to Gucci's Hobo, it's hard to tell the copy from the original. Rene carries all shapes, sizes and colors at attractive prices. Costume jewelry and belts also available.

Upper East Side   **212-987-4558**
1325 Madison Avenue   bet. 93/94th St.
NYC 10128   Mon.-Sat. 10-7, Sun. 12-6

Upper East Side   **212-327-3912**
1007 Madison Avenue   bet. 77/78th St.
NYC 10021   Mon.-Sat. 10-6:30, Sun. 12-5

René Lezard M/W
René Lezard, a German-based design house, is known for turning out confident lifestyle sportswear for men and women. Designs are clean, understated and stylish—a sort of Teutonic Armani. Elegant suitings, classic pants, cashmeres from the Loro Piana mills, shirts and accessories make up their ready-to-wear collection. Soft tailoring synthesized with urban sportiness define the Lezard label.
www.rene-lezard.com

SoHo 212-274-0700
417 West Broadway bet. Spring/Prince
NYC 10012 Mon.-Sat. 11-7, Sun. 12-6

René Mancini W
René Mancini sells refined, elegant shoes that are meticulously crafted in France. A Mancini design comes with perfect cap toes and delicate small heels. Although expensive, it's worth it. Best to stock up during their semi-annual sales.

Midtown East 212-308-7644
470 Park Avenue at 58th St.
NYC 10022 Mon.-Sat. 10-5:45

Replay Country Store M/W/C
"Heavy duty durable and dependable" is the tag line for this Italian purveyor of casual, outdoor clothing, which follows the fashion trends. The store's only label is Replay, found on their assortment of sportswear, jeans, underwear, shoes and even china. Grab a bite at their in-store eatery called The Replay Café. www.replay.it.com

SoHo 212-673-6300
109 Prince Street at Greene
NYC 10012 Mon.-Sat. 11-7, Sun. 11-6

☆ Resurrection Vintage M/W
Resurrection Vintage is an outpost for New York's fashionistas looking for an outfit that has probably graced a magazine page or two. Owner Katy Rodriguez focuses exclusively on clothes from the 60's and 70's. She searches far and wide for her merchandise, bringing back coveted labels and looks that are in mint condition and perennially fashionable. Find clothing, shoes, and accessories by Valentino, Yves St. Laurent, Pucci, Courreges, Ferragamo, Gucci, and Pierre Cardin. No bargain prices, but a great alternative to Madison Avenue boutiques.

NoLiTa 212-625-1374
217 Mott Street bet. Prince/Spring
NYC 10012 Mon.-Sat. 11-7, Sun. 11-7

East Village 212-228-0063
123 East 7th Street bet. 1st/Ave. A
NYC 10009 Mon.-Sat. 2-10, Sun. 2-9

Reva Mivasagar W
An extensive collection of made-to-order, matronly eveningwear that greets you upon entering, but the real

story at Reva Mivasagar is bridal gowns. This Australian designer's collection is feminine, traditional, and suitable for any type of wedding. Allow three to four months for special orders on bridalwear and one to two months for their evening collection. Off-the-rack samples are also for sale.

SoHo   **212-334-3860**
28 Wooster Street   at Grand Street
NYC 10013   Mon.-Fri. 11:30-7, Sat. 11-7, Sun. 12-6

Richard Metz Golf Equipment   M/W

Richard Metz's store is a golfer's paradise; he even has a practice cage and putting green for lessons. Find the latest in top-quality golf equipment by makers like Callaway, Taylor Made, Hogan and Titleist. Men's apparel includes wind shirts, vests, rain suits, socks, shoes, and hats.

Midtown East   **212-759-6940**
425 Madison Avenue, 3rd Floor   at 49th St.
NYC 10017   Mon.-Fri. 9-7, Sat. 11-6, Sun. 10-5

Ripplu   W

Shaping breasts and firming buttocks without surgery. Impossible, you say. Not for the folks at Ripplu, who will fit you with a series of custom bras and panties, which will actually lift and reshape these critical anatomical parts. If you find this hard to believe, just look at the sales help, who are Ripplu's latest advertising with their hourglass figures. They're also courteous and helpful.

Fifth Avenue   **212-599-2223**
575 Fifth Avenue, 2nd Fl.   bet. 46/47th St.
NYC 10017   Mon.-Sat. 11-7

Ritz Furs   W

Women come here to shop for "gently" pre-owned furs. For years Ritz has satisfied customers with their fine selection of mink, lynx, fox, sable and more. Ritz expertly restores these forlorn furs into new condition. In addition, find shearlings, fur-trimmed and lined outerwear, fur hats, and stoles. An attentive, polite sales staff and great prices are the key to Ritz's 70 successful years.

Midtown West   **212-265-4559**
107 West 57th Street   bet. 6/7th Ave.
NYC 10019   Mon.-Sat. 9-6

Robert Clergerie   M/W

The "in crowd" shops here for a taste of French luxury. Footwear fashionistas crave Clergerie's chic, stylish modern classics. Find a variety of looks, ranging from trendy wedges and platforms to femininely styled heels. Styles include pumps, boots, loafers, sandals and evening shoes in great colors and quality leathers. A Clergerie design is a foot-flattering finale to any outfit. A limited selection of men's oxfords, loafers, boots and sandals. Expensive.

Upper East Side   **212-207-8600**
681 Madison Avenue   bet. 61/62nd St.
NYC 10021   Mon.-Sat. 10-6

Rockport

Roberto Cavalli W
Roberto Cavalli's window displays always get us in a naughty mood. His mannequins are dressed in sexy, wild outfits: fur-trimmed jeans coupled with a metallic animal print top, for example. Known for his python and floral print jeans, Cavalli emphasizes body conscious designs in suede, leather and fur using bright colors and lots of print. Find faux pony skin pants, fur-trimmed knits, body-hugging tops, shearling coats and more. These are high energy, sassy, sultry fashions for women who want to affect the city's male testosterone level. www.robertocavallinyc.com

Upper East Side   **212-755-7722**
711 Madison Avenue   at 63rd Street
NYC 10021   Mon.-Sat. 10-6

Robert Talbott M
A California-based shirt shop for the fashion conscious. Choose from 40 ready-made styles or custom order from their selection of over 200 fabric swatches. Dress shirts are tailored in a full cut and manufactured in top quality cottons and broadcloths. Ties, cufflinks, cummerbunds and pocket squares make perfect accessories. Shirt prices average $150. 800-747-8778 www.roberttalbott.com

Upper East Side   **212-751-1200**
680 Madison Avenue   bet. 61/62nd St.
NYC 10021   Mon.-Sat. 10-6

Rochester Big & Tall M
Rochester Big & Tall is America's #1 source for the discriminating man in need of larger and lengthier sizes. A full service shop running the gamut from underwear to designer suits with labels like Zegna, Canali, Donna Karan and Versace. Sportswear, casual and active wear, and accessories round out the assortment. Shoes by Allen-Edmonds, Cole-Haan, Ferragamo, Bruno Magli, and others.
800-282-8200

Midtown West   **212-247-7500**
1301 Sixth Avenue   at 52nd St.
NYC 10019   Mon.-Fri. 9:30-6:30,
    Thurs. 9:30-8, Sat. 9:30-6

Lower Manhattan   **212-952-8500**
67 Wall Street   at Pearl St.
NYC 10005   Mon.-Fri. 9-6, Sat. 9-5

Rockport M/W
Rockport's mission statement is "to make the world more comfortable," and indeed they do. Find rugged hiking boots, sneakers, loafers, sandals, lace-ups, hearty pumps and nifty looking golf shoes. Foot soothing products like massagers and sprays are available, as well as reflexology treatments on weekends. 800-762-5767 www.rockport.com

Upper West Side   **212-579-1301**
160 Columbus Avenue   bet. 67/68th St.
NYC 10023   Mon.-Sat. 10-8, Sun. 12-6

Rodier W
Ultra-conservative knitwear is Rodier's speciality. Find coordinating suits, pants, sweaters, and dresses manufactured in a variety of fabrics like linen, wool blends, polyester acrylic and cottons.

Upper East Side 212-439-0104
1310 Third Avenue at 75th St.
NYC 10021 Mon.-Sat. 10-6, Thurs. 10-7, Sun. 12-5

Rosa Custom Ties M
Globe-trotting executives visit Rosa's while in New York to custom order luxurious cravats. Choose from over 5,000 Italian silks, in prints or solids, then wait two weeks for your tie to be hand-stitched and interlined to perfection. Prices ranging from $95 to $125. No minimum order required.

Midtown West 212-245-2191
30 West 57th Street, 6th Fl. bet. 5th/6th Ave.
NYC 10019 Mon.-Fri. 9:30-5:30, Sat. by appointment

Rosette Couturiere W
Brenda Barmore has taken over the helm of this woman's custom tailor founded by Rosette Harris. She will duplicate a design, add her own interpretation, or merely do alteration work. A 9-to-5 suit will run you $550 (fabric price not included), while dinner suits start at $650.

Upper West Side 212-877-3372
160 West 71st Street, 2nd Fl. bet. Columbus/B'way
NYC 10023 Tues.-Fri. 10-6, Sat. 10-5

☆ Sacco W
Sacco carries a footwear style for everyone. Designs run from classic to flirty and trendy. Find mules, pumps, loafers, mary-janes, platforms, slingbacks, sandals, boots and more. Labels include Cynthia Rowley, Nancy Nancy, Charles Jourdan, Bettye Muller, Gretel's Clogs and Sacco. Pay an average price of $130. 877-464-7771 www.sacco.com

Upper West Side 212-874-8362
2355 Broadway bet. 85/86th St.
NYC 10024 Mon.-Fri. 11-8, Sat. & Sun. 11-7

Upper West Side 212-799-5229
324 Columbus Avenue bet. 75/76th St.
NYC 10023 Mon.-Fri. 11-8, Sat. 11-7, Sun. 12-7

Chelsea 212-675-5180
94 Seventh Avenue bet. 15/16th St.
NYC 10011 Mon.-Fri. 11-8, Sat. 11-7, Sun. 12-7

SoHo 212-925-8010
111 Thompson Street bet. Spring/Prince
NYC 10012 Mon.-Fri. 11-8, Sat. 11-7, Sun. 12-7

☆ Saint Laurie, Ltd. M/W
If you're in search of traditional, made-to-measure menswear, then Saint Laurie is a good source. Select a Saint Laurie suit fabric or dress shirt style and have it tailored accordingly. Average suit price is $1,000, while dress shirts

Salvatore Ferragamo

run from $125 to $235. Off-the-rack suits, furnishings and tuxedos also available. For women find made-to-measure only. www.saintlaurie.com

Midtown East   **212-473-0100**
350 Park Avenue   bet. 51/52nd St.
NYC 10022   Mon.-Fri. 9:30-6:30,
Thurs. 9:30-8, Sat. 9:30-6

The Sak   W

It all started with one simple design: a casual shoulder bag (in Sak's signature "Tightweave") that was durable, attractive, and versatile. Years later Sak is still designing a range of fine quality products from pillows to shoes. Yet their strength remains in a selection of bags that includes Solar (a light-weight leather collection), bridal bags in pale pink or white "Tightweave," tote bags woven in water lily root and nylon, as well as a collection of wooden beaded styles. With prices that range from $30 to $140, The Sak is one of the city's best values. 888-THESAK-1 www.thesak.com

SoHo   **212-625-3200**
521 Broadway   bet. Spring/Broome
NYC 10012   Mon.-Sat. 10-7, Sun. 12-5

Saks Fifth Avenue   M/W/C

This quintessential New York City department store, housed in a landmark building, is currently undergoing a five-year, $100 million renovation aimed at improving floor space, beefing up designer labels and creating settings that clearly display their best-selling lines. By 2003, the scheduled completion date, Saks is sure to be one of the finest up-to-the-minute fashion emporiums in the city. Cosmetics, handbags, hosiery, and accessories occupy the main floor, while women's fashions take center stage with four floors devoted to ready-to-wear, evening wear and sportswear. Choose from designers like Celine, Gucci, Dolce & Gabbana, Michael Kors, Marc Jacobs, Samsonite, Max Mara, Piazza Sempione, Ellen Tracy, Emanuel and more. Other departments include women's shoes (designer and contemporary), bridal, furs, outerwear, lingerie, and children's. Gentlemen will find two complete floors devoted to American and European designer labels. Select from suits by Hickey Freeman, Alan Flusser, Armani, and Zegna. Also find men's furnishings, outerwear, formal wear, and shoes. Finally, visit the Elizabeth Arden Spa salon or grab a bite to eat in the café. 800-345-3454 www.saksfifthavenue.com

Fifth Avenue   **212-753-4000**
611 Fifth Avenue   bet. 49/50th St.
NYC 10022   Mon.-Sat. 10-7, Sun. 12-6

Salvatore Ferragamo   W

The Ferragamo name has always been associated with top quality shoes. Women, particularly, swear by their superb comfort and fit. Find classic styles manufactured in luxury leathers with sizes that range from 5AAA to 11B. Semi-annual sales are the best time to stock up. Ferragamo's cloth-

Salvatore Ferragamo

ing exudes the same polished and refined quality. Shop a ready-to-wear collection that includes nicely tailored suits, jackets, skirts, separates, and coats, all in luxurious fabrics and tasteful styling. In addition, find handbags, scarves, and accessories that also embrace the Ferragamo trademark of classic elegance. 800-572-6641
www.salvatoreferragamo.it.com

Fifth Avenue	**212-759-3822**
661 Fifth Avenue	bet. 52/53rd St.
NYC 10022	Mon.-Sat. 10-6, Thurs. 10-7

Salvatore Ferragamo M

Ferragamo's collection of suits, sportswear, shirts, and outerwear is perfect for office, travel, or play. Their fashion influence, however, is strongest in neckwear and shoes. Ties have whimsical patterns and rich colors. You simply need to own at least one. Footwear runs from business and formal to casual and sporty. The designers at Ferragamo continue to remain faithful to their classic standards, while never losing sight of modern trends. 800-572-6641
www.salvatoreferragamo.it.com

Fifth Avenue	**212-759-7990**
725 Fifth Avenue	bet. 56/57th St.
NYC 10022	Mon.-Sat. 10-6, Thurs. 10-7

Sample W

This pocket-sized boutique appeals to young and old with its collection of silk/cotton blend knitwear. Find sweaters, cardigans, shirts, skirts, and pants with modern, yet delicate cuts in a great selection of colors. Towels and bath products round out the assortment. www.samplestudio.com

NoLiTa	**212-431-7866**
268 Elizabeth Street	bet. Houston/Prince
NYC 10012	Tues.-Sat. 12-7, Sun. 12-5

Samuel's Hats W

Two blocks from the World Trade Center, Samuel's Hats sells a wide variety of women's hats by top-of-the-line milliners. Styles run from fancy dress to casual, and labels include Eric Javits, Kokin, Philip Tracey and Louise Green.

Lower Manhattan	**212-513-7322**
74 Nassau Street	bet. John/Fulton St.
NYC 10038	Mon.-Fri. 9-7, Sat. 10-5

San Francisco Clothing W/C

This long established Lexington Avenue shop sells fad-free sportswear and understated eveningwear under the San Francisco label. Find skirts, jackets, dresses, blouses, and tailored shirts in natural fabrics and straightforward designs. In addition, shop a lively and refreshing children's collection featuring labels like Flap Happy, Yams and Le Top. Adorable looks from newborn to 6X.

Upper East Side	**212-472-8740**
975 Lexington Avenue	bet. 70/71st St.
NYC 10021	Mon.-Sat. 11-6

Santoni
M/W

An Italian purveyor of conservative, handmade shoes predominately for men. Attention to style, shape, color and fit is the Santoni trademark. Find two collections designed to meet all your footwear needs, whether casual, dressy or corporate. Prices range from $235 to $1,045. Women can choose from a small selection of driving shoes, mules and loafers.

Upper East Side   212-794-3820
864 Madison Avenue   bet. 70/71st St.
NYC 10021   Mon.-Fri. 10-7, Sat. 10-6

Scandinavian Ski Shop
M/W/C

A convenient Midtown source for ski and winter sports apparel and equipment. Find clothing and accessories by Bogner, Low Alpine, Helly Hanson, Nevica, Killy and more. When the snow melts, Scandinavian outfits its customers for tennis, golf, hiking and competition swimming.
800-722-6754

Midtown West   212-757-8524
40 West 57th Street   bet. 5th/6th Ave.
NYC 10019   Mon.-Fri. 10-6:30, Sat. 10-6, Sun. 11-5

Scarlet & Sage
W

Comfortable, natural fabrics with an Indian flavor are the focus of the collection at Scarlet and Sage. Think elegant day-into-evening loungewear. Find caftans, slip dresses, coat dresses with frog closures, and simple tops in linen, silk charmeuse and light merino wools. S & S is perfect for layering pieces to create a clean, yet versatile, silhouette.
www.scarletandsage.com

NoLiTa   212-219-1290
7 Prince Street   bet. Elizabeth/Bowery
NYC 10012   Tues.-Sun. 12-7

Scoop
W

The scoop on Scoop goes like this: it's the hottest place to shop in town. Fashionistas come for up-to-the-minute looks that embrace the trends without being trendy. Owner Stefani Greenfield selects the best from each designer, paying particular attention to color. Choose from coats by Michael Kors, wrap dresses by Diane von Furstenberg, long flowing sheaths by Muriel Brandolini, embellished sweaters by Patty Shelabarger, pants by Theory and Chaiken, T-shirts by Charlotte Ronson, snug and sexy sweaters, and dresses by Tocca. A fabulous selection of handbags and jewelry, as well as shoes by Jimmy Choo. www.scoopnyc.com

Upper East Side   212-535-5577
1275 Third Avenue   bet. 73/74th St.
NYC 10021   Mon.-Fri. 11-8, Sat. 11-7, Sun. 12-6
SoHo   212-925-2886
532 Broadway   bet. Prince/Spring
NYC 10012   Mon.-Sat. 11-8, Sun. 11-7

Screaming Mimi's M/W

Screaming Mimi's sells vintage garb dating from the 1940s to the 80's. Although the clothing is from another era, the look is modern and cutting edge. Find men's pants from the 40's, leather jackets, vintage bras and bustiers, skirts, tops, shoes, and accessories. For a young, fearless and funky crowd whose fashion sense knows no boundaries.

NoHo   **212-677-6464**
382 Lafayette Street   bet. Great Jones/4th St.
NYC 10003   Mon.-Sat. 12-8, Sun. 12-6

Seam W

Owners/designers Joanna Garza and Dori Adler cater to professionals, local artists and tourists. Each design is cut to fit and "shaped for real women," who actually have hips and curves in all the right places. Sizes run from 4 to 16. Find dresses, pants, jackets, and shirt-dresses designed to be layered, mixed and matched, and, best of all, wearable season-after-season. Check out their georgette sheer coat paired with a pair of pants. In addition, find 3 Dot T-shirts, sweaters, sarongs, handbags, and jewelry.

TriBeCa   **212-732-9411**
117 West Broadway   bet. Duane/Reade
NYC 10013   Mon.-Sat. 12-7, Sun. 1-6

Sean M

Welcome to Sean's, your French connection to menswear. Find designer Emil Lafaurie's collection of suits, sportswear, casual painter's jackets, and shirts that are fashionable without being trendy. Lafaurie's shirts, in solid shades, will complement any tie, trouser or pair of jeans. The look: Ralph Lauren meets Agnes B. and "work day meets play day."

Upper West Side   **212-769-1489**
224 Columbus Avenue   bet. 70/71st St.
NYC 10023   Mon.-Sat. 11-8, Sun. 12-6

SoHo   **212-598-5980**
132 Thompson Street   bet. Houston/Prince
NYC 10012   Mon.-Sat. 11-8, Sun. 12-7

Searle Blatt M/W

In the last two years, Searle Blatt has introduced trendy clothing labels to their collection, which doesn't measure up to what they do best: versatile, quality outerwear. Find shearlings, microfiber reversibles, cashmere, alpaca and wool overcoats, as well as trench coats, available in a variety of colors, fabrics, and linings. Searle's best-selling storm coat sports reversible faux fur. Sportswear labels include Alice & Trixie, Betsey Johnson, Easel, and Tark. Accessories also available.

Upper East Side (W)   **212-988-7318**
1124 Madison Avenue   at 84th St.
NYC 10028   Mon.-Sat. 10-6, Thurs. 10-7, Sun. 12-5

Upper East Side (W)   212-717-4022
1035 Madison Avenue   at 79th St.
NYC 10021   Mon.-Sat. 10-6, Thurs. 10-7, Sun. 12-5

Upper East Side (W)   212-772-2225
860 Madison Avenue   bet. 70/71st St.
NYC 10021   Mon.-Sat. 10-6, Thurs. 10-7, Sun. 12-5

Upper East Side (W)   212-838-599 0
1051 Third Avenue   at 62nd St.
NYC 10021   Mon.-Sat. 10-6, Thurs. 10-7, Sun. 12-5

Midtown East   212-753-9021
605-609 Madison Avenue   bet. 57/58th St.
NYC 10022   Mon.-Fri. 10-7, Sat. 10-6

Second Act Childrenswear   B/G

There's no better place at which to drop off your children's outgrown clothing than at Second Act. Welcome to this kidswear consignment shop, which has been in business for over 37 years. Although some find the atmosphere claustrophobic, others dive right in to rummage through the incredible bargains. Find lots of merchandise from the Gap, Polo and Tommy Hilfiger, plus pretty dresses by European labels like Mona Lisa, Jacadi, Jean Bouget, and Mimi. From newborn to preteen.

Upper East Side   212-988-2440
1046 Madison Avenue, 2nd Floor   bet. 79/80th Street
NYC 10021   Tues.-Sat. 9-5

Seigo   M

Seigo sells limited edition, 100% handmade, silk ties using the same mills that manufacture Japan's traditional kimonos. Select from intricately colored ties to simple patterned ones. Seigo also features a large selection of bow-ties in vibrant colors. Bow-ties start at $45, while neckties retail for $80.

Upper East Side   212-987-0191
1248 Madison Avenue   bet. 89/90th St.
NYC 10128   Mon.-Sat. 10-6:30, Sun. 11:30-5:30

Seize sur Vingt (16/20)   M/W

Seize sur Vingt sells luxury ready-to-wear and custom made men's clothing. Find beautifully tailored Italian cotton shirts, cashmere sweaters, pants, jackets, and suits, as well as handmade boxers and accessories. While Seize sur Vingt has given themselves the French school grade of 16/20 (equivalent to an A-), we think they deserve a 20/20 (A+). Sophisticated clothing for urbanites. Great men's-styled collar shirts for women.

NoLiTa   212-343-0476
243 Elizabeth Street   bet. Houston/Prince
NYC 10012   Mon.-Sun. 12-7

Selia Yang   W

A high-end boutique selling feminine fashions for the contemporary woman. Find dresses in simple hourglass silhouettes, skirts, shirts, and knits that can be dressed up or dressed down. Her favorite fabrics are silk organza and beaded satin. Great coordinating accessories that include handbags, tiaras, and jewelry.

East Village   212-254-9073
328 East 9th Street   bet. 1st/2nd Ave.
NYC 10003   Tues.-Fri. 1-8, Sat. & Sun. 12-6

Sergio Rossi   M/W

Women have been rumored to buy a particular outfit just to match a pair of Sergio Rossi pumps. Known for his ultra-glamorous shoes, Rossi has broadened his designs to include trendy styles. Find classic pointy-toe pumps with curved heels, beaded satin mules, platforms, wedgies, and more. A limited selection of men's casual and dressy shoes.

Upper East Side   212-396-4814
835 Madison Avenue   bet. 69/70th St.
NYC 10021   Mon.-Sat. 10-6

Seven Boutique   W

Driven by skyrocketing SoHo rents, entrepreneurial retailers like Seven are flocking to Orchard Street and bringing a whole new kind of merchandise with them. Owned by a group of friends, Seven aspires to "a perfect combination of art and fashion where one foot is in retailing and the other in the art world." Shop a 1,000-sq. ft. "boutique-cum gallery" space, featuring an avant-garde women's collection of one-of-a-kind pieces. Seven's collection, represented by progressive New York-based young designers, is appreciated for its artistic appeal and form. Labels include Markus Huemer/Unit, Mark Kroeker, Rubin Chapelle, United Bamboo, and Claudia Hill.

Lower East Side   646-654-0156
180 Orchard Street   bet. Houston/Stanton
NYC 10002   Mon.-Sun. 12-9

Shack Inc.   W

Of the shops that have migrated south from retail-choked SoHo to laid-back TriBeCa, Shack is a highlight. Designer J. Morgan Puett takes her inspiration from nature, history and daily events to create unisex clothing that customers will "feel utterly at ease in." Most of her clothing is made in the shop, and her fabrics of choice are silk linen and cotton gauze in soft shades. Find dresses, skirts, drawstring pants, tops and jackets.

TriBeCa   212-267-8004
137 West Broadway   bet. Duane/Thomas
NYC 10013   Mon.-Fri. 11-6, Sat. & Sun. 12-6

Shambala   W

Although Shambala is mainly a jewelry store, it's also a terrific source for pashminas. Find 100% pashmina shawls and stoles, plain or beautifully embroidered in sumptuous colors, and expect to pay $170 for shawls and $128 for stoles. Don't miss designer Joseph Nagual's deerskin totes with sterling silver facets.

SoHo   212-941-6505
92 Thompson Street   bet. Prince/Spring
NYC 10012   Mon.-Sat. 12-7, Sun. 1-6

Shanghai Tang   W

Crushed by a $2 million rent tab on Madison and 61st Street, Shanghai Tang closed shop and rethought their retailing strategy. Well, they're back, and only a few doors up the street from their old digs. Despite a dark interior, there is still a blaze of color from Tang's Asian-inspired fashions and accessories. From traditional Mao jackets and long Cheongsam dresses to modern reproductions, Shanghai Tang blends Oriental chic with Western twists.
www.shanghaitang.com

Upper East Side   212-888-5262
714 Madison Avenue   bet. 63/64th St.
NYC 10021   Mon.-Sat. 10-7, Sun. 12-6

Sharagano   W

A limited selection of trendy, yet wearable and reasonably priced French designer sportswear. Find dresses, tops, sweaters, pants, and coats in sexy fabrics and form-fitted shapes. Fashions for those who want to show off their figures. Good prices.

SoHo   212-941-7086
529 Broadway   bet. Spring/Prince
NYC 10012   Mon.-Sat. 10-9, Sun. 11-8

Shen   W

If layering is your style (and money is no object), then sample Shen's gossamer-weight chiffon and silk skirts, tunic tops, comfortable pants, and loose-fitting dresses and sweaters. The ultimate cover-up shop.

Upper East Side   212-717-1185
1005 Madison Avenue   bet. 77/78th St.
NYC 10021   Mon.-Fri. 10-6:30, Sat. 10-6

Shin Choi   W

Korean designer Shin Choi works the trends without being trendy. Her line caters to women in search of chic basics at bridge prices. Find a modern and stylish collection that includes sheath dresses, 3/4-length jackets, skirts, shirts, and knits. Quality fabrics, clean lines and wearability define Choi's timeless and tasteful designs.

SoHo   212-625-9202
119 Mercer Street   bet. Prince/Spring
NYC 10012   Mon.-Sat. 11-7

☆ The Shirt Store   M/W

The stars of the Broadway hit "Kiss me Kate" get their stage shirts here, so why shouldn't you? The Shirt Store is a good destination for those seeking the perfect shirt. Request off-

Shoe

the-rack, made-to-measure or custom. Their "White Label" collection is priced between $40 and $125, while their higher-end line "Blue Label" retails at $120 to $185. Each shirt is finely tailored in Sea Island cotton, fits like a dream and is reasonably priced. Request any alteration, whether adding a pocket or shortening a sleeve. Custom shirts run from $125 to $240 with an eight-to-ten-week delivery. Ties, cufflinks, and suspenders complete the assortment. 1-800-buy-a-shirt www.shirtstore.com

Midtown East	**212-557-8040**
51 East 44th Street	at Vanderbilt Ave.
NYC 10017	Mon.-Fri. 8-6:30, Sat. 10-5
Midtown West	**212-371-4540**
7 West 56th Street	bet. Fifth/Sixth Ave.
NYC 10019	Mon.-Sat. 10-6:30
Lower Manhattan	**212-797-8040**
71 Broadway	bet. Rector/Exchange
NYC 10006	Mon.-Fri. 7:30-6:30

Shoe M/W

Remember the wooden-soled "earth shoe"? Well, it's back. Shoe's "Cydwoq" line is a cross between a clog and a nature shoe; designs are unusual, but comfortable. Shoe also carries dainty mules, pumps, and sandals, plus a selection of tote bags, leather handbags, beaded evening bags, and kidskin gloves in luscious colors.

NoLiTa	**212-941-0205**
197 Mulberry Street	bet. Spring/Kenmare
NYC 10012	Mon.-Sun. 12-7

★ Shoofly B/G

Shoofly carries a stylish, well-priced footwear assortment for your small fry. Find fashion forward styles with European labels like Aster, Mod 8, Miniebell, Vennetini, and Baby Botte. Sizes run from newborn to size 9. Great accessories like wild-print tights, summer and winter hats, jewelry, and cute beaded and faux-fur bags.

Upper West Side	**212-580-4390**
465 Amsterdam Avenue	bet. 82/83rd St.
NYC 10024	Mon.-Sat. 11-7, Sun. 12-6
TriBeCa	**212-406-3270**
42 Hudson Street	bet. Duane/Thomas
NYC 10013	Mon.-Sat. 11-7, Sun. 12-6

★ Sigerson Morrison W

This is where the fashion elite and "in crowd" get themselves shod. FIT graduates Kari Sigerson and Miranda Morrison continue to attract shoe mavens who eagerly await the arrival of their new collections. Find the latest looks in bright colors and girly silhouettes, from ballerina flats and sling-back sandals to skinny-heeled pumps and boots. No chunky heels or nosebleed stilettos here, just lots of flattering styles with sophisticated edge. Pay $200 to $300 for shoes and $600 for boots. Handbags also available with the same clean look.

Skella

NoLiTa   212-219-3893
28 Prince Street   bet. Mott/Elizabeth
NYC 10012   Mon.-Sat. 11-7, Sun. 12-6

Silverado   M/W

Strictly leather here. Silverado sells pants, jackets, outerwear, Western boots, briefcases, handbags, and accessories, manufactured in lambskin, cowhide, leather, and suede. Pay $500 for jackets and $550 for pants. Allow three to four weeks for custom made.

SoHo   212-966-4470
542 Broadway   bet. Spring/Prince
NYC 10012   Mon.-Fri. 11-8, Sat. 11-9, Sun. 11-8

Sisley   M/W

Sisley, Benetton's top-of-the-line label, is packed with well-priced, up-to-date clothing suitable for all times of day. Find suits, dresses, pants, sweaters, tops, and outerwear that give you a "total look" for urban or country living. Prices won't put a strain on your wallet.

SoHo   212-375-0538
469 West Broadway   bet. Prince/Houston
NYC 10012   Mon.-Sat. 11-8, Sun. 11-7

Skechers USA   M/W/C

This California-based company sells casual, edgy lifestyle footwear for the gen-x crowd. Find men's, women's, and children's shoes loaded with "hip-hop" attitude and mounted on impressive rubber platforms. Styles include utility rugged wear, casual basics, and sneakers. 800-shoe-411 www.skechers.com

Upper West Side   212-712-0539
2169 Broadway   bet. 76/77th St.
NYC 10024   Mon.-Sat. 10-8, Sun. 11-6

Flatiron   212-627-9420
150 Fifth Avenue   bet. 19/20th St.
NYC 10011   Mon.-Sat. 10-8, Sun. 11-6

West Village   212-253-5810
55 West 8th Street   bet 5th/6th Ave.
NYC 10011   Mon.-Thurs. 10-9,
   Fri. & Sat. 10-10, Sun. 11-7

SoHo   212-431-8803
530 Broadway   at Spring
NYC 10012   Mon.-Fri. 10:30-8:30,
   Sat. 10:30-9, Sun. 10:30-8

Skella   W

Basic, versatile clothing that owner/designer Deborah Skella believes "will flatter most figures." Skella emphasizes gauzy separates, natural fabrics, and designs that work well for layering. Find styles suitable for casual Fridays, as well as dresses for evening and formal occasions. Skella's clean lines and feminine styling are perfect for the 20-40 crowd. Some coordinating accessories and custom wedding dresses, too.

Lower East Side   212-505-0115
156 Orchard Street   bet. Rivington/Stanton
NYC 10002   Tues.-Sun. 10-6 or by appt.

Sleek on Bleecker   W
One of the few West Village shops to sell contemporary fashions. Find trendy sportswear that's urban chic for day and downtown hip for night. Find pants, dresses, shirts, sweaters, T-shirts, and jeans by trendy labels like Paul & Joe, Theory, Tibi, Rebecca Dannenberg, Chaiken, Spooner and Daryl K.

West Village   212-243-0284
361 Bleecker   bet. W. 10/Charles Street
NYC 10014   Mon.-Sat. 12-8, Sun. 12-6

Small Change   B/G
A children's shop packed with casual basics, dress wear, outerwear and accessories. Labels include Cacharel, Sonia Rykiel, Christian Dior and Le Petit Bateau. During the winter, shop their enormous outerwear selection for the perfect snowsuit, coat, hat, or pair of gloves. Shoes by Sonnet, Start-Rite and Babybot. From newborn to 14 years.

Upper East Side   212-772-6455
964 Lexington Avenue   bet. 70/71st St.
NYC 10021   Mon.-Fri. 10-5:45, Sat. 10-4:45

Soco   W
A trip to NoLiTa is not complete without a stop at Soco, a 70-year-old French company specializing in chic, sleek handbags and small leathergoods. Find their bags in a range of shapes, sizes, and colors with fabrications that include calfskin, patent leather, canvas, nylon, and raffia. Prices run from $19 to $395. Don't miss their collection of sandals topped with brightly patterned chiffon from Scarpet a Porter.

NoLiTa   212-625-0720
55 Spring Street   bet. Lafayette/Mulberry
NYC 10012   Mon.-Sat. 11-7, Sun. 12-6

SoHo Woman   W
This shop carries exquisite fabrics—100% cotton, linen, matte jersey, wool, crepe and silks featured in simple silhouettes for sizes 10 through 28. Find mandarin-styled tops in great colors, washable silks by URU, as well as year-round merchandise from labels like Flax and Coco and Juan. A good source for easy-to-wear clothing perfect for travel.

Midtown West   212-391-7263
32 West 40th Street   bet. Fifth/Sixth Ave.
NYC 10018   Mon.-Fri. 11-7, Sat. 12-5

SoHo Jeans   M/W
A small, well-stocked shop featuring new and vintage Levi jeans. Prices start at $30. If you're in the market for a pair of retro Levi's from the 50's, expect to pay $700.

Speedo Authentic Fitness

SoHo   212-505-5291
69 West Houston Street   bet. Wooster/W. B'way
NYC 10012   Mon.-Sat. 12-8, Sun. 12-7

Sonia Rykiel   W
Long known as the "Queen of Sweaters," Rykiel continues to please with her collection of liberated, unconstructed clothes. Find crepe and gabardine suits, knitwear, tunics, skirts, dresses and coats. Her velour line emphasizes comfort and coordination (no surprise here, as Rykiel invented the velour jogging suit). Swimwear and sarongs available in summer.

Upper East Side   212-396-3060
849 Madison Avenue   bet. 70/71st St.
NYC 10021   Mon.-Sat. 10-6

Space Kiddets   B/G
Space Kiddets carries everything from soup to nuts in children's clothing. Packed with European and American brand names, find adorable clothes for infants, as well as trendsetting fashions for those hard-to-please pre-teens. Labels include Naf Naf, My Boy Sam, Black Parrot, Fly Girls and Charlie Rocket. Looks range from classic to funky. From newborn to preteen.

Flatiron   212-420-9878
46 East 21st Street   bet. B'way/Park Ave. S.
NYC 10010   Mon., Tues & Fri. 10:30-6,
Wed. & Thurs. 10:30-7, Sat. 10:30-5:30

Speedo Authentic Fitness   M/W
Speedo, the official outfitter of the U.S. Olympic swim team, also outfits the everyday sports enthusiast in their Speedo Authentic fitness stores. Find athletic wear and swimwear for your workouts. Choose from bike shorts, leggings, bra tops, sweatshirts, unitards, polar fleece outerwear, and swimwear. Quality is good, and so are their prices.
800-577-3336 www.speedo.com

Upper West Side   212-501-8140
150 Columbus Avenue   bet. 66/67th St.
NYC 10023   Mon.-Fri. 9-9, Sat. 10-9, Sun. 11-7

Midtown East   212-688-4595
721 Lexington Avenue   at 58th St.
NYC 10022   Mon.-Fri. 9-9, Sat. 10-8, Sun. 10-6

Midtown East   212-838-5988
40 East 57th Street   bet. Park/Madison Ave.
NYC 10022   Mon.-Fri. 10-8, Sat. 11-7, Sun. 11-6

Midtown East   212-682-3830
90 Park Avenue (downstairs)   at 39th St.
NYC 10016   Mon.-Fri. 8-8, Sat. 10-6, Sun. 11-6

Fifth Avenue   212-768-7737
500 Fifth Avenue   at 42nd St.
NYC 10110   Mon.-Fri. 8-8, Sat. 10-8, Sun. 11-6

Sports Authority   M/W

Sports Authority caters to your family's sports needs. In dozens of departments, find apparel and equipment for skiing, skating, rollerblading, biking, tennis, and football. Pump yourself up with body-building equipment and fitness machines.

Midtown East 212-355-9725
845 Third Avenue at 51st St.
NYC 10022 Mon.-Fri. 8:30-8, Sat. 10-7, Sun. 11-6

Midtown West 212-355-6430
57 West 57th Street at 6th Ave.
NYC 10019 Mon.-Fri. 9-8, Sat. 10-7, Sun. 11-6

Midtown West 212-563-7195
401 Seventh Avenue at 33rd St.
NYC 10001 Mon.-Fri. 9:30-8, Sat. 10-7, Sun. 11-6

Chelsea 212-929-8971
636 Sixth Avenue at 19th St.
NYC 10001 Mon.-Fri. 10-8, Sat. 10-7, Sun. 11-6

Spring Flowers   B/G

A good alternative to Bonpoint. Venture inside to find casual and fancy European clothing at attractive prices, including Cacharel print dresses, outfits by Le Petit Bateau, and smocked dresses at a reasonable $100. From infant to pre-teen. Imported shoes up to age 6.

Upper East Side 212-717-8182
905 Madison Avenue bet. 72/73rd St.
NYC 10021 Mon.-Sat. 10-6, Sun. 11-6

Upper East Side 212-758-2669
1050 Third Avenue at 62nd St.
NYC 10021 Mon.-Sat. 10-6, Sun. 11-6

Stephane Kelian   M/W

Footwear designer Stephane Kelian is the master of hand-woven leather shoes. His collection includes platforms, wedges, boots, open-toed slings, pumps, sandals and loafers. His comfort line, a sneaker/loafer hybrid, is available in suede, leather, and nylon. A limited selection for men.

Upper East Side 212-980-1919
717 Madison Avenue bet. 63/64th St.
NYC 10021 Mon.-Sat. 10-6

SoHo 212-925-3077
158 Mercer bet. Houston/Prince
NYC 10012 Mon.-Sat. 11-7, Sun. 12-6

Steven Alan   M/W

Hard-core shoppers and trendsters come here first to check out what's new in the market. Owner Steven Alan discovers new fashion talent and scoops up the very best pieces. Shop the hippest and coolest labels like Rebecca Dannenberg, Paul & Joe, Built by Wendy, United Bamboo, SVO and 6 by Martin Margiela. Looks include fitted tops in a stretchy plastic-coated fabric, apron-wrap skirts, deconstructed pants, leather jeans and sexy lingerie. A great handbag selection featuring rectangular clutches, messenger bags, and sequined totes. Jewelry and belts round out the assortment.

SoHo (W)	212-334-6354
60 Wooster Street	bet. Broome/Spring
NYC 10012	Mon.-Sat. 11-7, Sun. 12-7
SoHo (M)	212-625-2541
558 Broome Street	bet. 6th Ave./Varick
NYC 10013	Thurs.-Sat. 12-7, Sun. 12-6

Steven Stolman W

Designer Steven Stolman has left the rat race of Seventh Avenue and directed his full attention to his exclusive boutiques. Find skirts, dresses, and pants in whimsical patterns, whether an elaborate toile scene or an amusing animal print—he has designed an entire collection with home furnishing fabrics! In addition, find taffeta ballgowns and skirts, silk faille blazers, sweater sets, shoes, and accessories. It's all wonderfully romantic and feminine.

Upper East Side	212-249-5050
22 East 72nd Street, #4A	bet. 5th/Madison Ave.
NYC 10021	Mon.-Fri. 10-6, Sat. 11-5

Steve Madden M/W

Some shoppers swear Madden's shoes are stylish, while others say they're plain wacky—you be the judge. In any case, it's all platforms all the time, whether it's a sneaker, maryjane, boot, sandal, pump, or loafer. Chunky and clunky, they can add six inches to your height! For the punkster set.
800-747-6233 www.stevemadden.com

Upper East Side	212-426-0538
150 East 86th Street	bet. Lex./Third Ave.
NYC 10028	Mon.-Fri. 11-8,
	Sat. 11:30-8:30, Sun. 11-7
Upper West Side	212-799-4221
2315 Broadway	at 84th St.
NYC 10024	Mon.-Thurs. 11-8,
	Fri. & Sat. 11-8:30, Sun. 11-7:30
Midtown West	212-736-3283
45 West 34th Street	bet. Fifth/Sixth Ave.
NYC 10001	Mon.-Fri. 10-9, Sat. 10-9:30, Sun. 10-6
SoHo	212-343-1800
540 Broadway	bet. Prince/Spring
NYC 10012	Mon.-Thurs. 11-8,
	Fri. & Sat. 11-8:30, Sun. 11-7:30
Chelsea	212-989-1120
84 7th Avenue	bet. 15/16th St.
NYC 10011	Mon.-Sat. 11-8, Sun. 12-7

St. John W

St. John is a good source for classic, wrinkle-free knitwear. Suits and dresses are ideal for travel and have desk-to-dinner versatility. Their Griffith & Grey label, catering to the young professional seeking contemporary looks, features suits, dresses, and jackets in updated designs and modern fabrics like stretch wool. Sizes from 2 to 14. Suits run an average price of $1,000.

Fifth Avenue   **212-755-5252**
665 Fifth Avenue   at 53rd St.
NYC 10022   Mon.-Sat. 10-7, Sun. 11-6

The Stork Club   B/G

Shopping at the Stork Club is like going back in time. This small shop, replete with old pedal cars and antique toys, is packed with unique and whimsical children's clothing. Find hand-loomed sweaters, dresses in vintage fabrics, hand-knit tops, T-shirts, hats and accessories. Wicker baskets, complete with three-piece baby sets (chenille blanket, hat, and toy), make wonderful baby shower gifts.

SoHo   **212-505-1927**
142 Sullivan Street   bet. Prince/Houston
NYC 10012   Mon.-Sat. 11-7, Sun. 12-6

Stream   W

Stream's shopping environment is meant to invoke the spiritual comfort of a gently flowing stream, a calming breeze, and a soothing light. Shop a three-level lifestyle store that includes an art gallery, an avant-garde clothing collection by designers Dirk Bikkembergs, Dirk Van Saene and Bernhard Willhelm, as well as footwear and accessories. A relaxing tea salon, offering 150 brands of tea and tablewares, is on the lower level. The merchandise is eclectic, creative, and perfect for those seeking individual expression. New this year: a menswear collection. www.streamsoho.com

SoHo   **212-226-2328**
69 Mercer Street   bet. Spring/Broome
NYC 10012   Mon.-Sat. 11-7, Sun. 12-6

Stuart Weitzman   W

Women shop here knowing that Weitzman has a shoe for every foot, small or large (size 2 to 12), narrow or wide (from AAAA to C). Styles run from casual to dressy, including made-to-order rhinestone pumps. Choose from over 40 bridal shoes. www.stuartweitzman.com

Midtown East   **212-750-2555**
625 Madison Avenue   bet. 58/59th St.
NYC 10022   Mon.-Fri. 10-6:30, Sat. 10-6, Sun. 12-5

Stubbs & Wootton   M/W

Whether it's in Palm Beach, the Hamptons or Manhattan, Stubbs & Wootton continues to shod today's socialites. Percy Steinhart's collection of needlepoint, velvet, and tapestry flat-soled shoes and slippers are handmade in Spain and wonderfully comfortable. Expect to pay $135 for needlepoint styles and $200 for a pair of embossed velvet slippers.
877-478-8227

Super Runners Shop

Upper East Side   212-249-5200
22 East 72nd Street   bet. 5th/Madison Ave
NYC 10021   Mon.-Fri. 10-6, Sat. 11-5

Studio 109   M/W

Musicians Keith Richards and Lauryn Hill are devoted fans of this custom leather establishment. Designer Patricia Adams works with a variety of skins, so whether you're in the market for a leather bra top, a pair of elk or deerskin pants, a python jacket, or a suede skirt, she's the woman to see. Choose from her book of swatches and expect a two-to-three-week delivery time. Custom leather pants start at $650, jackets at $700, and skirts at $475.
www.studio109.com

East Village   212-420-0077
115 St. Marks Place   bet. Ave. A/1st Ave.
NYC 10009   Mon.-Sun. 12-8

Sulka & Company   M

Long recognized for their opulent silk robes and pajamas, Sulka is catnip for the needs of the diligently affluent. Take perverse delight in spending $1,750 for an elegant smoking jacket or invest in a swank tuxedo shirt that will endure a lifetime of wear. Made-to-measure and custom suits are extravagantly priced at $2,450, while dress shirts run from $125 to $200. Find men's furnishings, sport jackets with 18-karat gold buttons, eight-ply cashmere cardigan sweaters, slacks, outerwear and accessories.

Upper East Side   212-452-1900
840 Madison Avenue   bet. 69/70th St.
NYC 10021   Mon.-Sat. 10-6

Midtown East   212-980-5200
430 Park Avenue   at 55th St.
NYC 10022   Mon.-Fri. 9:30-6, Sat. 10-6

Sunrise Ruby   W

Shop owner Allison Furman Norris travels far and wide—from a Hollywood film set to a Parisian flea market—for her collection of secondhand clothing. Choose from coveted labels like Prada, Gaultier, Anna Sui, and Kate Spade at bargain hunter prices.

TriBeCa   212-791-7735
141 Reade Street   bet. Greenwich/Hudson
NYC 10013   Tues.-Sat. 12-7 by appointment

Super Runners Shop   M/W

The serious runner shops here for shoes, clothing and accoutrements. Brand names include Nike, New Balance, Asics, Adidas, In Sport, and Moving Comfort. The sales staff are all super runners, too, so you'll get firsthand advice during your selection. www.super-runners.com

Upper East Side   212-369-6010
1337 Lexington Avenue   at 89th St.
NYC 10028   Mon.-Fri. 10-7, Thurs. 10-9,
    Sat. 10-6, Sun., 12-5

Suzanne

Upper East Side	212-249-2133
1244 Third Avenue	bet. 71/72nd St.
NYC 10021	Mon.-Fri. 10-7, Thurs. 10-9,
	Sat. 10-6, Sun. 12-5
Upper West Side	212-787-7665
360 Amsterdam Avenue	bet. 77/78th St.
NYC 10024	Mon.-Fri. 10-7, Thurs. 10-9,
	Sat. 10-6, Sun. 11-5

Suzanne W

Squeeze into this tiny millinery shop stuffed with every hat style imaginable. An excellent source for fancy dress or special occasion hats. If you're off to the Saratoga races, visit Suzanne for a memorable topper.

Upper East Side	212-593-3232
700 Madison Avenue	bet. 62/63rd St.
NYC 10021	Mon.-Sat. 11-6

Su-zen W

Located in a landmark, historic building, this tranquil space's pressed tin ceilings and cast iron columns serve as a perfect backdrop for Susan Hahn's collection. Her comfortable clothing is based on unique fabrics and quality craftsmanship. Find a full range of separates, suits, dresses, shirts, jackets, pants, and outerwear designed to be worn layered or singly. Unusual yarns, such as handspun wool and high-tech synthetics, make knitwear an important part of the Su-zen collection. Su-zen caters to a professional clientele looking to feel at ease in their clothes.

SoHo	212-925-3744
17 Greene Street	bet. Grand/Canal
NYC 10013	Mon.-Sat. 11-7, Sun. 12-6

Sylvia Heisel W

One reason Sylvia Heisel's customers are so devoted to her is that they can custom order just about anything. Custom-made comes in over forty fabric samples and boasts a two-week delivery. Off-the rack merchandise includes luxury sportswear, eveningwear, and accessories in looks that are a cross between dressy and casual. The Heisel label is about easy, comfortable clothing made to couture quality standards. Mother-of-the-bride designs are a Heisel speciality.

SoHo	646-654-6768
131 Thompson Street	bet. Houston/Prince
NYC 10012	Mon.-Sat. 11-7, Sun. 12-6

T. Anthony M/W

In 1946 T. Anthony's collection of sophisticated luggage catered to the world's social elite, including the Duke and Duchess of Windsor. Today the tradition continues. Find briefcases, handbags, small leathergoods, desk sets, photo albums, jewelry boxes, and, of course, their signature leather and canvas luggage. A good alternative to Louis Vuitton luggage. 888-722-2406 www.tanthony.com

Midtown East   212-750-9797
445 Park Avenue   at 56th St.
NYC 10022   Mon.-Fri. 9:30-6, Sat. 10-6

Tahari W

An ideal shop for the busy executive in search of tailored suits that go from the office to dinner. Find a dress-down-Friday casual line, suits, evening dresses, separates, and accessories. Pay $360 for jackets and $220 for pants. The look is feminine and classic.

Lower Manhattan   212-945-2450
225 Liberty Street   at 2 World Financial Center
NYC 10281   Mon.-Fri. 10-7, Sat. 11-5, Sun. 12-5

☆ Takashimaya M/W

If you don't have time to travel to Tokyo, visit Takashimaya on Fifth Avenue. This is a store that calmly caters to all of your senses as it recreates the tranquility and beauty of the Far East. Apart from a small and exclusive cosmetics department, the main attraction on the first floor is the exquisite Christian Tortu flower and garden shop. On four floors find elegant tabletop accessories, stationery, furniture, gifts, and bed and bath accessories. Men and women can choose from a small collection of European clothing lines. If you happen to be in the store during lunch, stop downstairs at the Tea Box, which features a Japanese menu of light and delicious food.

Fifth Avenue   212-350-0100
693 Fifth Avenue   bet. 54/55th St.
NYC 10022   Mon.-Sat. 10-7

Talbot's W

From their mail-order business to their nationwide chain of shops, Talbot's is an affordable source for classic career and casual clothing. Discover the head-to-toe essentials you need to build a conservative and sensible wardrobe. Misses and petites sizes also available. Shoes and accessories round out the assortment. 800-992-9010 www.talbots.com

Upper East Side   212-988-8585
1251 Third Avenue   at 72nd St.
NYC 10021   Mon.-Fri. 10-8, Sat. 10-7, Sun. 12-6

Upper West Side   212-875-8754
2289-2291 Broadway   bet. 82/83rd St.
NYC 10024   Mon.-Sat. 10-9, Sun. 12-6

Midtown East   212-838-8811
525 Madison Avenue   bet. 53/54th St.
NYC 10022   Mon.-Fri. 10-7, Sat. 10-6, Sun. 12-5

Lower Manhattan   212-425-0166
189-191 Front Street   at South Street Seaport
NYC 10038   Mon.-Sat. 10-9, Sun. 11-8

Talbot's Kids B/G

Talbot's Kids caters to your child's everyday needs. Unlike their women's collection, fashions for children are energetic and animated. Find pants, dresses, blazers, ties, skirts, dress shirts, T-shirts, sweatshirts, sleepwear, and even underwear. Looks run from classic to fashion forward with attractive price points. 800-992-9010 www.talbots.com

Upper East Side   212-570-1630
1523 Second Avenue   at 79th St.
NYC 10021   Mon.-Sat. 9-7, Thurs. 9:30-8, Sun. 12-5

Tanino Crisci   M/W

Tanino Crisci markets to the customer seeking conservative handmade shoes. From a well-crafted riding boot to a classic wing-tipped lace-up, each shoe is meticulously crafted in luxury leathers. Expect to pay from $390 to $2,000.

Upper East Side   212-535-1014
795 Madison Avenue   bet. 67/68th St.
NYC 10021   Mon.-Sat. 10-6

Tartine et Chocolat   B/G

For well-turned-out children, mothers have long turned to Tartine et Chocolat. After a brief absence, T & C is back in full swing again. Mothers-to-be can shop their signature layette collection of furniture, linens, and more. Sporty basics like pants, shirts, and sweaters will outfit your boy, while adorable smocked dresses will delight your girl. Pay $116 for dresses, $60 for boy's shirts, and $80 for onezies. In addition, find shoes and accessories that will coordinate with all your outfits. From newborn to 10 years.

Upper East Side   212-717-2112
1047 Madison Avenue   at 80th St.
NYC 10021   Mon.-Sat. 10-7, Sun. 12-5

Tatiana Resale Boutique   W

As the name suggests, Tatiana is a resale boutique that sells designer duds that are "slightly" used, "almost" new and, best of all, at "gentle" prices. Choose from a range of women's apparel, accessories, and shoes—a Moschino wool jacket, a Chanel suit, a Dolce & Gabbana frock, a pair of Prada flats or an Hermès or Gucci handbag. Remember, timing is everything.

Upper East Side   212-717-7684
860 Lexington Avenue, 2nd Fl.   bet. 64/65th St.
NYC 10021   Mon.-Fri. 11-7, Sat. 11-6, Sun. 12-5

Team Shoes   M/W/C

Team specializes in casual outdoor shoes. Find boots, hiking shoes, and loafers from labels like Cole Haan, Alden, and Timberland. A small children's selection.

SoHo   212-353-8333
480 West Broadway   bet. Houston/Prince
NYC 10012   Mon.-Sun. 11-8

Ted Baker London   M

A popular British label known for its modern collection of menswear, Ted Baker's main attraction is without doubt his shirts. Once you buy one, you'll want to try them all. Manufactured in high-tech fabrics and microfibers, his silky, soft shirts come long and short sleeved in a multitude of colors. Some men claim that donning a Ted Baker shirt is like "wearing lingerie." Contemporary-styled suits, knitwear, and trousers round out the assortment. New this year: the "Endurance," a 100% wool suit that's ideal for travel: fold it up, remove it from your suitcase, unfold it and wear it wrinkle-free straight to the office. Also, look out for Baker's new sun-resistant shirts in fabric with an SPF factor of 15(!).

SoHo   212-343-8989
107 Grand Street   bet. Mercer/B'way
NYC 10012   Mon.-Sat. 11:30-7, Sun. 12-6

Tehen   W

Owned by one of France's largest textile companies, Tehen's stock in trade is fabrics and textures. Find a color coordinated collection in no-nonsense shapes. Mix and match pants, jackets, skirts, oversized sweaters, and tops with looks that are relaxed, easy, and modern.

SoHo   212-925-4788
91 Greene Street   bet. Prince/Spring
NYC 10012   Mon-Sat. 11-7, Sun 12-6

Terra Plana   M/W

At Terra Plana, you can choose from a selection of shoes with sporty, casual looks. Find lace-up boots, oxfords, and step-ins in standard black and brown leathers and suedes. Footwear with a modern edge. Best for men.

NoLiTa   212-274-9000
260 Elizabeth Street   bet. Houston/Prince
NYC 10012   Tues.-Sat. 12-7, Sun. 12-6

Thomas Pink   M/W

Good news! You no longer have to cross the Atlantic for a Pink's shirt. He's come right to you with a spacious shop filled with an extraordinarily colorful selection of shirts and ties. Luxury shirtmaking is the name of the game here. Find a collection of ready-made shirts in quality fabrics, traditional British tailoring, and wonderful color and pattern assortments. Prices start at $100. Pay $10 for sleeve alterations and $12 for monogramming. Accessories include ties, cashmere sweaters, cufflinks, suspenders, pocket squares, and scarves. 888-336-1192 www.thomaspink.co.uk

Midtown East   212-838-1928
520 Madison Avenue   bet. 53/54th St.
NYC 10022   Mon.-Fri. 10-7, Thurs. 10-8,
    Sat. 10-6, Sun. 12-6

Midtown West   212-840-9663
1155 Sixth Avenue   at 44th Street
NYC 10036   Mon.-Fri. 10-7, Thurs. 10-8,
    Sat. 10-6, Sun. 12-5

TG-170   W

Owner Terri Gillis attracts uptown and downtown girls, who come to check out the fashion world's new designers.

Thread

She's successfully launched the careers of many name designers. Find up-to-the-minute, well-balanced selection of merchandise by labels like Rebecca Dannenberg, Pixie Yates, Living Doll, Libby McGinnis, and Liz Cohen. Shop for hipster pants, tight tops, shirts, knits, sweater sets, and dresses that are fun, wearable, and cutting edge.

Lower East Side	212-995-8660
170 Ludlow Street	bet. Houston/Stanton
NYC 10002	Mon.-Sun. 12-8

Thread W

Bridesmaids, fear not, your days of walking down the aisle in a frumpy bridesmaid dress are over, thanks to owners Beth Blake and Sophie Simmons. Thread also specializes in special occasion dress, from fancy cocktail dresses to eveningwear. Find feminine and modern silhouettes in luxury fabrics (silk, chiffon, satin, and velvet) that will have bridesmaids and others looking their best. Styles include long, flowy silk skirts paired with satin camisole tops ($125), taffeta and stretch georgette dresses, and separates. All under the Thread label at reasonable prices. Custom order by size, color, and fabric and expect a 4-to-8-week delivery.
www.threaddesign.com

Chelsea	212-414-8844
408 West 15th Street, 4th Floor	bet. Ninth/Tenth Ave.
NYC 10011	Wed.-Sat. 10-7 by appointment only

Tibet Arts & Crafts W

There's a touch of ethnicity, color, and freshness in this tiny boutique. Find raw silk, Tibetan-styled shirts at $68 (a favorite of actress Cameron Diaz), fabulous reversible pashmina scarves and shawls in dazzling color assortments, antique patched and brocade bags at a mere $12, 100% raw and patterned silk shawls, traditional ceremonial hats, and jewelry. Best Bet: pashmina shawls.
www.citysearch.com/nyc/tibetarts

SoHo	212-529-4344
144 Sullivan Street	bet. Houston/Prince
NYC 10012	Mon.-Sun. 11-8

West Village	212-260-5880
197 Bleecker Street	bet. MacDougal/Sixth Ave.
NYC 10012	Mon.-Fri. 11-9, Sat & Sun. 11-10

Tibet Bazaar W

A strong aroma of incense leads you into this speciality boutique featuring clothing and accessories direct from the Himalayas. Find traditional silk wrap skirts and mandarin styled tops manufactured in Shantung silks, brocade hats with fur trim, plain or beaded cashmere and wool shawls from India, and a collection of pashmina wraps priced at a reasonable $145.

Upper West Side	212-595-8487
473 Amsterdam Avenue	bet. 82/83rd St.
NYC 10024	Mon.-Sun. 11-7

Timberland Shoes M/W/C
Timberland sells outdoor footwear, apparel, and accessories. Any product you buy here is guaranteed to withstand the rigors of time, while providing excellent comfort. Styles run from casual shoes to rugged boots. Find hiking boots, driving moccasins, boating shoes, and weatherbucks. Men's outdoor apparel also available. Children's from size 5 toddler and up. 800-445-5545 www.timberland.com

Upper East Side **212-754-0434**
709 Madison Avenue at 63rd St.
NYC 10021 Mon.-Fri. 10-7, Sat. 10-6, Sun. 12-6

Timtoum M/W
Owner Erika Lively carries an eclectic selection of merchandise, from old records to clothing made out of vintage fabrics, including her own label Go-Global. Check out her unusual bag designs (made of jeep-top fabric) in fun shapes with handy side-pocket compartments. In addition, find denim and corduroy pants, skirts, shirts, and leathers, all slightly "bent with age."

Lower East Side **212-780-0456**
179 Orchard Street bet. Houston/Stanton
NYC 10002 Mon.-Sun. 1-8

TJ Maxx M/W/C
Off-price merchandise for the entire family, as well as a large selection of accessories for home, bed, and bath. If you're lucky, you might find a designer name like Polo, DKNY, or Yves Saint Laurent.

Chelsea **212-229-0875**
620 Sixth Avenue bet. 18/19th St.
NYC 10011 Mon.-Sat. 9:30-9, Sun. 11-7

Tocca W
Find Indian inspired sari fabrics used in a collection of contemporary sportswear and dresses. Alexandra White's sleek, feminine designs are for women who appreciate simplicity and ease more than they appreciate drama. Tocca's collection is predominately dresses and skirts in colorful fabrics, often embroidered and beaded, with sweet, flirty looks. Wonderful bedding selection is a must.

SoHo **212-343-3912**
161 Mercer Street bet. Houston/Prince
NYC 10012 Mon.-Sat. 11-7, Sun. 12-6

Today's Man M
Shop here for value-priced menswear that includes everything from socks to tuxedos. Find business attire, furnishings, sportswear, casual wear, shoes, and even underwear. Suit prices run from $159 to $400, and you may even come across the Fendi label (the only designer name they carry). 800-950-7848 www.todaysman.com

Fifth Avenue **212-557-3111**
529 Fifth Avenue at 44th St.
NYC 10017 Mon.-Fri. 9-7, Sat. 9-6, Sun. 12-5

Todd Oldham

Chelsea	**212-924-0200**
625 Sixth Avenue	bet. 18/19th St.
NYC 10011	Mon.-Sat. 9:30-9, Sun. 11-7

Todd Oldham M/W
Now that Todd Oldham has licensed his name to Jones New York, he appears to have tamed his free-spirited act. Gone are the days of mixing clashing, colorful prints, and here instead is a collection of casual weekend clothing. Find sensible basics that include jeans, khakis, T-shirts, sweats, skirts and halter dresses. A good choice for the younger set.
www.toddoldham.com

SoHo	**212-219-3531**
123 Wooster Street	bet. Spring/Prince
NYC 10012	Mon.-Sat. 11-7, Sun. 12-6

Tod's M/W
There's no business like shoe business, and Tod's founder, Diego Delle Valle, would probably agree as his flat-heeled, high-style footwear caress the famous feet of Hollywood stars. Society fashionistas also stock up on his signature collection of stylish, comfortable pebble car shoes with prices starting at $245. You'll also find a selection of Italian slides, smart-looking mules, and boots. The status symbol in handbags is still Tod's structured leather D bag, named after the late Princess Diana; pay up to $1,400 for one of these calfskin beauties. New this year: Watch for Tod's newest shoe style "Vertigo," a mini-heeled pump, and an updated version of Tod's triangular-shaped "City Bag." 800-457-TODS
www.tods.com

Midtown East	**212-644-5945**
650 Madison Avenue	bet. 59/60th St.
NYC 10022	Mon.-Sat. 10-6, Thurs. 10-7, Sun. 12-5

Toga Bike Shop M/W/C
Voted one of the top 100 bicycle shops in the country, Toga is the oldest and largest cycling retailer in New York. Find bikes by Cannondale, Bianchi, Specialized, Lite-speed, and Santa Cruz, as well as a good selection of accessories. Their specialty: designing men's and women's saddles for ultimate comfort and fit. Repair classes, bike tours, and bike rentals at $35 per day also available.

Upper West Side	**212-799-9625**
110 West End Avenue	at 64th St.
NYC 10023	Mon.-Fri. 11-7, Thurs. 11-8,
	Sat. 10-6, Sun. 11-6

Tokio 7 M/W
This consignment shop's dingy interior shouldn't deter young bargain hunters. While it's serious hit or miss depending upon the condition of the clothing, find a collection of avant-garde designer labels priced according to designer popularity, style and, of course, condition. On a good day, you might come across a $200 Yohji Yamamoto suit or pair of $120 Helmut Lang pants, as well as an item by Gaultier,

Paul Smith, or Betsey Johnson. It's affordable, trendy, hand-me-down clothing in generally fair condition.

East Village	212-353-8443
64 East 7th Street	bet. First/Second Ave.
NYC 10003	Mon.-Sun. 12-8:30

Tokyo Joe   M/W

Another consignment shop featuring hip designer labels at moderate prices. Every day the merchandise changes, so scoop something up when you see it. Find designer clothing, shoes, bags, and accessories by labels like Gucci, Marc Jacobs, Prada, Comme des Garcons, Miu Miu, and Donna Karan. Items are generally in good condition, and the prices can't be beat.

East Village	212-473-0724
334 East 11th Street	bet. 1st/2nd Ave.
NYC 10003	Mon.-Sun. 12-9
Midtown East	212-532-3605
240 East 28th Street	bet. 2nd/3rd Avenue
NYC 10016	Mon.-Sat. 11-7:30

Tootsi Plohound   M/W

Who would guess that a footwear retailer with such a bizarre name would attract New York's shoenoscenti? Find a large selection of hip designer labels like Freelance, Patrick Cox, Miu Miu, Todd Oldham, Costume National, Granello, and Clone, as well as their "Otto" private label. Tootsi Plohound is for fashion test pilots seeking the very latest in footwear trends.

Midtown East	212-231-3199
38 East 57th Street	bet. Park/Madison Ave.
NYC 10022	Mon.-Wed. 11:30-7:30,
	Thurs. & Fri. 11-8, Sat. 11-7, Sun. 12-6
Flatiron	212-460-8650
137 Fifth Avenue	bet. 20/21st St.
NYC 10010	Mon.-Fri. 11:30-7:30, Sat. 11-8, Sun. 12-7
SoHo	212-925-8931
413 West Broadway	bet. Prince/Spring
NYC 10012	Mon.-Sat. 11:30-7:30, Sat. 11-8, Sun. 12-7

Tracey Tooker Hats   W

This tiny corner shop is filled to the rafters with Tooker's latest looks in hats. She handmakes her creations, from off-the-rack to custom, in fashion's latest fabrics including fleece, fur, felt, and straw. A Tooker topper travels from the beach to the Derby.

Upper East Side	212-472-9603
1211 Lexington Avenue	at 82nd St.
NYC 10028	Mon.-Sat. 11-7, Sun. 12-5

☆ Tracy Feith   W

American designer Tracy Feith outfits both uptown and downtown girls with his collection of feminine, delicate fashions based on fabric, color, and detail. Shop in a serene, uncluttered space and find two separate collections. His higher-end line features dresses, skirts, shirts, and corset tops designed in fashion forward fabrics like new wave denim, embroidered fleece, silks, and perforated suede. Yet inspired fashion sleuths come here for Feith's "Raj" collection of ethnic and exotic print dresses, skirts, and pants where pretty meets modern-day flirtatious. Shoes, handbags, and jewelry also available.

NoLiTa 212-334-3097
209 Mulberry Street bet. Spring/Kenmare
NYC 10012 Mon.-Sat. 11-7, Sun. 12-7

Training Camp M/W

Owner Udi Avshalom says, "Footwear is my addiction…the only thing I like more than footwear is my wife." Training Camp has a cult following, which includes rapper Puff Daddy. Shop here for the latest in brand name sneakers (Nike, Reebok, Air Jordans, and Bo Jacksons), and hip, "street vibe" looks by Avirex, Phat Farm and Royal Elastics. Prices run from $30 to $100.

Midtown West 212-840-7842
25 West 45th Street bet. Fifth/Sixth Ave.
NYC 10036 Mon.-Sat. 9-7:30, Sun. 10-6:30

Midtown West 212-921-4430
1079 Sixth Avenue at 41st Street
NYC 10036 Mon.-Sat. 9-7:30, Sun. 10-6:30

Transfer International M/W

A consignment shop that caters to younger customers (high school to college) in search of designer duds at reasonable prices. Labels include Gucci, Prada, Hermès, Miu Miu, and Chanel. Some outfits have never even been worn.

SoHo 212-355-4230
594 Broadway bet. Prince/Houston
NYC 10012 Tues.-Sun. 1-8 and by appointment

TriBeCa Luggage & Leather W/M

Never judge a suitcase by its cover, or something like that, because there is, in fact, very little luggage here—just a fabulous selection of handbags. Find straw totes, leather everyday bags, crocheted and beaded pieces, knapsacks, messenger bags, briefcases, weekend and travel bags, and carry-on luggage. Labels include Longchamp, Utility Canvas, Un Après Midi de Chien (Dog-Day-Afternoon), Rafe, Francesco Brasia, Gun-Makie, and Diesel. Prices run from $100 to $300. Check out the new trend in handbags: a stamped ostrich, dog-shaped bag for $175. Wallets, toilet kits, photo albums, and umbrellas complete the assortment.

TriBeCa 212-732-6444
295 Greenwich Street bet. Chambers/Warren
NYC 10007 Mon.-Fri. 10-7:30,
  Sat. 11-6, Sun. 12-5

Tristan & America M/W
Tristan & America, a Canadian import, caters to the young professional in search of career and casual clothing at reasonable prices. Styles are simple, classic, and sporty. Ample selection of suits. Pay $350 for men's suits, while women's jackets run $130 and skirts average $58.

Midtown West **212-246-2354**
1230 Sixth Avenue at 49th St.
NYC 10020 Mon.-Sat. 9-8, Sun. 12-6

SoHo **212-965-1810**
560 Broadway bet. Prince/Spring
NYC 10012 Mon.-Sat. 10-8, Sun. 11-7

Trufaux W
Trufaux sells edgy fashions made from entirely synthetic materials. Find pressed crocodile rain jackets, python print pants, ultra-suede skirts and jackets, leopard print dresses, waxed nylon skirts, slim-fitted tops, nylon overcoats with faux fur, and mink ponchos. Trufaux's creations look so real, you may still be ambushed by PETA's red paint brigades, but don't despair, these synthetic beauties are all machine washable. Other labels include Trina Turk, Emma Black, and Tark. Handbags also available.

SoHo **212-334-4545**
301 West Broadway bet. Grand/Canal
NYC 10013 Mon.-Sat. 11-7, Sun. 12-6

Tse Cashmere M/W/C
A purveyor of luxury knitwear offering comfort, style, and versatility. Find sweaters, cardigans, turtleneck, twin sets, sportswear, and coats in modern, clean, and sophisticated designs. If you thought cashmere was just for adults, think again! For infants, find baby jumpers, tops, and blankets, while children can stay snuggly and warm in Tse's cashmere outfits and separates. Robes, blankets, mufflers, and gloves also available. Expensive.

Upper East Side **212-472-7790**
827 Madison Avenue at 69th St.
NYC 10021 Mon.-Sat. 10-6, Thurs. 10-7

TseSurface W
TseSurface is a more affordable version of Tse. Shop for hooded cashmere sweatshirts, cardigans, skirts, backless halter tops, and tank top shells in bright colors, black, and the occasional pattern. The TseSurface collection emphasizes modern cuts, trim fits and younger looks for the 18 to 35 crowd. Prices run from $150 to $450.

NoLiTa **212-343-7033**
226 Elizabeth Street bet. Prince/Houston
NYC 10012 Mon.-Sat. 12-7, Sun. 12-6

Tupli M
At Tupli, men can shop a modern footwear collection that will have them walking the streets in urban style. Find

Turnbull & Asser

Italain made suede and leather loafers, lace-ups, an updated '40's soccer shoe, and Prada look-a-likes. Labels include MOMA, Calvin Klein, Sky Wrek, Alberto Guardiani and GFF.

West Village   212-620-0305
378 Bleecker Street   bet. Charles/Perry
NYC 10014   Mon.-Fri. 11-7:30, Sat. & Sun. 12-6

Turnbull & Asser   M/W
Since 1885, Turnbull & Asser have dressed England's aristocrats, moguls, and movie stars. Today, you can shop London's finest haberdasher right here in New York. Find traditional suits, men's furnishings, formal wear, sportswear, outerwear, sleepwear, shoes, and accessories. Their specialty is a bespoke shirt department, which boasts over 600 shirting fabrics, from bold stripes to scores of checks and patterns. 877-887-6284 www.turnbullandasser.com

Midtown East   212-319-8100
42 East 57th Street   bet. Park/Madison Ave.
NYC 10022   Mon.-Sat. 9:30-6

Unisa   W
Fashionable, fun, and well-priced shoes fill this well-stocked shop. Find mules, sandals, driving moccasins, pumps, and boots under the Unisa label. It's nice to find a hip and trendy shoe retailer on Madison Avenue that doesn't cost an arm and a "foot." 800-327-3619

Upper East Side   212-753-7474
701 Madison Avenue   bet. 62/63rd St.
NYC 10021   Mon.-Sat. 10-7, Thurs. 10-8, Sun. 12-5

Untitled   M/W
Untitled carries a terrific selection of avant-garde clothing by trendy, fashion forward designers. Find Helmut Lang's jean and shirt collection, as well as garb by Moschino, Iceberg, Alexander McQueen, Gaultier, and Plein Sud. Styles run from casual street smart to evening chic.

West Village   212-505-9725
26 West 8th Street   bet. 5th/6th Ave.
NYC 10011   Mon.-Sat. 11:30-9, Sun. 12-9

Urban Outfitters   M/W
Urban Outfitters is for the young and trendy in search of the latest urban trends. Find a collection of jeans, T-shirts, tank tops, jackets, accessories, gifts and a make-up line perhaps too honestly named "Urban Decay." Labels include Bulldog, Lux, Henna, Diesel, Free People, Mooks and their own label Urban Outfitters. www.urbn.com

Upper West Side   212-579-3912
2081 Broadway   at 72nd St.
NYC 10023   Mon.-Sat. 11-7, Sun. 12-5

East Village   212-375-1277
162 Second Avenue   bet. Tenth/Eleventh Ave.
NYC 10002   Mon.-Wed. 12-10,
    Thurs.-Sat. 11-11, Sun. 12-9

West Village   212-677-9350
374 Sixth Avenue   bet. Waverly/Wash. Pl.
NYC 10011   Mon.-Sat. 10-10, Sun. 12-9

NoHo   212-475-0009
628 Broadway   bet. Houston/Bleecker
NYC 10012   Mon.-Sat. 10-10, Sun. 12-8

Utility Canvas   M/W

Canvasianados will be thrilled by this store's collection of practical, versatile all-American clothing manufactured in canvas, from heavy-duty industrial weights to light as air soft-brushed textures. Find canvas-lined wool jackets, shirts, pants and shorts, as well as a few non-canvas pieces, such as anoraks and nylon jackets by the Artist in Orbit label. Best bet is their line of canvas bags, from a boxy "Market" bag to a $30 utility sac.

SoHo   212-673-2203
146 Sullivan Street   bet. Houston/Prince
NYC 10012   Mon.-Fri. 11-7, Sat. 11-8, Sun. 12-6

Valentino   M/W

The famous Valentino name conjures images of elegance and luxury, and those who shop here expect no less. Every design is cut haute couture, and makes you feel like royalty. Collections are distinctive, sensuous and rich in feeling. For her, find a ready-to-wear collection that includes suits in all shapes, pants, separates and "look-at-me" leathers, as well as high glam, embellished eveningwear. For him, choose from a line of smart-looking suits, shirts, casual wear, and Oscar night tuxedos. A Valentino design embodies effortless chic and opulence. Prices are over-the-top, but for a taste of Roman luxury it's well worth the investment, especially for women who wear red—they will adore Valentino's trademark red. Accessories also available.
877-360-0864

Upper East Side   212-772-6969
747 Madison Avenue   at 65th St.
NYC 10021   Mon.-Sat. 10-6

Vamps   M/W

This neighborhood shoe shop is best for comfort footwear. Find labels like Aerosoles, Rockport, Mephisto, Hush Puppies, Via Spiga, Dr. Scholl's, and Kenneth Cole. Moderately priced bridal shoes also available.

Upper East Side   212-734-3967
1420 Second Avenue   at 74th St.
NYC 10021   Mon.-Fri. 10-7:30, Sat. 10-7, Sun. 12-6

Vanessa Noel   W

"My shoes don't wear you, you wear them," says footwear designer Vanessa Noel. After years of shodding celebrities, socialites, and her regular customers through department store sales, Vanessa has plans to go retail with a swank townhouse shop. Find three different collections featuring mules, sling-backs, pumps and boots in sumptuous leathers,

lizards, suedes and crushed velvets, all finished with a range of heels from 1/4" heels to 4 1/2" stilettos. Ultra-feminine looks, tapering shapes and ultimate comfort define the Noel label. A large selection of bridal shoes also available.
www.vanessanoel.com

Upper East Side   Opening Spring 2001   212-906-0054
158 East 64th Street   bet. Lexington/Third Ave.
NYC 10021   Mon.-Sat. 10-6

Varda M/W

Varda features Italian handmade shoes in one-width sizing. Although the sales staff claims their shoes will fit narrow or wide feet, you will have to be the judge. Find classic designs that make the transition from day to evening as easy as one-two-three.

Upper East Side   212-472-7552
786 Madison Avenue   bet. 66/67th St.
NYC 10021   Mon.-Sat. 10-7

Upper West Side   212-873-6910
2080 Broadway   bet. 71/72 St.
NYC 10023   Mon.-Sat. 10-7:30, Sun. 12-7

SoHo   212-941-4990
149 Spring Street   bet. Wooster/W. B'way
NYC 10012   Mon.-Sun. 10-7:30

Variazioni W

An Italian clothing chain featuring edgy, contemporary clothing. From business suits and eveningwear to sporty and casual wear, find labels by Rebecca Dannenberg, Icon, Vivienne Tam, Easel, and Philosophy.

Upper West Side   212-874-7474
309 Columbus Avenue   bet. 74/75th St.
NYC 10023   Mon.-Sat. 11-8, Sun. 11-7

Midtown West   212-980-4900
37 West 57th Street   bet. 5th/6th Ave.
NYC 10019   Mon.-Sat. 10-7:30, Sun. 12-6

Ventilo W

Designer Armand Ventilo fuses Asian/Indian influences with French sophistication to create clothing that ranges from simple layered outfits in cool linens, silk and organzas to well-tailored suits in gabardine and tweed. The shop's Zen-like atmosphere makes it easy to spend hours perusing his wares, including special "finds" in his home collection.

SoHo   212-625-3660
69 Greene Street   bet. Spring/Broome
NYC 10012   Mon.-Sat. 11-7, Sun. 12-6

Vera Wang Bridal House, Ltd. W

This heavenly bridal salon will have the bride bathed in a luminous glow. Sheer elegance, fabulous styling, and beautiful craftsmanship define a Wang design. Choose from a sophisticated collection that runs from simple to elaborate, from an up-to-the-minute fashionable gown or one with old-fashioned frills. Also find evening stunners like long beaded dresses and feminine column dresses.

Upper East Side 212-628-3400
991 Madison Avenue at 77th St.
NYC 10021 Mon.-Sat. 9-6 by appointment only

Vera Wang Maids on Madison W

Across the street from her bridal salon, Vera Wang has set up a new shop exclusively for bridesmaids. According to Wang, "The entire bridal party should be as beautiful as the bride." Discover dresses, skirts, separates, camisoles, blouses and sweaters in wonderful shades of champagne, lilac, maize, soft pink and navy.

Upper East Side 212-628-9898
980 Madison Avenue, 3rd Fl. bet. 76/77th St.
NYC 10021 Tues.-Thurs. 11-7, Fri. 10-6,
Sat. 10-6 by appointment only, Sun. 11-5

Veronique W

Veronique's mission is "to provide clothes that are designed to be like the ones you're used to wearing when you're not pregnant." Find exclusive collections imported from Paris and Milan, which are functional, comfortable, and fashionable. Maternity wear that expectant mothers can wear with effortless style at the office, at home or an evening night out. Expensive, but worth it.

Upper East Side 212-831-7800
1321 Madison Avenue at 93rd St.
NYC 10128 Mon.-Sat. 10-6, Thurs. 10-7

Vertigo W

A French clothing retailer favored by young professional women in search of street-smart career wear. Find a collection of suits that go from desk to dinner, cashmere sweaters, shirts, handbags, and belts. The look: slim-fitted European classics with a fashion edge.

Upper East Side 212-439-9626
755 Madison Avenue bet. 65/66th St.
NYC 10021 Mon.-Sat. 10-7, Sun. 12-6

Verve W

The owner claims he carries over 125 different lines in his tiny West Village shop, from handbag and hat styles to sunglasses, jewelry and watches. Basic leather day bags and beaded purses make up his handbag collection, while hat designs go from the streets to the beach. Labels include Cynthia Rowley, Kazuyo Nakano, Isabella Fiore, Leyla, and Adrienne Vittadini.

West Village 212-691-6516
353 Bleecker bet. W. 10th/Charles St.
NYC 10014 Mon.-Sat. 11-7:30, Sun. 12-6

☆ Via Spiga M/W
An Italian footwear company that sells three lines of moderately priced shoes for all times of day. Looks range from casual and classic to funky and trendy. Find wedges, slide mules, sling-backs, thongs, pumps, and boots. It's fashionable, well-made footwear for urbanites. A small selection of men's shoes.

Upper East Side   212-988-4877
765 Madison Avenue   bet. 65/66th St.
NYC 10021   Mon.-Sat. 10-6, Sun. 12-5

SoHo   212-431-7007
390 West Broadway   bet. Spring/Broome
NYC 10013   Mon.-Sat. 11-7, Sun. 12-6

Victoria's Secret W
Every man and woman alive knows that Victoria's Secret is the source for sexy, eye-catching lingerie, regardless of their income bracket. Kudos to this lingerie retailer, which markets romance and allure at reasonable prices. Find lingerie, sleepwear, and slinky accessories in bright colors and soft feminine prints. He'll throw away his copy of their famous catalogue (Frederique who?) when he sees you wearing Victoria's Secret. 800-888-1500 www.victoriassecret.com

Upper East Side   212-717-7035
1240 Third Avenue   bet. 71/72nd St.
NYC 10021   Mon.-Sat. 10-8, Sun. 12-6

Upper West Side   Opening Fall 2000
1981 Broadway   at 67th St.
NYC 10023   Mon.-Sat. 10-8, Sun 12-6

Midtown East   212-758-5592
34 East 57th Street   bet. Park/Madison Ave.
NYC 10022   Mon.-Fri. 10-8, Sat. 10-7, Sun. 12-6

Flatiron   212-477-4118
115 Fifth Avenue   bet. 18/19th St.
NYC 10003   Mon.-Sat. 10-8, Sun. 12-6

SoHo   212-274-9519
565 Broadway   at Prince St.
NYC 10012   Mon.-Sat. 10-9, Sun. 12-7

Lower Manhattan   212-962-8122
South Street Seaport   Pier 17
NYC 10038   Mon.-Sat. 10-9, Sun. 11-8

☆ Vilebrequin M/B
This French purveyor of swimwear has landed in New York, and what better neighborhood than chic SoHo. Men and boys alike will delight in a colorful selection of swim trunks, featuring classic drawstring styles and surfer trunks. Choose from wonderful florals, stripes, checks, and solids in a myriad of colors. Pay $109 for adult swimwear and $55 for boys. From 2 years to adult.

SoHo   212-431-0673
436 West Broadway   bet. Spring/Prince
NYC 10012   Mon.-Sun. 11-7

Vincent and Edgar M

Overheard the other day: "There is Lobb, there is Cleverley, and then there is Vincent and Edgar." V & E is New York's finest custom-made shoe establishment. Shoemaker Roman Vaingauz labors for 40 hours to produce a single pair of his extremely bespoke shoes. Men's shoes start at $1,500 and women's at $1,100, with an additional $575 for a pair of wooden shoe lasts. Ten-to-twelve-week delivery.

Upper East Side 212-753-3461
972 Lexington Avenue at 71st St.
NYC 10021 by appointment

Vincent Nicolosi M/W

A high-end tailor of classic suits for "chairman of the board" types. Expect six-to-eight-week delivery. Will not quote prices over the phone.

Midtown East 212-486-6214
510 Madison Avenue at 53rd St.
NYC 10022 Mon.-Sat. 9-5

Vivaldi Boutique W

An Upper East Side boutique selling day and eveningwear with French and Italian designer labels like Claude Montana, Christian Lacroix, Sonia Rykiel, and Thierry Mugler. Find cocktail dresses, day and evening suits, special occasion dress, and formal gowns. A good source for ladies who need personalized attention when choosing their wardrobe. Accessories include jewelry, handbags, hats, and scarves.

Upper East Side 212-734-2805
1288 Third Avenue at 74th St.
NYC 10021 Mon.-Sat. 11-7, Thurs. 11-8, Sun. 12-5

Vivienne Tam W

Designer Vivienne Tam sticks to her formula for slinky, feminine pieces with just the right amount of edge. Inspired by her love of arts and crafts, Tam marries beading and embroidery with traditional fabrics. Design and fabric motifs uniquely blend elements of East and West. Find beautiful sheer floral dresses, pinstriped suits, embroidered skirts, jackets, printed nylon mesh tops, and separates.

SoHo 212-966-2398
99 Greene Street bet. Spring/Prince
NYC 10012 Mon.-Fri. 11-7, Sat. 11:30-7:30, Sun. 12-7

Vivienne Westwood M/W

When today's fashion divas are long gone, this iconoclastic British designer's epitaph will read, "Vivienne created and others followed." Welcome to Vivienne Westwood, the "Queen of Punk," who wants us all to look like naughty school girls. Collections are colorful, scandalous and campy. These are wild, non-conforming fashions where wearability takes a back seat to pure fantasy.

SoHo 212-334-5200
71 Greene Street bet. Spring/Broome
NYC 10012 Mon.-Sat. 11-7, Sun. 12-6

Walter Steiger M/W

When you treat yourself to a pair of Walter Steiger shoes, consider yourself well-heeled. Known for their unusual heel shapes, Walter Steiger features a variety of looks. Find sexy stilettos, mid-heeled pumps, platforms, sandals, loafers, and even a treaded walking shoe. Designs are soft, feminine, and easy-to-wear. His two-toned golf shoes will inspire you to head for the links. Men's shoes feature pointy-toed loafers, boots, sleek sneakers, and golf shoes.
www.waltersteiger.com

Upper East Side (W) 212-570-1212
739 Madison Avenue bet. 64/65th St.
NYC 10021 Mon.-Sat. 10-6

Midtown East 212-826-7171
417 Park Avenue at 55th St.
NYC 10022 Mon.-Fri. 10-6, Sat. 10-5

Wang W

The Wang sisters design practical, feminine fashions with desk-to-dinner versatility. Find a collection of coordinating skirts, dresses, and jackets with tailored cuts at moderate price points.

NoLiTa 212-941-6134
166 Elizabeth Street bet. Spring/Kenmare
NYC 10012 Mon.-Sat. 12-7, Sun. 12-6

Warehouse W

British fashions for the 18 to 35 crowd. Find contemporary sportswear with updated looks. Choose from casual suits, skirts, jackets, tops, jeans and accessories. Street-smart clothes for the young and trendy. Moderate prices.

Flatiron 212-243-7333
150 Fifth Avenue bet. 19/20th St.
NYC 10011 Mon.-Thurs. 10-8, Fri. & Sat. 10-9, Sun. 12-6

SoHo 212-941-0910
581 Broadway bet. Houston/Prince
NYC 10012 Mon.-Fri. 11-8, Sat. 10-9, Sun. 12-8

Warren Edwards M/W

Flying solo without longtime partner Susan Bennis, Warren Edwards is back with his signature collection of exotic and luxurious footwear. His designs incorporate three elements: creativity, femininity and fashion sensibility. Women can choose from glamorous evening pumps, mules, wedges, animal print suede loafers, driving moccasins, sandals, and boots. Men will take delight in the collection of suede and crocodile loafers, dress shoes, boots, and weekend wear. Prices run from $325 to $1,800. Warren Edwards is clearly for those who can afford to indulge themselves.

Upper East Side 212-223-4374
107 East 60th Street bet. Park/Lex.
NYC 10022 Mon.-Sat. 10-6

Waterwear W

Waterwear caters to all your swimwear needs. Choose from a variety of looks, from string and low-waisted bikinis to one-piece suits. Labels include Karla Colletto, Rosa Ferrer, Shan, Speedo and Gortex. Accessorize your suit with a coordinating cover-up or sarong. Bathing caps, sandals, and visors also available.

Upper East Side 212-570-6606
1349 Third Avenue at 77th St.
NYC 10021 Mon.-Fri. 10-8, Sat. 10-6, Sun. 12-6

Wathne M/W

Wathne offers a luxury sportswear collection designed for country life. Find sporting attire, separates, silk-screened scarves, boots, and accessories that embody a romantic style of bucolic living. Buyer beware: With prices this steep, perhaps you should buy the real McCoy at Hermès.
888-592-8463

Midtown West 212-262-7100
4 West 57th Street bet. 5th/6th Ave.
NYC 10019 Mon.-Sat. 10-6

Wearkstatt W

Brides-to-be will rejoice at the choices available in this SoHo bridal boutique. German designer Jonas Hegewish designs gowns to fit the personality of each bride, whether she wants simple and romantic or sleek and sculpted. Other bridal labels include Sanchez, and Bonnillo. Best to make an appointment.

SoHo 212-334-9494
33 Greene Street at Grand
NYC 10013 Tues.-Fri. 11-7, Thurs. 11-8, Sat. 10-6

Wet Seal M/W

This California-based company markets ultra-hip clothing for the junior set. Find everything from jeans, T-shirts, and club wear to underwear, sleepwear, and accessories. Sexy, tight-fitting little numbers for girls and street smart looks for guys. Shoes also available.

Midtown West 212-216-0622
901 Sixth Avenue at 33rd St.
NYC 10001 Mon.-Sat. 10-8, Sun. 11-7

NoHo 212-253-2470
670 Broadway at Bond
NYC 10012 Mon.-Sat. 10-9, Sun. 12-7

What Comes Around Goes Around M/W

A vintage shop selling clothing that's truly been around—from Victorian tops, eveningwear from the 30's, and polyester from the 70's to an Edwardian dust jacket, Hawaiian

shirts, and Pucci prints. Also, find an impressive denim collection, military jackets, leather, suede, shoes, and scarves. The merchandise at What Comes Around Goes Around is a good alternative to today's high-priced trends. Sales staff is knowledgeable and eager to please.
www.nyvintage.com

SoHo   212-343-9303
351 West Broadway   bet. Broome/Grand
NYC 10013   Mon.-Thurs. 11-8,
Fri. & Sat. 11-midnight, Sun. 12-7

The Wicker Garden B/G
This neighborhood shop offers everything your baby needs under one roof. Proud new mothers and mothers-to-be can shop Wicker Garden's enormous assortment, ranging from layette selections to adorable, hand-painted furniture and cribs. From 0-12 months.

Upper East Side   212-410-7001
1327 Madison Avenue bet.   93/94th St.
NYC 10128   Mon.-Sat. 10-6

William Fioravanti M
This popular bespoke tailor has a waiting list just to get an appointment. Once you've got a foot in the door, choose from luxurious English and Italian fabrics, and customize a suit, shirt, or topcoat. Suits start at $4,250. Expect a 10-to-12 week delivery.

Midtown West   212-355-1540
45 West 57th Street   bet. 5th/6th Ave.
NYC 10019   Mon.-Fri. 9-5 by appointment

★ Wolford Boutique W
Long considered the Rolls-Royce of hosiery, Wolford boasts advanced legwear and bodywear fashions. Find novelty hose, sheers, thigh-highs, opaques, and knee-highs in wonderful color shades. For the silkiest sheers, ask for the "Aura 5 Collection," and for a great run-resistant hose, ask for their best-selling "Individual 10." In addition, check out Wolford's line of brightly colored, multi-functional sheer tubes that can be worn as either a skirt or a dress (long or short). Bodysuits, swimwear, and fabulous men's socks round out the assortment.

Upper East Side   212-327-1000
996 Madison Avenue   bet. 77/78th St.
NYC 10021   Mon.-Sat. 10-6

Midtown East   212-688-4850
619 Madison Avenue   bet. 58/59th St.
NYC 10021   Mon.-Sat. 10-6

NoHo   212-358-1617
52 University Place   bet. 9/10th St.
NYC 10003   Mon.-Sat. 11-7

SoHo   212-343-0808
122 Greene Street   at Prince
NYC 10012   Mon.-Sat. 11-7, Sun. 12-6

Yohji Yamamoto

Women by Peter Elliot W

Women by Peter Elliot extends Elliot's tradition of classic clothing to the fairer sex, fusing masculine tailoring with feminine styling. Find handsome cashmere jackets, traditional men's shirts (adapted for women), four-ply cashmere sweater sets from Scotland and outerwear in luxury fabrics. Elliot even recommends Italian Borsalino hats for his female clientele.

Upper East Side 212-570-5747
1067 Madison Avenue bet. 80/81st St.
NYC 10028 Mon.-Sat. 10-6, Sun. 1-5

World of Golf M/W/C

This small store sells an enormous volume of golf equipment. World of Golf offers brand names like Callaway, Spaulding, Top-Flite, Cobra, Ping, Mizuno, and Taylor Made. Limited selection of clothing.

Midtown East 212-755-9398
147 East 47th Street bet. Third/Lex. Ave.
NYC 10017 Mon.-Sat. 9-7, Sun. 11-5

X.O.X.O. W

A good source for teenagers in search of trendy clothing at affordable price points. Mix and match to create a variety of looks. Find skirts, jackets, dresses, pants, snug tops, jeans and T-shirts in a junior cut. Hip and cool, but not built to last. www.xoxo.com

NoHo 212-995-5858
732 Broadway bet. Waverly/Astor Pl.
NYC 10003 Mon.-Sat. 11-9, Sun. 12-8

SoHo 212-334-9450
426 West Broadway bet. Prince/Spring
NYC 10012 Mon.-Thurs. 11-8, Fri. & Sat. 11-9, Sun. 11-7

Yaso W

Turkish owner Janan Tomko launches the careers of many undiscovered design talents from Europe and LA. Choose from a large dress selection, special occasion frocks, sportswear and casual wear. Labels include Monah Li, Buzz 18, Michael Stars, The Wonder-Tee, Jane Booke and their newest design talent Bahar Korcan. Find shoes by Graye (made in the same factory as Prada) and hats by Eric Javits and Louise Green.

SoHo 212-941-8506
62 Grand Street bet. Wooster/W. B'way
NYC 10012 Mon.-Sun. 11-7

Yohji Yamamoto M/W

Yohji Yamamoto continues to rock fashion's foundations with his modern and practical design inventions. Yamamoto's trademarks: dramatically sculpted designs, a neutral color palette and luxurious fabrics. Find a ready-to-wear collection that includes dressy suits, inventively cut and draped, fabulous white shirts, sweaters, coats, shoes and accessories. Although Yamamoto's designs are architectural, simplicity and femininity are never compromised.

SoHo   **212-966-9066**
103 Grand Street   at Mercer
NYC 10013   Mon.-Sat. 11-7, Sun. 12-6

Young's Hat Corner   M

Since 1890, Young's Hat Corner has catered to gents in search of the appropriate hat style. Styles run from casual to dressy, including fancy toppers, English caps, baseball hats, and straw hats for summer.

Lower Manhattan   **212-964-5693**
139 Nassau Street   at Beekman
NYC 10038   Mon.-Fri. 9-5:30, Sat. 10-2:30

Yumi Katsura   W

This upscale bridal salon has an extensive selection of dreamy gowns. Erisa, who designs for Yumi Katsura and The Erisa Collection, says she wants "to shatter the mold of traditional bridal dressing." Find modern silhouettes in a variety of looks, from simple to elaborate embroideries. Three to four months delivery time.

Upper East Side   **212-772-3760**
907 Madison Avenue   bet. 72/73rd St.
NYC 10021   Mon.-Fri. 11-6, Sat. 10-5

Yves Saint Laurent   W

Just how far can fashion wizard Tom Ford spread his wings? Apparently all the way from Italy to France. In addition to his duties with Gucci, Ford is the new director of YSL and the sole designer of their women's and men's collection. A Saint Laurent design continues to be the epitome of reliable chic. Clean lines, classic simplicity, strong silhouettes, and a superb color sense distinguish the label. Find a collection of precision-cut suits, separates, eveningwear and outerwear that reflects Ford's fresh approach to YSL's tradition of fashion. 800-424-8600 www.yslonline.com

Upper East Side   **212-988-3821**
855 Madison Avenue   bet. 70/71st St.
NYC 10021   Mon.-Sat. 10-6

Yves Saint Laurent Rive Gauche Hommes   M

Designer Hedi Slimane is out, and Tom Ford is in. Ford has long admired Saint Laurent, and with his appointment as creative director, his dream has come true. The Rive Gauche collection now heads in a new fashion direction appealing to a hipper audience. Ford has successfully taken original drawings by the master himself and added a modern edge. Find a line of ready-to-wear featuring classic suits, dress shirts, men's furnishings, casual sportswear, leather, outerwear, accessories, and a limited shoe selection. Modern, luxurious fabrics paired with urban elegance define the Rive Gauche label. 800-424-8600

Zara International

SoHo   212-274-0522
88 Wooster Street   bet. Spring/Broome
NYC 10002   Mon.-Sat. 11-7, Sun. 12-6

Yvone Christa   W

You can't open a fashion magazine these days without seeing Hollywood's latest "it" girl wearing a piece of jewelry or carrying a handbag from Yvone Christa. Bags come in all shapes, colors, sizes and textures, but are primarily for evening; priced from $50 to $500. Also, a vast selection of delicate, feminine jewelry that will complement daytime or evening outfits. www.yvonechrista.com

SoHo   212-965-1001
107 Mercer Street   bet. Prince/Spring
NYC 10012   Mon.-Fri. 12-7, Sat. 12-8. Sun. 1-7

Zabari   W

Perfect for the teenager seeking trendy clothes meant to last one season. This cavernous shop stocks all the latest clothes looks, from capri pants and skimpy tops to slip dresses, jeans, and jackets. Zabari's bright fabrics look great from a distance, tend to feel flimsy up close. Labels include Alice & Trixie, Lotta, Zabari, The Wrights, and Anna Kuan.

SoHo   212-431-7502
506 Broadway   bet. Spring/Broome
NYC 10012   Mon.-Sun. 11-8

Zao   M/W

This futuristic, new-age shop encompasses a total techno-lifestyle concept. Start with the art gallery in the back then move onto the retail store in the front featuring the latest in high-tech houseware and gifts from Japan and Italy. And, yes, finally you notice the clothes. From ready-to-wear to relaxed couture, Zao urges the customer to blend the high-end with the low-end. Designers include Maurizio Galante, Theory, Christian Weber, and Ato Japan. Although the message at Zao's is mixed, it's well worth experiencing this futuristic shopping environment at least once.

Lower East Side   212-505-0500
175 Orchard Street   bet. Houston/Stanton
NYC 10002   Mon.-Sun. 11-7

Zara International   M/W

This trendy Spanish chain is aggressively expanding its business throughout the city with constant store openings. Zara's huge success with tourists is partly based on a currency conversion chart attached to every article of clothing. Young professionals will find modern suitings, shirts, sweaters, and coats for work, and trendier styles like snakeskin print pants, knits, leather biker jackets, and nylon ponchos. Zara will let you dress with confidence and style without putting a dent in your wallet. Shoes and accessories also available.

Z'Baby Company

Midtown East (W)	**212-754-1120**
750 Lexington Avenue	at 59th St.
NYC 10022	Mon.-Sat. 10-8, Sun. 12-6
Midtown West	**212-868-6551**
39 West 34th Street	bet. Fifth/Sixth Ave.
NYC 10001	Mon.-Fri. 10-9, Sat. & Sun. 10-8
Flatiron	**212-741-0555**
101 Fifth Avenue	bet. 17/18th St.
NYC 10003	Mon.-Sat. 10-8, Sun. 12-7
SoHo	**212-343-1725**
580 Broadway	at Prince
NYC 10012	Mon.-Sat. 10-8, Sun. 12-7

Z'Baby Company B/G

A children's store packed with trendy domestic and imported clothing for cutting-edge progeny from newborn to size 7. Expect to find fun play clothes, pretty dresses, sweaters, T-shirts and underwear from designers like Cacharel, Kenzo, Missoni, Laura Lynn, Giesswein and Cake Walk. Newborn to size 7.

Upper East Side	**212-472-2229**
996 Lexington Avenue	at 72nd St.
NYC 10021	Mon.-Sat. 10-7, Sun. 11:30-5
Upper West Side	**212-579-2229**
100 West 72nd Street	at Columbus
NYC 10023	Mon.-Sat. 10:30-8, Sun. 11-6:30

Zeller Tuxedo M

At Zeller Tuxedo, rent or purchase men's formalwear. Find a good selection of designer names like Pierre Cardin and Christian Dior for rentals. Choose Calvin Klein, Lord West, Joseph Abboud, Mani, as well as less expensive brands for purchases. Rental prices start at $120, while buying runs from $400 to $1,000. Shirts and black tie accessories available.

Upper East Side	**212-688-0100**
1010 Third Avenue	bet. 60/61st St.
NYC 10021	Mon.-Fri. 9-6:30, Sat. 10-5:30, Sun. 11-4:30

Zero W

Maria Cornejo goes out on her own by showcasing her modern, comfortable clothes in her shop/design studio. Find a small collection of pants, dresses, skirts and tops in fabrics from denim Lycra to waterproof, sueded poly seatex. Wearable clothes with urban looks.

NoLiTa	**212-925-3849**
225 Mott Street	bet. Prince/Spring
NYC 10012	Mon.-Fri. 12:30-7:30, Sat.& Sun. 12:30-6:30

Zion W

The professional shops here for a secure, tailored look with desk-to-dinner versatility. Find racks of suits and matching separates in dozens of colors. The look is understated, fad-free and easy-to-wear. Ask Joan Lunden, she's one of their loyal customers.

SoHo   **212-966-4634**
367 West Broadway   at Broome
NYC 10013   Mon.-Sat. 11- 7:30

Zitomer
M/W/C

A mini-department store stocked with every beauty, bath and health product imaginable. Cosmetics, fragrances, pashminas, beach scarves, cashmere shawls, jewelry and a wide assortment of hair accessories are on display. Zitomers even boasts a second floor complete with children's clothing and toy department. During the winter, cashmere wraps and faux mink neck warmers are worth a look. 888-219-2888

Upper East Side   **212-737-4480**
969 Madison Avenue   bet. 75/76th St.
NYC 10021   Mon.-Fri. 9-8, Sat. 9-7, Sun. 10-6

Stores by Category

Women's

Men's

Unisex

Children's

"When women are depressed, they eat or go shopping. Men invade another country. It's a whole different way of thinking." —*Elayne Boosler*

"I feel like I'm having a fashion orgasm. I just put this one on and it fits likes a glove. This is a bit surreal. I feel like I'm acting and playing me." —*Cate Blanchett in a gown by John Galliano*

Which designer started his empire with the money he made selling his Volkswagon in 1975, and 25 years later his deconstructed, soft-shoulder suit is an institution that changed the way men look at clothing and at their own bodies? *Answer: Giorgio Armani*

Stores by Category

Women's Accessories

Add
Alexandre de Paris
Alexia Crawford Accessories
Anthropologie
Barneys New York
Bergdorf Goodman
Bloomingdale's
Boyd's Pharmacy
Calypso St. Barths
Catherine
Clyde's on Madison
En Soie
Frederic Fekkai
Gamine
Henri Bendel
Hermès
Language
Lord & Taylor
Macy's
Orva
Portantina
Precision
Saks Fifth Avenue
Shambala
Yvone Christa
Zitomer

Women's Ballet/Dance & Work-Out Apparel

Capezio
Champs
Crunch
Danskin
Freed of London
Lady Footlocker
Niketown

Women's Bridal

Barneys New York
Bergdorf Goodman
Bloomingdale's
The Bridal Party-
  Dresses for Bridesmaids
Carolina Herrera
Cosa Bella
Kenneth Cole (shoes only)
Kleinfeld & Sons
Manolo Blahnik
  (shoes only)
Michael's Resale
Michelle Roth & Co.
Mika Inatome
Morgane Le Fay
Nicole Miller
Peter Fox (shoes only)
Pilar Rossi
Reva Mivasagar
Saks Fifth Avenue
Stuart Weitzman
  (shoes only)
Thread (bridesmaid only)
Vanessa Noel (shoes only)
Vera Wang Maids
  on Madison
Vera Wang
Wearkstatt
Yumi Katsura

Stores by Category

Women's Career
Anik
Ann Taylor
Barami
Barneys New York
Bergdorf Goodman
Bloomingdale's
Brooks Brothers
Country Road Australia
Dana Buchman
Episode
J. McLaughlin
Jaeger
Joan & David
Liz Claiborne
Lord & Taylor
Paul Stuart
St. John
The New York Look
Tahari
Talbot's
Tristan & America
Vertigo
Zara International
Zion

Women's Cashmere/Knitwear
Alberene Cashmere
Bergdorf Goodman
Berk
Best of Scotland
Bloomingdale's
Cashmere, Cashmere
Cashmere New York
Jennifer Tyler
Jennifer Tyler Too
Laura Biagiotti
Loro Piana
M-A-G
Malo
Manrico
N. Peal
Saks Fifth Avenue
Sample
Tse Cashmere
TseSurface

Women's Casual
Abercrombie & Fitch
American Colors
American Eagle Outfitters
Ann Taylor Loft
Anthropologie
A Perfect Day in Paradise
April Cornell
A/X Armani Exchange
Banana Republic
Barneys New York
Basic/Basic
Benetton
Bloomingdale's
Canal Jean Co.
Diesel
Eddie Bauer
Express
Forreal Basics
Gap
Granny-Made
Guess?
Henry Lehr
J. Crew
Lacoste
Leggiadro
Levi Strauss
The Limited
Lord & Taylor
Lucky Brand Dungarees
Macy's
Old Navy Clothing Co.
Quiksilver
Replay Country Store
Saks Fifth Avenue
Todd Oldham
Utility Canvas

Stores by Category

Women's Classic

Arleen Bowman
Beretta
Bottega Veneta
Burberrys
Cosa Bella
Davide Cenci
En Soie
Entre Nous
Etro
Geiger
Hermès
Holland & Holland
Hunting World
J. McLaughlin
Klein's of Monticello
Laura Ashley
Loro Piana
Luca Luca
Noriko Maeda
Paul & Shark
Polo Ralph Lauren
Rodier
Saks Fifth Avenue
San Francisco Clothing
Scarlet & Sage
Shen
Steven Stolman
St. John
Su-zen
Sylvia Heisel
Wathne
Women by Peter Elliot

Women's Consignment

Alice Underground
Allan & Suzi
Bis
Encore
Fan Club
Fisch for the Hip
Ina
Kavanagh's Designer Resale
Michael's Resale
New and Almost New (NAAN)
Out of Our Closet
Sunrise Ruby
Tatiana Resale Boutique
Tokio 7
Tokyo Joe
Transfer International

Women's Custom Tailoring

Akiue-Go
Arthur Gluck Shirtmakers
Cheo Tailors
Couture by Jennifer Dule
House of Dormeuil
Lee Anderson
John Anthony
Ménage À Trois
Piccione
Pierre Garroudi
Rosette Couturiere

Stores by Category

Women's Contemporary

A. Cheng
A Détacher
Agnes B.
Alpana Bawa
Alskling
Anna
Anik
Anthropologie
Antique Boutique
The Apartment
A.P.C.
Assets London
Atrium
Bagutta
Barneys New York
BCBG by Max Azria
Bebe
Bebesh
Bergdorf Goodman
Betsey Bunky Nini
Big Drop
Bissou Bissou
Bloomingdale's
Bond 07
Calypso St. Barths
Catherine
Christine Ganeaux
Christopher Totman
Cinco
Claire Blaydon
Club Monaco
C.P. Shades
Daang Goodman
Daryl K
Darryl's
Deborah Moorfield
Detour
Diana & Jeffries
DieselStyleLab
DKNY
D/L Cerney
Dosa
The Dressing Room
Eileen Fisher
Emporio Armani
Episode
Epperson Studio
Equipment
Erica Tanov
February Eleventh
Final Home
Find Outlet
Fiona Walker
Foley + Corinna
Forreal
Fragile
Franceska
French Connection
Gamine
Ghost
Hedra Prue
Heun
Hennes & Mauritz
Henri Bendel
Himaya
Iceberg
If
Intermix
Institut
In the Black
Janet Russo
Jeffrey New York
Jill Anderson
Jimin Lee/Translatio

Stores by Category

Women's Contemporary (continued)

- Joseph
- Katayone Adeli
- Kirna Zabête
- La Gallerie la Rue
- Language
- Laundry, by Shelli Segal
- Laundry Industry
- Lina Tsai
- Linda Dresner
- Louie
- Lucy Barnes
- Margie Tsai
- Mark Montano
- Martier
- Max Studio
- Mayle
- Meghan Kinney Studio
- Montmartre
- Nanette Lepore
- Nellie M.
- New Frontier
- Nicole Vaughn
- Oasis
- Oilily for Women
- Olive & Bette's
- The Open Door Gallery
- Parke & Ronen
- Pleats Please
- Plein Sud
- Precision
- Product
- Rampage
- Red Tape by Rebecca Dannenberg
- Roberto Cavalli
- Saks Fifth Avenue
- Scoop
- Seam
- Selia Yang
- Shack
- Shanghai Tang
- Sharagano
- Shin Choi
- Sisley
- Skella
- Sleek on Bleecker
- Steven Alan
- Stream
- Tehen
- TG - 170
- Tocca
- Tracy Feith
- Trufaux
- Untitled
- Variazioni
- Ventilo
- Vertigo
- Wang
- Warehouse
- Yaso
- Zabari
- Zao
- Zara International
- Zero

Stores by Category

Women's Designer

Anna Sui
Atsuro Tayama
Barbara Bui
Betsey Johnson
Calvin Klein
Carolina Herrera
Celine
Cerutti
Chanel
Chloe
Christian Dior
Commes Des Garçons
Costume National
Cynthia Rowley
D & G
Dolce & Gabbana
Donna Karan
Emilio Pucci
Emmanuel Ungaro
Enrique Martinez
Escada
Fendi
Genny
Geoffrey Beene
Gianfranco Ferre
Gianni Versace
Giorgio Armani
Givenchy
Gucci
Hanae Mori
Helmut Lang
Issey Miyake
Jill Stuart
Kenzo
Krizia
Laura Biagiotti
Les Copains
Louis Féraud
Louis Vuitton
Marc Jacobs
Max Mara
Michael Kors
Missoni
Miu Miu
Morgane Le Fay
Moschino
Nicole Farhi
Nicole Miller
Norma Kamali
Philosophy by Alberta Feretti
Polo Ralph Lauren
Prada
René Lezard
Salvatore Ferragamo
Sonia Rykiel
Valentino
Vera Wang
Vivienne Tam
Vivienne Westwood
Yohji Yamamoto
Yves Saint Laurent

Women's Discount

Bolton's
Burlington Coat Factory
Century 21
Daffy's
Filene's Basement
Forman's
Fuchsia
Loehman's
TJ Maxx

Women's Ethnic

Do Kham
Hello Sari
Jungle Planet
Kinnu
Pearl River
Tibet Arts & Crafts
Tibet Bazaar

Women's Evening & Special Occasion

Alicia Mugetti
Bebesh
Bergdorf Goodman
Bloomingdale's
Caché
Clifford Michael Design
Giorgio Armani
John Anthony
Lee Anderson
Lord & Taylor
Luca Luca
Makola
Marianne Novobatzky
Morgane Le Fay
Pierre Garroudi
Pilar Rossi
Reva Mivasagar
Saks Fifth Avenue
Sylvia Heisel
Thread
Valentino
Vera Wang
Vivaldi Boutique

Women's Furriers

Alexandros Furs
Alixandre
Ben Thylan Furs
Bergdorf Goodman
Bloomingdale's
Christie Brothers Furs
Denimax
Fendi
J. Mendel
Ritz Furs
Saks Fifth Avenue

Women's Hats

Add
Amy Downs Hats
Barbara Feinman Millinery
Barneys New York
Bergdorf Goodman
Bloomingdale's
Calypso St. Barths
Eugenia Kim
The Hat Shop
Hatitude
Kelly Christy
Language
Lisa Shaub
Lord & Taylor
Macy's
Saks Fifth Avenue
Samuel's Hats
Suzanne
Tracey Tooker Hats

Stores by Category

Women's Handbags & Leathergoods

Add
Amy Chan
Anya Hindmarch
Bally
Barneys New York
Barry Kieselstein-Cord
Bergdorf Goodman
Bill Amberg
Bloomingdale's
Blue Bag
Bottega Veneta
Calypso St. Barths
Celine
Chanel
Coach
Crouch & Fitzgerald
Deco Jewels
Dooney & Burke
Fendi
Fine & Klein
Furla
Gabriel Ichak
Ghurka
Gucci
Hans Koch
Hermès
Hunting World
Il Bisonte
Jamin Puech
J.S. Suarez
Judith Lieber
Kate Spade
Kazuyo Nakano
Lana Marks
Language
Lederer
LeSportSac
Longchamp
Lord & Taylor
Louis Vuitton
Macy's
Max Fiorentino
Peter Hermann
Prada
René Collection
The Sak
Saks Fifth Avenue
Salvatore Ferragamo
Seeger
Soco
T. Anthony
Tod's
Tribeca Luggage & Leather
Verve
Yvone Christa

Women's Hosiery

Barneys New York
Bergdorf Goodman
Bloomingdale's
Fogal
Legs Beautiful
Lord & Taylor
Macy's
M. Steuer Company
Orva
Saks Fifth Avenue
Wolford

Stores by Category

Women's Juniors
Abercrombie & Fitch
American Eagle Outfitters
Bloomingdale's
Doll House
Express
Forreal Basics
Gap
Hennes & Mauritz
Infinity
Lester's
Levi Strauss
The Limited
Lord of the Fleas
Macy's
Marsha D.D.
Reminiscence
Wet Seal
X.O.X.O.

Women's Leather
Bridge
Buffalo Chips USA
Denimax
Leather Corner
The Leather and Suede Workshop
Leather Rose
North Beach Leather
NYC Custom Leather
Original Leather
Silverado
Studio 109

Women's Lingerie & Sleepwear
Allure
Barneys New York
Bergdorf Goodman
Bloomingdale's
Bloomers
Bra Smythe
Brief Encounters
D. Porthault
Enerla
Franceska
Inside Story
Joovay
La Perla
La Petite Coquette
Le Corset
Lingerie on Lex
Lord & Taylor
Macy's
Makie
Martier
Nocturne
Only Hearts
Ripplu
Saks Fifth Avenue
Takashimaya
Victoria's Secret

Maternity
A Pea in the Pod
Barneys New York
Liz Lange Maternity
Madison Ave. Maternity & Baby
Maternity Work
Mimi Maternity
Mom's Night Out
Motherhood Maternity
Veronique

Stores by Category

Women's Petite Size
Ann Taylor
Bloomingdale's
Dana Buchman Petites
Liz Claiborne
Lord & Taylor
Macy's
Saks Fifth Avenue
Tahari
Talbot's

Women's Plus Size
Ashanti
August Max
Bloomingdale's
Lord & Taylor
Macy's
Marina Rinaldi
Saks Fifth Avenue
Soho Woman

Women's Shirts
Agnes B.
Anne Fontaine
A.P.C.
Banana Republic
Barneys New York
Bergdorf Goodman
Bloomingdale's
Brooks Brothers
Custom Shop
Equipment
J. Crew
Leggiadro
Polo Ralph Lauren
Saks Fifth Avenue
Scoop
Seize sur Vingt
The Shirt Shop
Thomas Pink
Turnbull & Asser

Womens Shoe's
Aerosoles
Aldo
Antoin
Arche
A. Testoni
Avitto
Bally
Barbara Shaum
Barneys New York
Bati
Belgian Shoes
Bergdorf Goodman
Bloomingdale's
Bottega Veneta
Botticelli
Bruno Magli
Camper
Cesare Piaciotti
Chanel
Charles Jourdan
Christian Louboutin
Chuckies
CK Calvin Klein Shoes and Bags
Cole-Haan
David Aaron
Easy Spirit
Enzo Angiolini
Eric Shoes

228

Stores by Category

Womens Shoe's (continued)

- Fortuna Valentina
- Fratelli Rosetti
- French Sole
- Galo
- Giordano's
- Giraudon
- Goffredo Fantini
- Gucci
- Helene Arpels
- Iramo
- Jeffrey New York
- Jenny B.
- Jimmy Choo
- J.M. Weston
- Joan & David
- John Fluevog
- Juno
- Jutta Neumann
- Kenneth Cole
- Kerquelen
- Lord & Taylor
- Luichiny
- Macy's
- Make 10
- Manolo Blahnik
- Maraolo
- Mark Schwartz
- Mare
- Martinez Valero
- Milen Shoes
- Nancy Geist
- Nine West
- Omari
- Orva
- Overland Trading Co.
- Peter Fox Shoes
- Petit Peton
- Plus Nine Footwear for Women
- Prada
- Rapax
- René Mancini
- Robert Clergerie
- Rockport
- Sacco
- Saks Fifth Avenue
- Salvatore Ferragamo
- Santoni
- Sergio Rossi
- Shoe
- Sigerson Morrison
- Skechers USA
- Soco
- Stephane Kelian
- Steve Madden
- Stuart Weitzman
- Stubbs & Wooten
- Tanino Crisci
- Team Shoes
- Terra Plana
- Timberland
- Tod's
- Tootsi Plohound
- Unisa
- Vamps
- Vanessa Noel
- Varda
- Via Spiga
- Vincent & Edgar (custom only)
- Walter Steiger
- Warren Edwards

Stores by Category

Women's Swimwear

Barneys New York
Bergdorf Goodman
Bloomingdale's
Bra Smythe
Calypso St. Barths
Canyon Beachwear
J. Crew
Keiko's
La Perla
Leggiadro
Liza Bruce
Lord & Taylor
Macy's
Malia Mills
Martier
Norma Kamali
Polo Sport
Prada Sport
Quiksilver
Saks Fifth Avenue
Speedo Authentic Fitness
Waterwear

Women's Vintage & Retro

Alice Underground
Andy's Chee-pees
Anna
Canal Jeans
Cherry
Harriet Love
Keni Valenti
Legacy
Mary Efron
The 1909 Company
99X
Reminiscence
Resurrection Vintage
Screaming Mimi's
Timtoum
What Comes Around Goes Around

Women's Wearable Art

Gallery of Wearable Art
Julie Artisan's Gallery
MarcoArt

Women's Young & Trendy

Barneys New York
Bloomingdale's
DDC Lab
Detour
Hennes & Mauritz
Hotel Venus
Lord of the Fleas
Macy's
99X
Patricia Field
Urban Outfitters

Men's Shoes

Aerosoles
Aldo
Allen Edmonds
A. Testoni
Avitto
Bally
Barbara Shaum
Barneys New York
Belgian Shoes
Bergdorf Goodman Men
Bloomingdale's
Bostonian
Botticelli
Bottega Veneta
Bruno Magli
Camper
Cesare Piaciotti
Church's English Shoes
Citishoes
CK Calvin Klein Shoes and Bags
Cole-Haan
Fratelli Rossetti
Giraudon
Goffredo Fantini
Gucci
Iramo
Jenny B.
J.M. Weston
John Fluevog
John Lobb
Johnston & Murphy
Juno
Jutta Neumann
Kenneth Cole
Kerquelen
Lord & Taylor
Macy's
Make 10
Maraolo
Mare
Milen Shoes
99X
Omari
Overland Trading Co.
Petit Peton
Prada
Robert Clergerie
Rockport
Saks Fifth Avenue
Salvatore Ferragamo
Santoni
Sergio Rossi
Shoe
Skechers USA
Stephane Kelian
Steve Madden
Stubbs & Wooten
Tanino Crisci
Team Shoes
Terra Plana
Timberland
Tod's
Tootsi Plohound
Tupli
Vamps
Varda
Via Spiga
Vincent & Edgar (custom only)
Walter Steiger
Warren Edwards

Men's Sleepwear
Makie

Stores by Category

Men's Sportswear—Traditional

- Barneys New York
- Bergdorf Goodman Men
- Beretta
- Brooks Brothers
- Burberrys
- Davide Cenci
- Etro
- H. Herzfeld
- Hermès
- Holland & Holland
- Hunting World
- Jay Kos
- J. McLaughlin
- Lord & Taylor
- Loro Piana
- Paul & Shark
- Paul Stuart
- Peter Elliot
- Polo Ralph Lauren
- Purdey
- Saks Fifth Avenue
- Wathne

Men's Swimwear

- Barneys New York
- Bergdorf Goodman Men
- Bloomingdale's
- Franceska
- J. Crew
- Lord & Taylor
- Macy's
- Polo Sport
- Prada Sport
- Quiksilver
- Saks Fifth Avenue
- Speedo Authentic Fitness
- Vilebrequin

Men's Ties

- Alfred Dunhill
- Barneys New York
- Bergdorf Goodman Men
- Bloomingdale's
- Brioni
- Brooks Brothers
- Burberrys
- Ermenegildo Zegna
- Etro
- Façonnable
- Ferragamo
- Hèrmes
- J. Press
- Jay Kos
- Joseph A. Banks
- Lord & Taylor
- Macy's
- Men's Wearhouse
- Paul Stuart
- Robert Talbott
- Saks Fifth Avenue
- Seigo
- Sulka
- Today's Man
- Thomas Pink
- Turnbull & Asser

Stores by Category

Men's Vintage & Retro

Alice Underground
Andy's Chee-pees
Canal Jeans
Cherry
99X
Reminiscence
Resurrection Vintage
Screaming Mimi's
Timtoum
What Comes Around Goes Around

Men's Young & Trendy

Bloomingdale's
DDC Lab
Hennes & Mauritz
Hotel Venus
Lord of the Fleas
Macy's
99X
Patricia Field
Swish
Urban Outfitters

Unisex Athletic

Athlete's Foot
Athletic Style
Champs
Crunch
Foot Locker
Modell's
New Balance
Niketown
Paragon
Polo Sport
Prada Sport
Reebok
Speedo Authentic Fitness
Sports Authority
Super Runners Shop
Training Camp

Unisex Department Stores

Barneys New York
Bergdorf Goodman
Bergdorf Goodman Men
Bloomingdale's
Brooks Brothers
Henri Bendel (women only)
Lord & Taylor
Macy's
Saks Fifth Avenue
Takashimaya

Unisex Golf

Champs
Lacoste
New York Golf Center
Niketown
Polo Sport
Prada Sport
Reebok Golf Shop
Richard Metz Golf Equipment
Walter Steiger (shoes only)
World of Golf

Stores by Category

Unisex Jeans

Abercrombie & Fitch
American Jean
A/X Armani Exchange
Barneys New York
Bloomingdale's
Canal Jean Company
Chuck Roaste
Diesel
Gap
Guess?
Levi Strauss
Lucky Brand Dungarees
Old Navy Clothing Co.
O.M.G.
Replay Country Store
Soho Jeans

Unisex Outerwear

Barneys New York
Bergdorf Goodman
Bloomingdale's
Brooks Brothers
Burberrys
Davide Cenci
Denimax
Lord & Taylor
Macy's
Paul Stuart
Saks Fifth Avenue
Searle Blatt

Unisex Outdoor Sports Equipment & Apparel

Athlete's Foot (shoes only)
Bicycle Habitat
Bicycle Renaissance
Blades Board and Skate
Champs
Conrad's Bike Shop
Diesel
Eastern Mountain Sports
Gerry Crosby & Co.
Lacoste
Lady Foot Locker
Masons Tennis
Metro Bicycle
Millers Harness Shop
Modell's
Niketown
Orvis
Paragon Sporting Goods
Patagonia
Polo Sport
Powers Court Tennis Outlet
Prada Sport
Princeton Ski Shop
Reebok
Scandinavian Ski Shop
Sports Authority
Toga Bike Shop

Unisex Tennis

Champs
Mason's Tennis Mart
Modell's
Niketown
Paragon Sporting Goods
Polo Sport
Powers Court Tennis Outlet
Reebok
Sports Authority

Stores by Category

Unisex Western
Billy Martin
Buffalo Chips USA

Children's Clothing
April Cornell
Au Chat Botté
The Baby Collection
Bambini
Barneys New York
Bebe Thompson
Bloomingdale's
Bonpoint
Bu and the Duck
Calypso Enfant
Catimini
The Children's Place
Coco & Z
Erica Tanov
Gap Kids & Baby Gap
Granny-Made
Greenstones Too
Gymboree
Jacadi
Julian & Sara
Kids are Magic
Koh's Kids
La Layette
La Petite Etoile
Laura Ashley
Laura Beth's Baby Collection
Lester's
Lilliput/SoHo Kids
Lord & Taylor
Macy's
Magic Windows
Miss Pym (custom only)
Nursery Lines
Oilily
Old Navy Clothing Co.
Osh Kosh B'Gosh
Patagonia
Peanutbutter & Jane
Saks Fifth Avenue
San Fransico Clothing
Second Act Childrenswear
Small Change
Space Kiddets
Spring Flowers
Tartine et Chocolat
The Stork Club
Talbot's Kids
The Wicker Garden
Vilebrequin
Z'Baby Company
Zitomer

Children's Discount
Century 21
Daffy's
TJ Maxx

Children's Shoes
Bambini
East Side Kids
Galo
Great Feet
Jacadi
Kids Footlocker
Lester's
Little Eric Shoes
Shoofly
Skechers USA
Spring Flowers
Timberland
Tod's

Stores by Neighborhood

Manhattan Walking Maps

Upper East Side

Upper West Side

Midtown East

Midtown West

Fifth Avenue

Flatiron

Chelsea

East Village / Lower East Side

NoHo / West Village

SoHo / NoLiTa

Lower Manhattan / TriBeCa

Brooklyn

"A woman's dress should be like a barbed-wired fence—
serving its purpose without obstructing the view."
—*Sophia Loren*

The story goes that in 1846, Lieutenant Henry Lumsden of the British Army was stationed in Punjab, India and couldn't bear to wear his felt uniform, so he dyed his 100 percent cotton jammies brown to look just like it. Since that time khaki-colored cottons have dressed everyone from Einstein to JFK to Picasso to Indiana Jones.

The sports company Nike was created by University of Oregon track coach Bill Bowerman and student athlete Phil Knight, who each pitched in $500. They paid another student $35 to design the swoosh. And the rest is history.

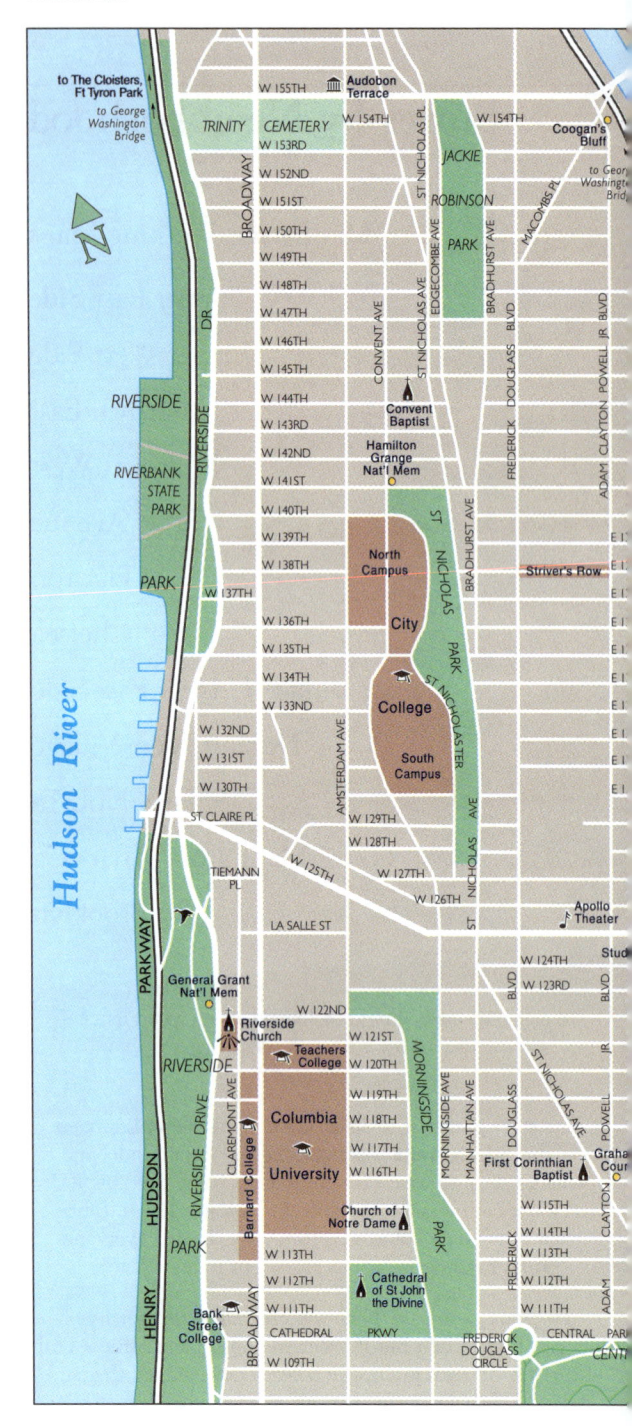

Manhattan Walking Maps
Harlem

Manhattan Walking Maps
East Harlem, Spanish Harlem

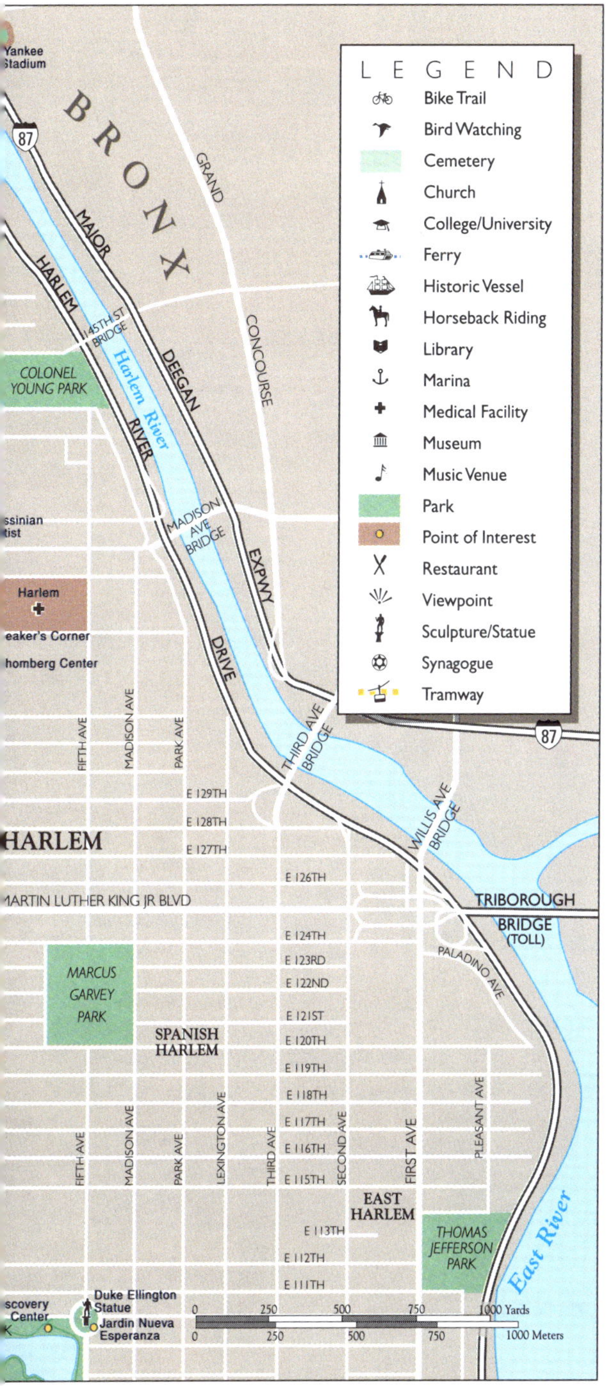

LEGEND
- 🚴 Bike Trail
- 🦅 Bird Watching
- Cemetery
- ⛪ Church
- 🎓 College/University
- Ferry
- 🚢 Historic Vessel
- 🐎 Horseback Riding
- 📖 Library
- ⚓ Marina
- ✚ Medical Facility
- 🏛 Museum
- ♪ Music Venue
- Park
- ⊙ Point of Interest
- ✕ Restaurant
- ☀ Viewpoint
- 👤 Sculpture/Statue
- ✡ Synagogue
- 🚡 Tramway

Yankee Stadium
BRONX
87
MAJOR DEEGAN EXPWY
HARLEM RIVER DRIVE
145TH ST BRIDGE
COLONEL YOUNG PARK
GRAND CONCOURSE
MADISON AVE BRIDGE
Abyssinian Baptist
Harlem +
Speaker's Corner
Schomberg Center
THIRD AVE BRIDGE
WILLIS AVE BRIDGE
87
FIFTH AVE
MADISON AVE
PARK AVE
E 129TH
E 128TH
E 127TH
HARLEM
E 126TH
MARTIN LUTHER KING JR BLVD
E 124TH
E 123RD
TRIBOROUGH BRIDGE (TOLL)
MARCUS GARVEY PARK
E 122ND
PALADINO AVE
E 121ST
SPANISH HARLEM
E 120TH
E 119TH
E 118TH
LEXINGTON AVE
E 117TH
SECOND AVE
E 116TH
FIRST AVE
E 115TH
PLEASANT AVE
EAST HARLEM
E 113TH
E 112TH
E 111TH
THOMAS JEFFERSON PARK
East River
Discovery Center
Duke Ellington Statue
Jardin Nueva Esperanza

0   250   500   750   1000 Yards
0   250   500   750   1000 Meters

Stores by Neighborhood

243

Manhattan Walking Maps
Upper West Side

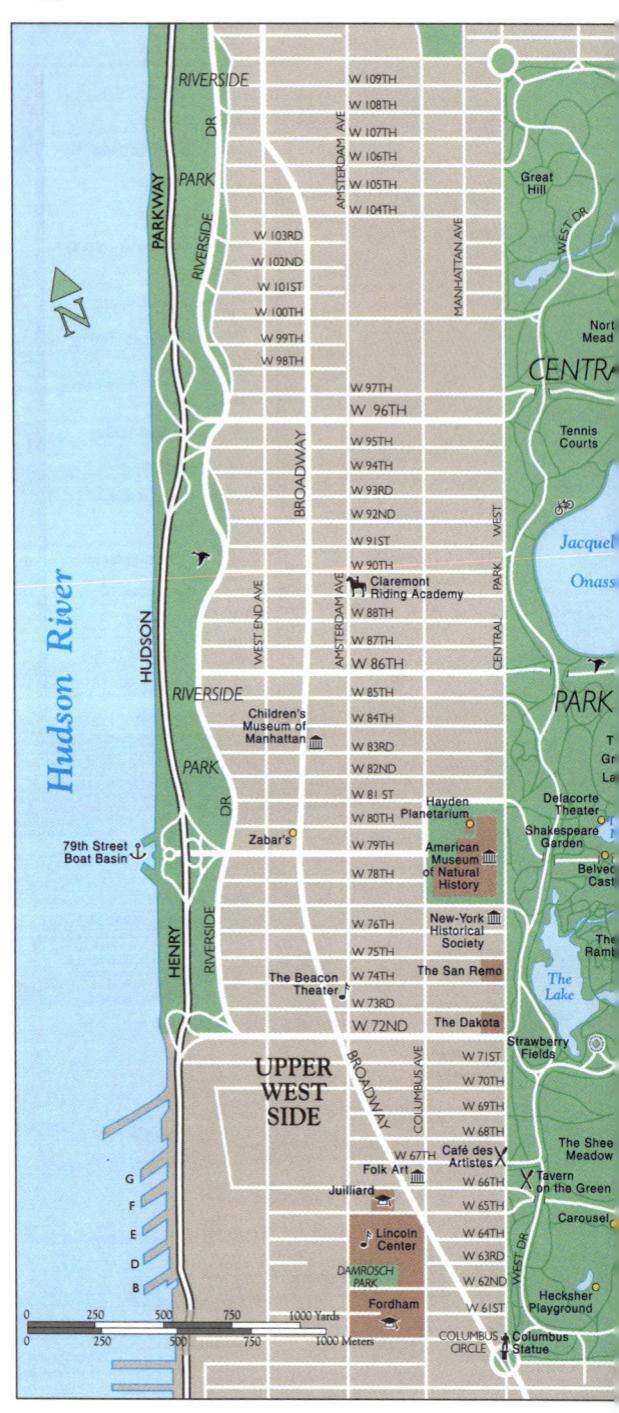

Manhattan Walking Maps
Upper East Side

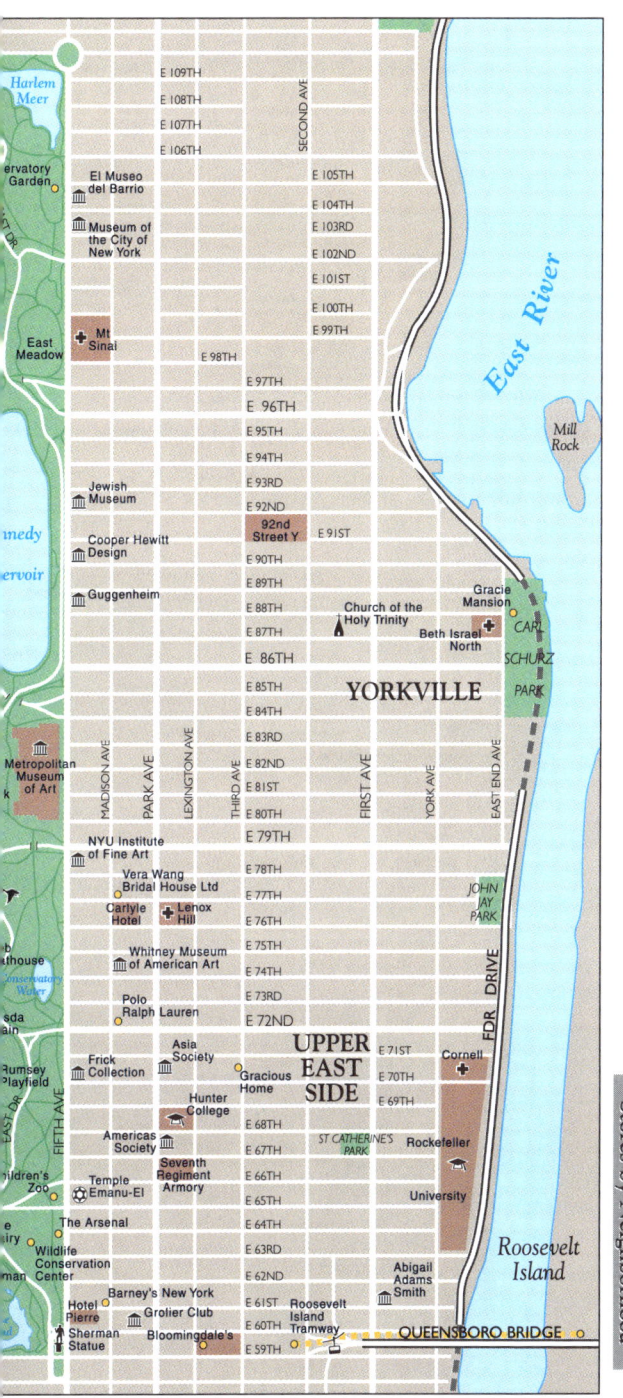

Manhattan Walking Maps
Midtown West, Chelsea

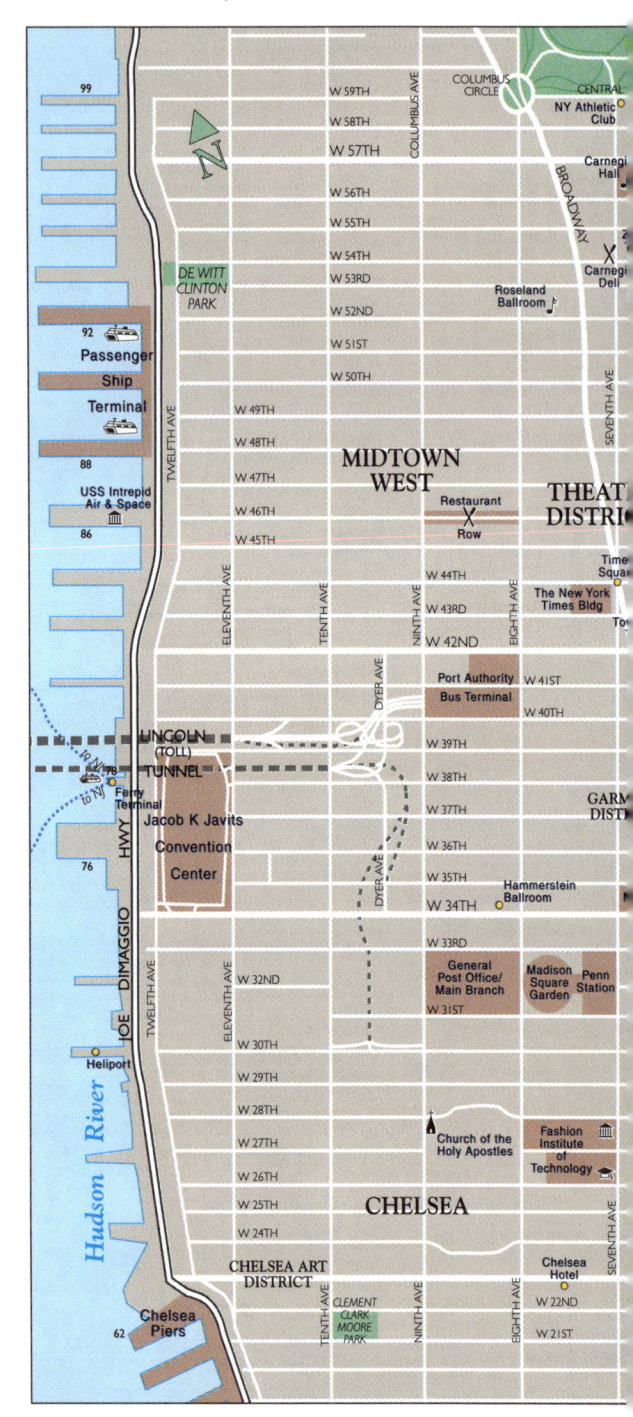

Manhattan Walking Maps
Midtown East, Fifth Avenue

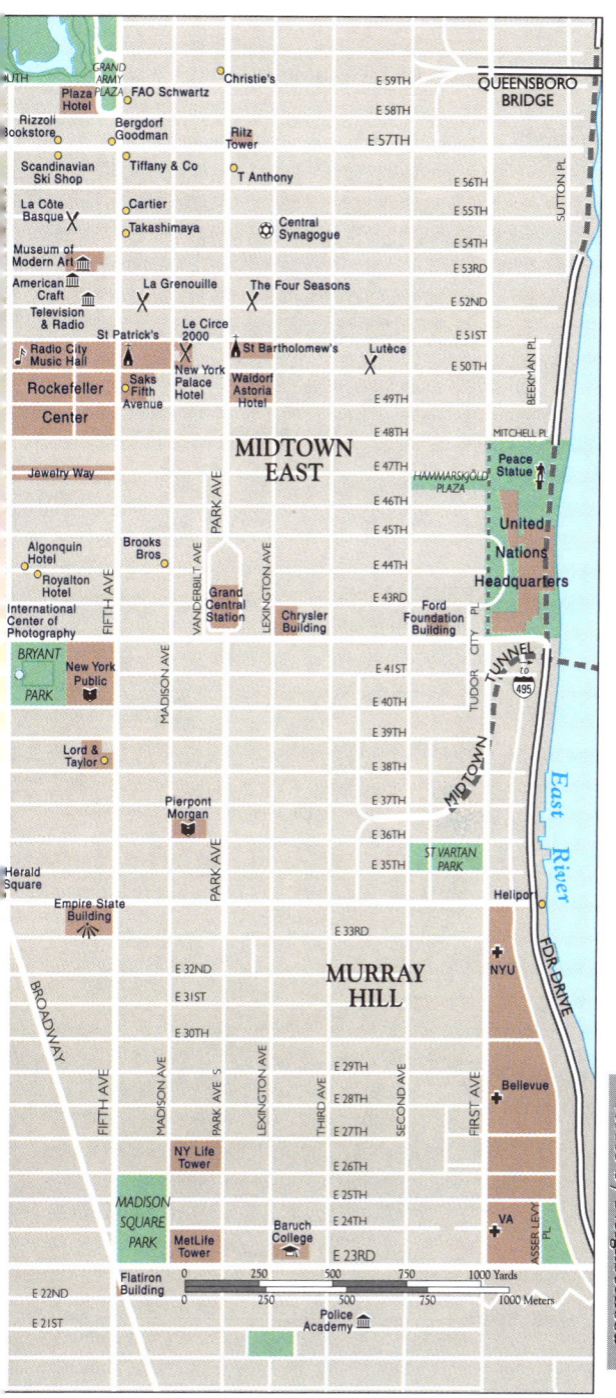

Manhattan Walking Maps
Chelsea, Flatiron, West Village, SoHo

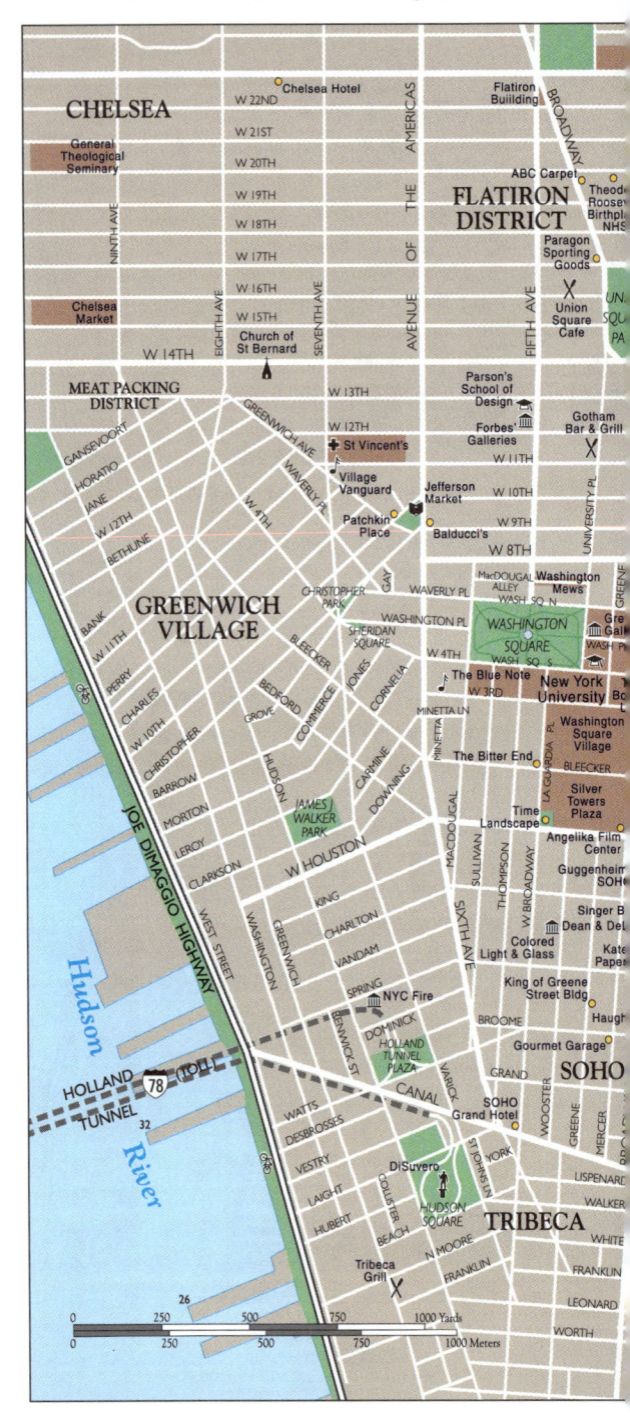

Manhattan Walking Maps
East Village, NoHo, NoLiTa, Lower East Side

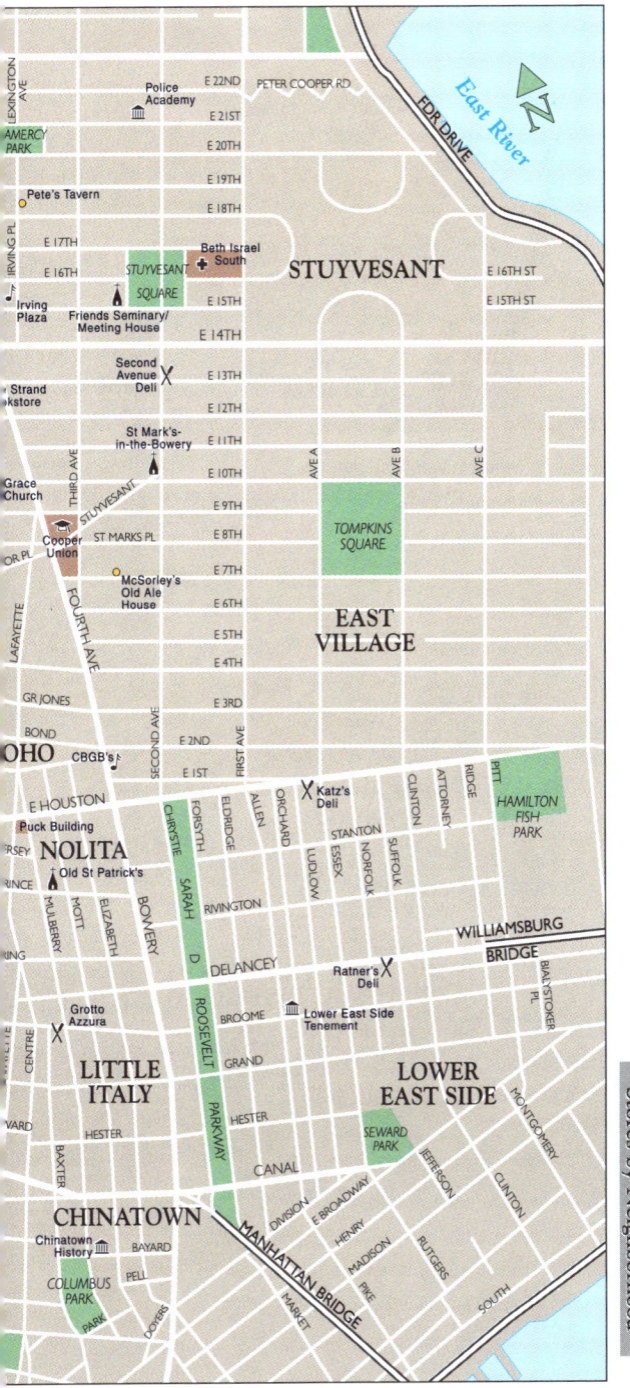

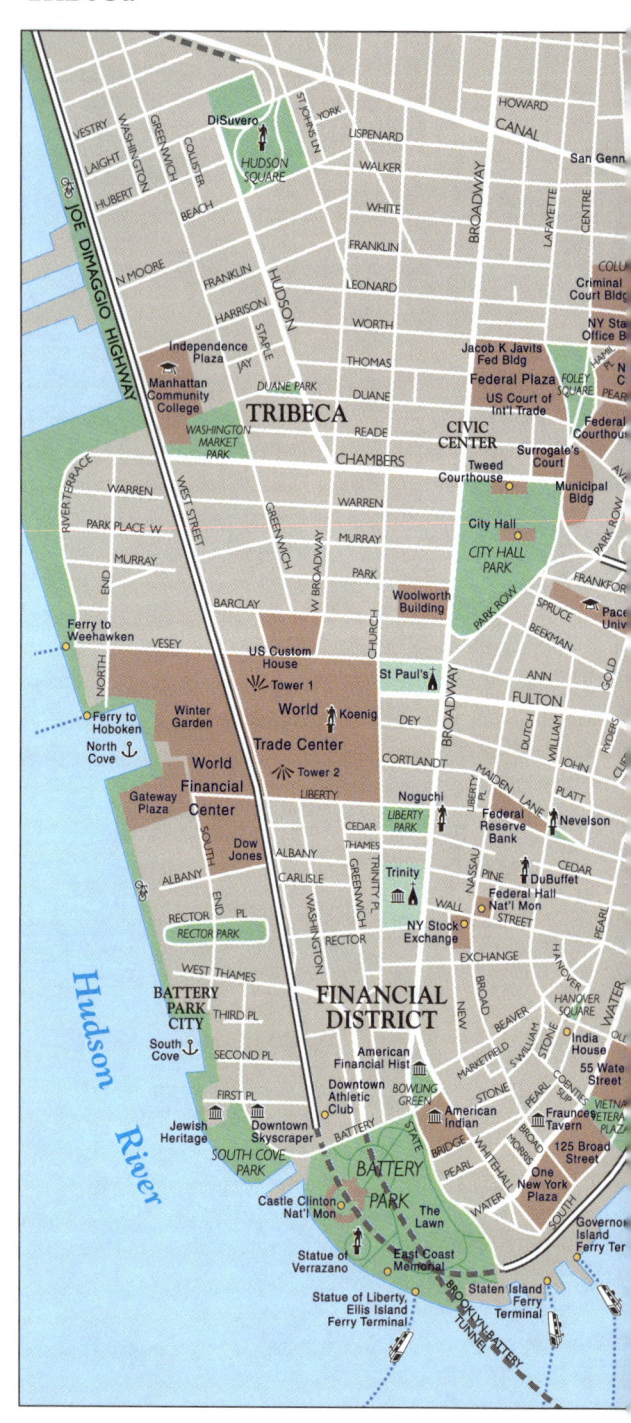

Manhattan Walking Maps
TriBeCa

Manhattan Walking Maps
Lower Manhattan

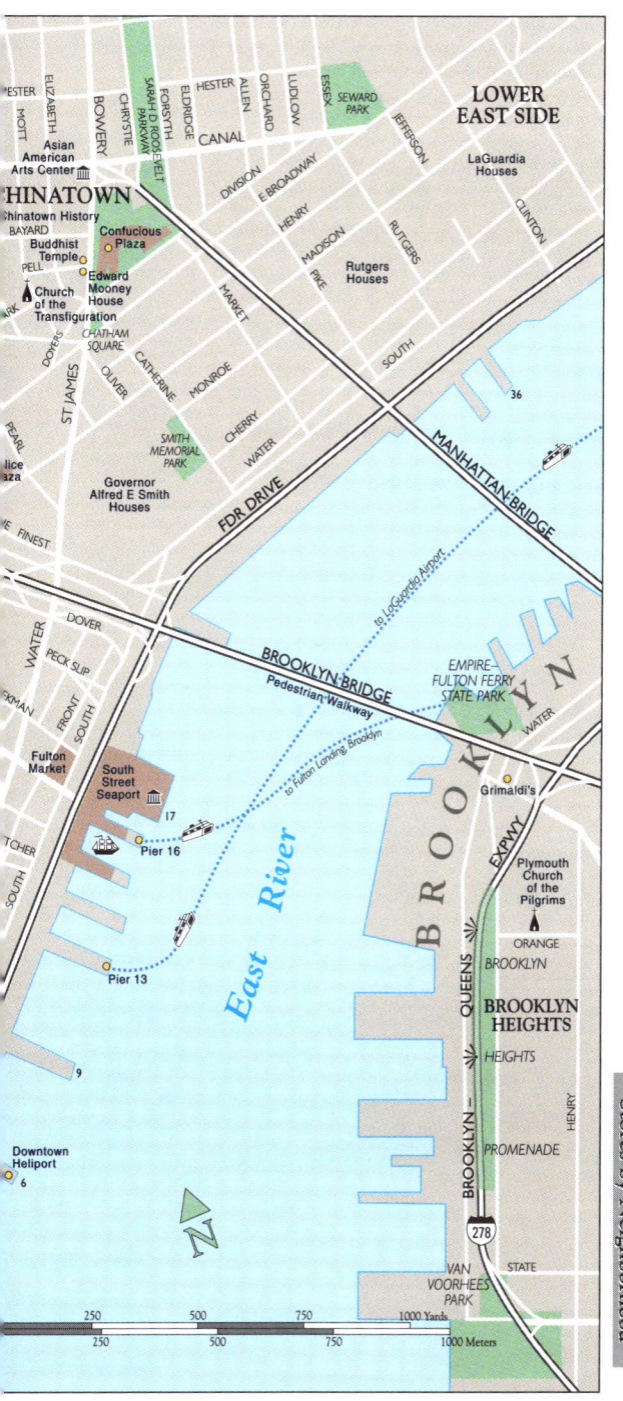

Upper East Side

Upper East Side *See map pages 244–245.*

East 90's

The Baby Collection	1384 Lexington bet. 91/92 St.
Bonpoint	1269 Madison at 91st
Capezio	1651 Third bet. 93/94 St.
Catimini	1284 Madison bet. 91/92 St.
East Side Kids	1298 Madison at 92nd
Jacadi	1281 bet. 91/92 St.
J. McLaughlin	1311 Madison bet. 92/93 St.
Rene Collection	1325 Madison bet. 93/94 St.
Veronique	1321 Madison at 93rd
Wicker Garden	1327 Madison bet. 93/94 St.

East 80's

Agnes B.	1063 Madison bet. 80/81 St.
Aldo	157 E. 86 bet. Third/Lex. Ave.
Allure	1324 Lexington bet. 88/89 St.
Anik	1122 Madison bet. 83/84 St.
Ann Taylor Loft	1492 Third bet. 84/85 St.
Au Chat Botté	1192 Madison bet. 87/88 St.
Banana Republic	1136 Madison bet. 84/85 St.
Bebe Thompson	1216 Lexington bet. 82/83 St.
Betsey Johnson	1060 Madison bet. 80/81 St.
Bis	1134 Madison bet. 84/85 St.
Blades Board and Skate	160 E. 86 bet. Third/Lex. Ave.
Bolton's	1180 Madison at 86th St.
Bolton's	161 E. 86 bet. Lex/Third Ave.
The Bridal Party- Dresses for Bridesmaids	243 E. 82 bet. Second/Third Ave.
Cashmere New York	1100 Madison bet. 82/83 St.
The Childrens Place	173 E. 86 bet. Lex./Third Ave.
Diana & Jeffries	1145 Madison at 85th
Easy Spirit	1518 Third bet. 85/86 St.
Encore	1132 Madison bet. 84/85 St.
Eric Shoes	1222 Madison at 88th
Foot Locker	159 E. 86 St. bet. Third/Lex. Ave.
Forreal	1200 Lexington bet. 81/82 St.
Franceska	1070 Madison at 81st
Gap	1511 Third at 85th
Gap Kids and Baby Gap	1535 Third bet. 86/87 St.
Gap	1164 Madison at 86th
Gap Kids and Baby Gap	1164 Madison at 86th
Great Feet	1241 Lexington at 84th
Greenstones & Cie	1184 Madison bet. 86/87 St.
Gymboree	1120 Madison bet. 83/84 St.
Infinity	1116 Madison at 83rd

Upper East Side

Little Eric Shoes	1118 Madison at 83rd
Magic Windows	1186 Madison bet. 86/87 St.
Marsha D.D.	1342 Lexington bet. 88/89 St.
Metro Bicycle	1311 Lexington at 88th
Mimi Maternity	1125 Madison at 84th
Miss Pym	1025 Fifth bet. 83/84 St.
Modell's	1535 Third bet. 86/87 St.
Motherhood Maternity	1449 Third at 82nd
Nellie M.	1309 Lexington at 88th
Nine West	184 E. 86 bet. Lex./Third
Original Leather	1100 Madison bet. 86/83 St.
Orva	155 E. 86 bet. Lex./Third
Peter Elliot	1070 Madison at 81st
Rapax	1100 Madison bet. 82/83 St.
Searle Blatt	1124 Madison at 84th
Steve Madden	150 E. 86 bet. Lex./Third Ave.
Super Runners Shop	1337 Lexington at 89th
Tartine et Chocolat	1047 Madison at 80th
Tracey Tooker Hats	1211 Lexington at 82nd
Women by Peter Elliot	1067 Madison bet. 80/81 St.

East 70's

Alexandre de Paris	971 Madison bet. 75/76 St.
Alicia Mugetti	999 Madison bet. 77/78 St.
Anik	1355 Third bet. 77/78 St.
Ann Taylor	1320 Third bet. 75/76 St.
Antoin	1110 Lexington bet. 77/78 St.
A Perfect Day In Paradise	153 E. 70 bet. Lex./Third Ave.
Arche	995 Madison at 77th
Bambini	1367 Third at 78th
Barami	1404 Second Ave. at 73rd
Bebe	1044 Madison bet. 79/80 St.
Betsey Bunky Nini	980 Lexington bet. 71/72 St.
Big Drop	1321 Third bet. 75/76 St.
Blades Board and Skate	1414 Second Ave. bet. 72/73 St.
Bloomers	1042 Lexington bet. 74/75 St.
Bra Smythe	905 Madison bet. 72/73 St.
Calypso St. Barths	935 Madison bet. 74/75 St.
Carolina Herrera	954 Madison at 74th
Cashmere-Cashmere	965 Madison bet. 75/76 St.
Christian Louboutin	941 Madison bet. 74/75 St.
Chloe	850 Madison at 70th
Cinco	960 Lexington at 70th
Clyde's on Madison	926 Madison bet. 73/74 St.
Eileen Fisher	1039 Madison bet. 79/80 St.
En Soie	988 Madison bet. 76/77 St.
Equipment	872 Madison at 71st
Eric Shoes	1333 Third at 76th

Upper East Side

Foot Locker	1345 First at 72nd
Forreal	1369 Third bet. 78/79 St.
Forreal Basics	1335 Third Ave. bet. 76/77 St.
Frederic Fekkai	874 Madison bet. 71/72 St.
French Sole	985 Lexington bet. 71/72 St.
Gamine	1322 Third bet. 75/76 St.
Gap	1066 Lexington at 75th
Gap Kids and Baby Gap	1037 Lexington at 74th
Gianfranco Ferre	845 Madison at 70th
Gymboree	1332 Third at 76th
Hanae Mori	27 E. 79 bet. Fifth/Mad.
Intermix	1003 Madison bet. 77/78 St.
Issey Miyake	992 Madison at 77th
Jay Kos	986 Lexington bet. 72/73 St.
Jennifer Tyler	854 Madison bet. 70/71 St.
J. McLaughlin	1343 Third at 77th
Judith Leiber	987 Madison bet. 76/77 St
Kids Footlocker	1504 Second bet. 78/79 St.
Lady Footlocker	1504 Second Ave. bet. 78/79 St.
Laura Beth's Baby Collection	300 E. 75 at Second Ave.
Lester's	1522 Second at 79th
Little Eric Shoes	1331 Third at 76th
Liz Lange Maternity	958 Madison bet. 75/76 St.
Luca Luca	1011 Madison at 78th
Madison Ave. Maternity & Baby	1043 Madison bet. 79/80 St.
Make 10	1227 Third bet. 70/71 St.
Makola	1045 Madison bet. 79/80 St.
Maraolo	1321 Third bet. 75/76 St.
Michael Kors	974 Madison at 76th
Michael's Resale	1041 Madison bet. 79/80 St.
Missoni	1009 Madison at 78th
Mom's Night Out	147 E. 72 bet. Lex./Third Ave.
Noriko Maeda	985 Madison bet. 76/77 St.
Nursery Lines	1034 Lexington at 74th
Oilily	870 Madison bet. 70/71 St.
Polo Ralph Lauren	867 Madison at 72nd
Polo Sport	888 Madison at 72nd
Portantina	895 Madison at 72nd
Prada	841 Madison at 70th
Precision	1310 Third at 75th
Rene Collection	1007 Madison bet. 77/78 St.
Rodier	1310 Third at 75th
San Francisco Clothing	975 Lexington bet. 70/71 St.
Santoni	864 Madison bet. 70/71 St.
Scoop	1275 Third bet. 73/74 St.
Searle Blatt	860 Madison bet. 70/71 St.
Searle Blatt	1035 Madison at 79th
Second Act Childrenswear	1046 Madison bet. 79/80 St.

Stores by Neighborhood

Upper East Side

Shen	1005 Madison bet. 77/78 St.
Small Change	964 Lexington bet. 70/71 St.
Sonia Rykiel	849 Madison bet. 70/71 St.
Spring Flowers	905 Madison bet. 72/73 St.
Steven Stolman	22 E. 72 bet. Fifth/Mad.
Stubbs & Wooten	22 E. 72 bet. Fifth/Mad.
Super Runners Shop	1244 Third bet. 71/72 St.
Talbot's	1251 Third at 72nd
Talbot's Kids	1523 Second at 79th
Vamps	1420 Second at 74th
Vera Wang	991 Madison at 77th
Vera Wang Maids on Madison	980 Madison bet. 76/77 St.
Victoria's Secret	1240 Third bet. 71/72 St.
Vincent and Edgar	972 Lexington at 71st
Vivaldi Boutique	1288 Third at 74th
Waterwear	1439 Third at 77th
Wolford	996 Madison bet. 77/78 St.
Yumi Katsuri	907 Madison bet. 72/73 St.
Yves Saint Laurent	855 Madison bet. 70/71 St.
Z' Baby & Co.	996 Lexington at 72nd
Zitomer	969 Madison bet. 75/76 St.

East 60's

Addison On Madison	698 Madison bet. 62/63 St.
Aerosoles	1555 Second at 61st
Alfred Dunhill	846 Madison bet. 69/70 St.
Ann Taylor	645 Madison at 60th
Ann Taylor Loft	1155 Third at 68 St.
Anne Fontaine	791 Madison at 67th
Anya Hindmarch	29 E. 60 bet. Madison/Park
Arche	1045 Third Ave. bet. 61/62 St.
Ashanti	872 Lexington bet. 65/66 St.
Athlete's Foot	1031 Third Ave. at 61st
Banana Republic	1131 Third at 67th
Barneys New York	660 Madison at 61st
BCBG by Max Azria	770 Madison at 66th
Bebe	1127 Third at 66th
Beretta	718 Madison bet. 63/64 St.
Berk	781 Madison bet. 66/67 St.
Betsey Johnson	251 E. 60 bet. Second/Third Ave.
Billy Martins	220 E. 60 at Third Ave.
Bogner	821 Madison bet. 68/69 St.
Bonpoint	811 Madison at 68th
Boyds	655 Madison bet. 60/61 St.
Calvin Klein	654 Madison at 60th
Canyon Beachwear	1136 Third bet. 66/67 St.
Capezio	136 E 61 bet. Lex./Park Ave.
Celine	667 Madison bet. 60/61 St.
Cerutti	789 Madison at 67th

Upper East Side

Cesare Paciotti	833 Madison bet. 69/70 St.
Charles Jourdan	777 Madison bet. 66/67 St.
Cheo Tailors	30 E. 60 bet. Mad./Park Ave.
Chuckies	1073 Third bet. 63/64 St.
Clifford Michael Design	45 E. 60 bet. Mad./Park Ave.
Club Monaco	1111 Third at 65th
Coach	710 Madison at 63rd
Cole-Haan	667 Madison at 61st
Cose Bella	7 E. 81 bet. Madison/Fifth Ave.
Country Road Australia	1130 Third bet. 66/67 St.
C.P. Shades	1119 Third bet. 65/66 St.
Davide Cenci	801 Madison bet. 67/68 St.
Diesel	770 Lexington at 60th
DKNY	665 Madison at 60th
Dolce & Gabbana	825 Madison bet. 68/69 St.
Donna Karan	819 Madison bet. 68/69 St.
Dooney & Burke	759 Madison bet. 65/66 St.
D. Porthault	11 E. 69 bet. Mad./Fifth Ave.
Eddie Bauer	1172 Third bet. 68/69 St.
Emanual Ungaro	792 Madison at 67th
Emilio Pucci	24 E. 64 bet. Mad./Fifth Ave.
Enrique Martinez	785 Madison bet. 66/67 St.
Entre Nous	1124 Third bet. 65/66 St
Etro	720 Madison bet. 63/64 St.
Fogal	680 Madison bet. 61/62 St.
Foot Locker	1187 Third at 69th
Furla	727 Madison bet. 63/64 St.
Gallery of Wearable Art	34 E. 67 bet. Mad./Park Ave.
Galo	692 Madison bet. 21/63 St.
Galo	825 Lexington at 63rd
Gap	1131-49 Third at 66th
Gap Kid and Baby Gap	1131-49 Third at 66th
Genny	831 Madison bet. 69/70 St.
Gianni Versace	815 Madison bet. 68/69 St.
Giordano's	1150 Second bet. 60/61 St.
Giorgio Armani	760 Madison at 65th
Givenchy	710 Madison at 63rd
Gymboree	1049 Third bet. 61/62 St.
Hermès	691 Madison bet. 62/63 St.
House of Dormeuil	21 E. 67 bet. Madison/Fifth Ave.
Iceberg	722 Madison at 66th
Il Bisonte	22 E. 65 bet. Fifth/Madison Ave.
Jacadi	781 Madison bet. 66/67 St.
Jaeger	818 Madison at 68/69 St.
John Lobb	680 Madison bet. 61/62 St.
J. Mendel	723 Madison bet. 63/64 St.
J.M. Weston	812 Madison at 68th
Joan & David	816 Madison bet. 68/69 St.

Upper East Side

Joseph	804 Madison bet. 67/68 St.
Joseph (pants)	796 Madison bet. 67/68 St.
Julie Artisans' Gallery	762 Madison bet. 65/66 St.
Kenzo	805 Madison bet. 67/68 St.
Krizia	769 Madison bet. 65/66 St.
La Layette	170 E. 61 bet. Third/Lex. Ave.
LaPerla	777 Madison bet. 66/67 St.
La Petite Etoile	746 Madison bet. 64/65 St.
Lee Anderson	23 E. 67 bet. Mad./Fifth Ave.
Leggiadro	700 Madison bet. 62/63 St.
Legs Beautiful	1025 Third at 61st
Les Copains	807 Madison bet. 67/68 St.
Lingerie on Lex.	831 Lexington bet. 63/64 St.
Longchamp	713 Madison bet. 63/64 St.
Loro Piana	821 Madison bet. 68/69 St.
Luca Luca	690 Madison at 62nd
Malo	814 Madison at 68th
Manrico	802 Madison bet. 67/68 St.
Maraolo	782 Lexington bet. 60/61 St.
Maraolo	835 Madison bet. 69/70 St.
Marina Rinaldi	800 Madison bet. 67/68 St.
Martier	1010 Third at 60th
Martinez Valero	1029 Third at 61st
Max Fiorentino	1024 Third bet. 60/61 St.
Max Mara	813 Madison at 68th
Menagé À Trois	799 Madison bet. 67/68 St.
Mimi Maternity	1021 Third bet. 60/61 St.
Morgane Le Fay	746 Madison bet. 64/65 St.
Moschino	803 Madison bet. 67/68 St.
Nicole Farhi	10 E. 60 bet. Madison/Fifth Ave.
Nicole Miller	780 Madison bet. 66/67 St.
Nine West	1195 Third bet. 69/70 St.
Nocturne	698 Madison bet. 62/63 St.
Oilily For Women	820 Madison bet. 68/69 St.
Olive & Bette's	1070 Madison bet. 81/82 St.
Paul & Shark	772 Madsion at 66th
Pilar Rossi	790 Madison bet. 66/67 St.
Purdey	844 Madison bet. 69/70 St.
Roberto Cavalli	711 Madison at 63rd
Robert Clergerie	681 Madison bet. 61/62 St.
Robert Talbott	680 Madison bet. 61/62 St.
Searle Blatt	1051 Third at 62nd
Sergio Rossi	835 Madison bet. 69/70 St.
Shanghai Tang	714 Madison at 63rd
Spring Flowers	1050 Third at 62nd
Stephane Kelian	717 Madison bet. 63/64 St.
Sulka	840 Madison bet. 69/70 St.
Suzanne	700 Madison bet. 62/63 St.

Upper West Side

Tanino Crisci	795 Madison bet. 67/68 St.
Tatiana Resale Boutique	860 Lexington bet. 64/65 St.
Timberland Shoes	709 Madison at 63rd
Tse Cashmere	827 Madison at 69th
Unisa	701 Madison bet. 62/63 St.
Valentino	747 Madison at 65th
Vanessa Noel	158 E. 64 bet. Lex./Third
Varda	786 Madison bet. 66/67 St.
Vertigo	755 Madison bet. 65/66 St.
Via Spiga	765 Madison bet. 65/66 St.
Walter Steiger	739 Madison bet. 64/65 St.
Warren Edwards	107 E. 60 bet. Park/Lex.
Zeller Tuxedo	1010 Third bet. 60/61 St.

Upper West Side *See map pages 244–245.*

Aerosoles	310 Columbus bet. 74/75 St.
Allan & Suzi	416 Amsterdam at 80th
Alskling	228 Columbus bet. 70/71 St.
Ann Taylor	2380 B'way at 87th
Ann Taylor	2015-17 B'way at 69th
April Cornell	487 Columbus bet. 83/84 St.
Assets London	464 Columbus bet. 82/83 St.
Athlete's Foot	2265 B'way bet. 81/82 St.
Athlete's Foot	2563 B'way bet. 96/97 St.
Banana Republic	215 Columbus bet. 69/70 St.
Banana Republic	2360 B'way at 86th
Barami	1879 B'way at 62nd
Barbara Gee Danskin Center (outlet)	2282 $1/2$ B'way bet. 82/83 St.
Barbara Gee Danskin Center (outlet)	2487 B'way bet. 92/93 St.
Bati	2323 B'way bet. 84/85 St.
Betsey Johnson	248 Columbus bet. 71/72 St.
Bicycle Renaissance	430 Columbus at 81st
Blades Board and Skate	120 W. 72 bet. Columbus/B'way
Brief Encounters	239 Columbus at 71st
Canyon Beachwear	311 Columbus bet. 74/75 St.
The Children's Place	2187 B'way at 77th
The Children's Place	2039 bet. B'way/Amsterdam Ave.
Club Monaco	2376 B'way at 87th
Coach	2321 B'way at 84th
Coco & Z	222 Columbus bet. 70/71 St.
CP Shades	300 Columbus at 74th
Crunch	162 W. 83 bet. Columbus/Amsterdam
Danskin	159 Columbus bet. 67/68 St.
Darryl's	492 Amsterdam bet. 83/84 St.
Diana & Jeffries	2062 B'way bet. 70/71 St.

Stores by Neighborhood

Upper West Side

Eastern Mountain Sports	20 W. 61 bet. B'way/Ninth Ave.
Easy Spirit	2251 B'way bet. 80/81 St.
Eddie Bauer	1978 B'way at 67th
Eileen Fisher	341 Columbus bet. 76/77 St.
Express	321 Columbus bet. 75/76 St.
Filene's Basement	2222 B'way at 79th
Frank Stella	440 Columbus at 81st
French Connection	304 Columbus bet. 74/75 St.
Furla	159A Columbus at 67th
Gap	1988 B'way at 67th
Gap Kids and Baby Gap	1988 B'way at 67th
Gap Kids and Baby Gap	341 Columbus bet. 76/77 St.
Gap	2109 B'way at 73rd
Gap	2551 B'way at 96th
Gap	2373 B'way at 86th
Gap (Women)	335 Columbus at 76th
Gap Kid and Baby Gap	2300 B'way at 83rd
Granny-Made	381 Amsterdam bet. 78/79 St.
Greenstones & Cie	442 Columbus bet. 81/82 St.
Gymboree	2271 B'way at 82nd
Gymboree	2015 B'way bet. 68/69 St.
Inside Story	198 Columbus at 69th
Kenneth Cole	353 Columbus at 77th
Kids are Magic	2293 B'way bet. 82/83 St.
Laura Ashley	398 Columbus at 79th
Lord of the Fleas	2142 B'way bet. 75/76 St.
Maraolo (outlet)	131 W. 72 bet. Amsterdam/Columbus Ave.
Mimi Maternity	2005 B'way bet. 68/69 St.
Montmartre	247 Columbus bet. 71/72 St.
Montmartre	2212 B'way bet. 78/79 St.
Nautica	216 Columbus at 70th
New Frontier	230 Columbus bet. 70/71 St.
The New York Look	30 Lincoln Plaza bet. 62/63 St.
The New York Look	2030 B'way bet. 69/70 St.
Nine West	2305 B'way bet. 83/84 St.
Olive & Bette's	252 Columbus bet. 71/72 St.
Only Hearts	386 Columbus bet. 78/79 St.
Original Leather	256 Columbus at 72nd
Patagonia	426 Columbus bet. 80/81 St.
Reebok	160 Columbus bet. 67/68 St.
Rockport	160 Columbus bet. 67/68 St.
Rosette Couturiere	160 W. 71 bet. Columbus/B'way
Sacco	324 Columbus bet. 75/76 St.
Sacco	2355 B'way bet. 85/86 St.
Sean	224 Columbus bet. 70/71 St.
Shoofly	465 Amsterdam bet. 82/83 St.
Skechers USA	2169 B'way bet. 76/77 St.
Speedo Authentic Fitness	150 Columbus at 66th

Steve Madden	2315 B'way at 84th
Super Runners Shop	360 Amster. bet. 77/78 St.
Talbots	2289-2291 B'way bet. 82/83 St.
Tibet Bazaar	473 Amsterdam bet. 82/83 St.
Toga Bike Shop	110 West End Ave. at 64th
Varda	2080 B'way bet. 71/72 St.
Variazioni	309 Columbus bet. 74/75 St.
Victoria's Secret	1981 B'way at 67th St.
Z'Baby Company	100 W. 72 at Columbus Ave.

Midtown East *See map pages 246–247.*

Aldo	730 Lex. bet. 58/59 St.
Alfred Dunhill	450 Park at 57th
Allen-Edmonds	551 Madison bet. 55/56 St.
Allen-Edmonds	24 E. 44 bet. Mad./Fifth Ave.
Alexandros Furs	5 E. 57 bet. Mad./Fifth Ave.
Ann Taylor	850 Third at 52nd
Ann Taylor Loft	150 E. 42 at Lexington
Ann Taylor loft	488 Madison at 52nd
AT Harris	11 E. 44 bet. Mad./Fifth Ave.
Athlete's Foot	41 E. 42 bet. Mad./Vanderbilt
Athlete's Foot	655 Lexington at 55th
Athletic Style	118 E. 59 bet. Park/Lex. Ave.
Bally	628 Madison at 59th
Bally	347 Madison bet. 44/45 St.
Banana Republic	130 E. 59 at Lexington
Barami	136 E. 57 at Lexington
Bebe	805 Third Ave. at 50th
Belgian Shoes	110 E. 55 bet. Park/Lex. Ave.
Bloomingdale's	1000 Third bet. 59/60 St.
Bolton's	4 E. 34 bet. Fifth/Mad. Ave.
Bostonian	515 Madison at 53rd
Bostonian	363 Madison at 43rd
Bottega Veneta	635 Madison bet. 59/60 St.
Brioni	57 E. 57 bet. Mad./Park Ave.
Brioni	55 E. 52 bet. Mad./Park Ave.
Brooks Brothers	346 Madison bet. 44/45 St.
Burberrys	9 E. 57 bet. Fifth/Mad. Ave.
Cache	805 Third bet. 49/50 St.
Chanel	15 E. 57 bet. Fifth/Mad. Ave.
Christian Dior	19 E. 57 bet. Fifth/Madison
Church's English Shoes	428 Madison at 49th
Citishoes	445 Park bet. 56/57 St.
Coach	342 Madison bet. 43/44 St.
Coach	595 Madison at 57th
Conrad's Bike Shop	25 Tudor City Pl. at 41st
Country Road Australia	335 Madison bet. 43/44 St.

Stores by Neighborhood

Midtown East

Crouch & Fitzgerald	400 Madison bet. 47/48 St.
Crunch	1109 Second Ave. bet. 58/59 St.
Custom Shop	338 Madison at 44th
Daffy's	335 Madison at 44th
Daffy's	125 E. 57 bet. Lex./Park Ave.
Dana Buchman	65 E. 57 bet. Mad./Park Ave.
Dana Buchman Petites	57 E. 57 bet. Mad./Park
Denimax	444 Madison bet. 49/50 St.
Easy Spirit	555 Madison at 56th
Eddie Bauer	711 Third bet. 44/45 St.
Eileen Fisher	521 Madison bet. 53/54 St.
Emporio Armani	601 Madison bet. 57/58 St.
Enzo Angiolini	714 Lexington bet. 57/58 St.
Enzo Angiolini	551 Madison at 55th
Enzo Angiolini	331 Madison at 43rd
Episode	625 Madison bet. 58/59 St.
Escada	7 E. 57 bet. Fifth/Mad. Ave.
Express	477 Madison bet. 51/52 St.
Express	722-728 Lexington bet. 58/59 St.
Express	733 Third at 46th
Fogal	510 Madison at 53rd
Foot Locker	150 E. 42 bet. Lex./Third Ave.
Forman's	145 E. 42 bet. Lex./Third Ave.
Frank Shattuck	18 E. 53 bet. Fifth/Mad. Ave.
Fratelli Rossetti	625 Madison at 58th
Gap	549 Third Ave. bet. 36/37 St.
Gap Kids and Baby Gap	549 Third Ave. bet. 36/37 St.
Gap	657-659 Third at 42nd
Gap Kids and Baby Gap	657-659 Third at 42nd
Gap	900 Third at 54th
Gap	734 Lexington bet. 58/59 St.
Gap	545 Madison at 55th
Gap Kids and Baby Gap	545 Madison at 55th
Gap Kids and Baby Gap	757 Third at 47th
Gap	757 Third at 47th
Geiger	505 Park at 59th
Ghurka	41 E. 57 bet. Mad./Park Ave.
H. Herzfeld	507 Madison at 52nd
Helene Arpels	470 Park bet. 57/58 St.
Holland & Holland	50 E. 57 bet. Madison/Park
Hunting World	16 E. 53 bet. Mad./Fifth Ave.
Jennifer Tyler, Two	705 Lexington at 57th
John Anthony	153 E. 51 bet. Lex./Third Ave.
Johnston & Murphy	520 Madison at 54th
Johnston & Murphy	345 Madison bet. 44/45 St.
J. Press	7 E. 44 bet. Mad./Fifth Ave.
Joseph A. Banks	366 Madison bet. 46/47 St.
J. S. Suarez	450 Park bet. 56/57 St.

Midtown East

Kavanagh's Designer Resale Shop	146 E. 49 bet. Third/Lex. Ave.
Lacoste	543 Madison bet. 54/55 St.
Lana Marks	645 Madison bet. 59/60 St.
The Leather and Suede Workshop	107 E. 59 bet. Lex./Park Ave.
Lederer	457 Madison at 51st
Legs Beautiful	153 E. 53 at Lexington Ave.
Legs Beautiful	200 Park Ave. bet. 44/45 St.
Levi Strauss	750 Lexington bet. 59/60 St.
Levi Strauss	3 E. 57 bet. Fifth/Mad. Ave.
Lexington Formalwear	12 E. 46 bet. Fifth/Mad. Ave.
Leonard Logsdail	9 E. 53 bet. Fifth/Mad. Ave.
Linda Dresner	484 Park at 58th
Louis Vuitton	49 E. 57 bet. Mad./Park Ave.
Maraolo	551 Madison at 55th
Mason's Tennis Mart	56 E. 53 bet. Madison/Park Ave.
Men's Wearhouse	380 Madison at 46th
Modell's	51 E. 42 bet. Vanderbilt/Mad. Ave.
New Balance	821 Third at 50th
Niketown	6 E. 57 bet. Fifth/Mad. Ave.
Nine West	750 Lexington bet. 58/59 St.
Nine West	757 Third bet. 47/48 St.
O.M.G.	850 Second at 45th
Overland Trading Company	712 Lexington bet. 57/58 St.
Oxxford Clothes	36 E. 57 bet. Park/Mad. Ave.
Paul Stuart	Madison at 45th
A Pea in the Pod	625 Madison bet. 58/59 St.
Plus Nine Footwear for Women	11 E. 57 bet. Madison/Fifth Ave.
Precision	522 Third at 35th
Prada	45 E. 57 St. bet. Park/Mad. Ave.
Rene Mancini	470 Park at 58th
Richard Metz Golf Equipment	425 Madison at 49th
Saint Laurie, Ltd.	350 Park Ave. bet. 51/52 St.
Searle Blatt	609 Madison bet. 57/58 St.
Seeger	400 Madison bet. 47/48 St.
The Shirt Store	51 E. 44 at Vanderbilt Ave.
Speedo Authentic Fitness	721 Lexington at 58th
Speedo Authentic Fitness	40 E. 57 bet. Park/Mad. Ave.
Speedo Authentic Fitness	90 Park Ave. at 39th
Sports Authority	845 Third Ave. at 51st
Stuart Weitzman	625 Madison bet. 58/59 St.
Sulka	430 Park at 55th
Talbot's	525 Madison bet. 53/54 St.
T. Anthony	445 Park at 56th
Thomas Pink	520 Madison bet. 53/54 St.
Tod's	650 Madison bet. 59/60 St.

Stores by Neighborhood

Midtown West

Tokyo Joe	240 E. 28 bet. Second/Third Ave.
Tootsi Plohound	38 E. 57 bet. Park/Mad. Ave.
Turnbull & Asser	42 E. 57 bet. Park/Mad. Ave.
Victoria's Secret	34 E. 57 bet. Park/Mad. Ave.
Vincent Nicolosi	510 Madison at 53rd
Walter Steiger	417 Park at 55th
Wolford	619 Madison bet. 58/59 St.
World of Golf	147 E. 47 bet. Third/Lex. Ave.
Zara International	750 Lexington at 59th

Midtown West *See map pages 246–247.*

Aldo	29 W. 34 bet. Fifth/Sixth Ave.
Alixandre	150 W. 30 bet. Sixth/Seventh Ave.
American Jean	142 W. 57 bet. Sixth/Seventh Ave.
Arche	128 W. 57 bet. Sixth/Seventh Ave.
Arthur Gluck Shirtmakers	47 W. 57 bet. Fifth/Sixth Ave.
Ascot Chang	7 W. 57 bet. Fifth/Sixth Ave.
Athlete's Foot	46 W. 34 bet. Fifth/Sixth Ave.
Athlete's Foot	1568 B'way at 47th
Banana Republic	17 W. 34 bet. Fifth/Sixth Ave.
Baldwin Formalwear	52 W. 56 bet. Fifth/Sixth Ave.
Barami	37 W. 57 bet. Fifth/Sixth Ave.
Barami	901 Sixth Ave. bet. 33/34 St.
Blades Board and Skate	901 Sixth Ave. at 32nd
Capezio	1776 B'way at 57th
Capezio	1650 B'way at 51st
Bolton's	27 W. 57 bet. Fifth/Sixth Ave.
Bolton's	110 W. 51 at Sixth Ave.
Bolton's	1700 B'way at 54th
Champs	1381-1399 Sixth at 56th
The Children's Place	1460 B'way bet. 41/42 St.
The Children's Place	901 Sixth bet. 32/33 St.
Crunch	144 W. 38 bet. B'way/ Seventh Ave.
Crunch	560 W. 43 at Eleventh Ave.
Christie Brothers Furs	333 Seventh bet. 28/29 St.
Daffy's	1311 B'way bet. 33/34 St.
Easy Spirit	1166 Sixth at 46th
Enzo Angiolini	901 Sixth bet. B'way/33 St.
Express	7 W. 34 bet. Fifth/Sixth Ave.
Express	901 Sixth bet. B'way/33 St.
Fiona Walker	451 W. 46 bet. Ninth/Tenth Ave.
Foot Locker	120 W. 34 bet. Sixth/Seventh Ave.
Foot Locker	43 W. 34 bet. Fifth/Sixth Ave.
Frank Stella	921 Seventh Ave. at 58th
Freed of London	922 Seventh Ave. at 58th
French Connection	1270 Sixth Ave. at 51st
Gap	60 W. 34 St. at B'way

Midtown West

Gap	1212 Sixth Ave. bet. 47/48 St.
Gap Kids and Baby Gap	1212 Sixth Ave. bet. 47/48 St.
Gap	1466 B'way at 42nd
Gap Kids and Baby Gap	1466 B'way at 42nd
Gap	250 W. 57 bet. B'way/Eighth Ave.
Gerry Cosby & Co.	3 Penn Plaza at MSG
H&M (Hennes & Mauritz)	34 St. bet. Fifth/Sixth Ave.
Jack Silver Formal Wear	1780 B'way bet. 57/58 St.
Keni Valenti	247 W. 30 bet. Seventh/Eighth Ave.
Lady Footlocker	901 Sixth bet. B'way/33 St.
Laura Biagiotti	4 W. 57 bet. Fifth/Sixth Ave.
Louis Féraud	3 W. 56 bet. Fifth/Sixth Ave.
Macy's at Herald Sq.	at B'way at 34 St.
Make 10	1386 Sixth bet. 56/57 St.
Manolo Blahnik	31 W. 54 bet. Fifth/Sixth Ave.
Maternity Work	16 W. 57 bet. Fifth/Sixth Ave.
Metro Bicycle	360 W. 47 at Ninth Ave.
Michelle Roth & Co.	24 W. 57 bet. Fifth/Sixth Ave.
Modell's	901 Sixth at 32nd
Motherhood Maternity	901 Sixth at 33rd
M. Steuer Company	31 W. 32 bet. Fifth/B'way
New Balance	51 W. 42 bet. Fifth/Sixth Ave.
New York Golf Center	131 W. 35 bet. B'way/Seventh Ave.
The New York Look	570 Seventh at 41st
Nine West	1230 Sixth at 49th
Norma Kamali	11 W. 56 bet. Fifth/Sixth Ave.
N. Peal	5 W. 56 bet. Fifth/Sixth Ave.
Old Navy Clothing Co.	150 W. 34 bet. Sixth/Seventh Ave.
Piccione	7 W. 56 bet. Fifth/Sixth Ave.
Ritz Furs	107 W. 57 bet. Sixth/Seventh Ave.
Rochester Big & Tall	1301 Sixth Ave. at 52nd
Rosa Custom Ties	30 W. 57 bet. Fifth/Sixth Ave.
Scandinavian Ski Shop	40 W. 57 bet. Fifth/Sixth Ave.
The Shirt Store	7 W. 56 bet. Fifth/Sixth Ave.
Soho Woman	32 W. 40 bet. Fifth/Sixth Ave.
Sports Authority	401 Seventh Ave. at 33rd
Sports Authority	57 W. 57 at Sixth Ave.
Steve Madden	45 W. 34 bet. Fifth/Sixth Ave.
Thomas Pink	1155 Sixth at 44th
Training Camp	25 W. 45 bet. Fifth/Sixth Ave.
Training Camp	1079 Sixth at 41st
Tristan & America	1230 Sixth at 49th
Variazioni	37 W. 57 bet. Fifth/Sixth Ave.
Wathne	4 W. 57 bet. Fifth/Sixth Ave.
Wet Seal	901 Sixth at 33rd
William Fioravanti	45 W. 57 bet. Fifth/Sixth Ave.
Zara International	39 W. 34 bet. Fifth/Sixth Ave.

Fifth Avenue

Fifth Avenue *See map pages 246–247.*

Alberene Cashmere	435 Fifth Ave. bet. 38/39 St.
Alan Flusser	611 Fifth Ave. bet. 49/50 St.
Ann Taylor	575 Fifth Ave. at 47th
A.Testoni	665 Fifth Ave. bet. 52/53 St.
A/X Armani Exchange	645 Fifth Ave. at 51st
Banana Republic	655 Fifth Ave. at 52nd
Banana Republic	626 Fifth Ave. at Rockefeller Ctr.
Benetton	597 Fifth Ave. bet. 48/49 St.
Bergdorf Goodman Men	745 Fifth Ave. at 58th
Bergdorf Goodman Women	754 Fifth Ave. bet. 57/58 St.
Best of Scotland	581 Fifth Ave. bet. 47/48 St.
Botticelli	666 Fifth Ave. at Rockefeller Ctr.
Botticelli	522 Fifth Ave. bet. 43/44 St.
Botticelli (women only)	620 Fifth Ave. bet. 49/50 St.
Brooks Brothers	666 Fifth Ave. bet. 52/53 St.
Bruno Magli	677 Fifth Ave. at 53rd
Club Monaco	699 Fifth Ave. bet. 54/55 St.
Coach	620 Fifth at Rockefeller Ctr.
Cole-Haan	620 Fifth Ave. at 50th
Custom Shop	618 Fifth Ave. at 49th
Dooney and Burke	725 Fifth Ave. bet. 56/57 St.
Ermenegildo Zegna	743 Fifth Ave. bet. 57/58 St.
Façonnable	689 Fifth Ave. at 54th
Fendi	720 Fifth Ave. at 56th
Forman's	560 Fifth Ave. at 46th
Gant	645 Fifth Ave. bet. 51/52 St.
Gap	680 Fifth Ave. at 54th
Geoffrey Beene	783 Fifth Ave. bet. 59/60 St.
Gianni Versace	647 Fifth Ave. bet. 51/52 St.
Gucci	685 Fifth Ave. at 54th
H&M (Hennes & Mauritz)	640 Fifth Ave. at 51st
Henri Bendel	712 Fifth Ave. at 56th
Jimmy Choo	645 Fifth Ave. at 51st
Liz Claiborne	650 Fifth Ave. at 52nd
Lord & Taylor	424 Fifth Ave. bet. 38/39 St.
Make 10	366 Fifth Ave. bet. 34/35 St.
The New York Look	551 Fifth Ave. at 45th
Nine West	675 Fifth Ave. bet. 53/54 St.
Orvis	522 Fifth at 44th
Oshkosh B'Gosh	586 Fifth Ave. bet. 47/48 St.
Prada	724 Fifth Ave. bet. 56/57 St.
Ripplu	575 Fifth Ave. bet. 46/47 St.
Saks Fifth Avenue	611 Fifth Ave. bet. 49/50 St.
Salvatore Ferragamo Men	725 Fifth Ave. bet. 56/57 St.
Salvatore Ferragamo Women	661 Fifth Ave. bet. 52/53 St.
Speedo Authentic Fitness	500 Fifth Ave. at 42nd

Flatiron / Chelsea

St. John	665 Fifth Ave. at 53rd
Takashimaya	693 Fifth Ave. bet. 54/55 St.
Today's Man	529 Fifth Ave. at 44th

Flatiron *See map pages 248–249.*

Anthropologie	85 Fifth Ave. at 16th
Banana Republic Women	89 Fifth Ave. bet. 16/17 St.
Banana Republic Men	122 Fifth Ave. at 18th
Barami	119 Fifth Ave. at 19th
Bebe	100 Fifth Ave. at 15th
The Childrens Place	36 Union Sq. East at 16th
Club Monaco	160 Fifth Ave. bet. 20/21 St.
Country Road Australia	156 Fifth Ave. bet. 20/21 St.
Couture by Jennifer Dule	133 Fifth Ave. at 20th
Crunch	54 E. 13 bet. B'way/Univ. Pl.
Daffy's	111 Fifth Ave. at 18th
Eileen Fisher	103 Fifth Ave. bet. 17/18 St.
Emporio Armani	110 Fifth Ave. at 16th
Express	130 Fifth Ave. at 18th
Foot Locker	252 First Ave. at 15th
Gap	122 Fifth Ave. bet. 17/18 St.
Gap Kids and Baby Gap	122 Fifth Ave. bet. 17/18 St.
Harry Rothman's	200 Park Ave. South at Union Sq.
Himaya	551 Fifth Ave. at 45th St.
Intermix	125 Fifth Ave. bet. 19/20 St.
J. Crew	91 Fifth Ave. bet. 16/17 St.
J. Crew	30 Rockefeller Ctr. at 50th
Joan & David	104 Fifth Ave. bet. 15/16 St.
Juno	170 Fifth Ave. at 22nd
Kenneth Cole	95 Fifth Ave. at 17th
La Gallerie la Rue	12 W. 23 bet. Fifth/Sixth Ave.
Miller's Harness Company	117 E. 24 bet. Park/Lex. Ave.
Moe Ginsburg	162 Fifth Ave. at 21st
Nine West	115 Fifth Ave. at 19th
Paragon Sporting Goods	867 B'way at 18th
Paul Smith	108 Fifth Ave. at 16th
Princeton Ski Shop	21 E. 22 bet. B'way/Park Ave. South
Skechers USA	150 Fifth Ave. bet. 19/20 St.
Space Kiddets	46 E. 21 bet. B'way/Park Ave.
Tootsi Plohound	137 Fifth Ave. bet. 20/21 St.
Victoria's Secret	115 Fifth Ave. bet. 18/19 St.
Warehouse	150 Fifth Ave. bet. 19/20 St.
Zara International	101 Fifth Ave. bet. 17/18 St.

Chelsea *See maps pages 246–247, 248–249.*

Agnes B.	13 E. 16 bet. Fifth Ave./Union Sq. West
Alexandros Furs	213 W. 28 bet. Seventh/Eighth Ave.

East Village / Lower East Side

Banana Republic (M)	111 Eighth Ave. bet. 15/16 St.
Ben Thylan Furs	345 Seventh Ave. bet. 29/30 St.
Burlington Coat Factory	707 Sixth Ave. at 23rd
Camouflage	139/141 Eighth Ave. at 17th
Comme des Garçons	520 W. 22 bet. Tenth/Eleventh Ave.
Eisenberg & Eisenberg	16 W. 17 bet. Fifth/Sixth Ave.
Fan Club	22 W. 19 bet. Fifth/Sixth Ave.
Find Outlet	361 W. 17 bet. Eighth/Ninth Ave.
Fisch for the Hip	153 W. 18 bet. Sixth/Seventh Ave.
Filene's Basement	620 Sixth Ave. bet. 18/19 St.
Gilcrest Clothing Co.	900 B'way at 20th
Giraudon	152 Eighth Ave. bet 17/18 St.
Jeffrey New York	449 W. 14 bet. Ninth/Tenth Ave.
Loehmann's	101 Seventh Ave. bet. 16/17 St.
Lucy Barnes	422 W. 15 bet. Ninth/Tenth Ave.
Metro Bicycle	546 Sixth Ave. at 15th
Motherhood Maternity	641 Sixth Ave. at 20th
Old Navy Clothing Co.	610 Sixth Ave. bet. 17/18 St.
Original Leather	84 Seventh Ave. bet 15/16 St.
Out Of Our Closet	136 W. 18 bet. Sixth/Seventh Ave.
Parke & Ronen	176 Ninth Ave. at 21st
Powers Court Tennis Outlet	132 1/2 W. 24 bet. Sixth/Seventh Ave.
Reebok Golf Shop	Chelsea Pier 59 at 23rd
Reminiscence	50 W. 23 bet. Fifth/Sixth Ave.
Sacco	94 Seventh Ave bet. 15/16 St.
Sports Authority	636 Sixth at 19th
Thread	408 W. 15 bet. Ninth/Tenth Ave.
TJ Maxx	620 Sixth Ave. bet. 18/19 St.
Today's Man	625 Sixth Ave. bet. 18/19 St.

East Village / Lower East Side *See map pages 248–249.*

A. Cheng	443 E. 9 bet. Ave. A/First Ave.
Akiue-Go	445 E. 9 bet. Ave. A/First Ave.
Amy Downs Hats	103 Stanton bet. Orchard/Ludlow
Anna	150 E. 3 bet. Ave. A/B
Barbara Feinman Millinery	66 E. 7 bet. First/Second Ave.
Barbara Shaum	60 E. 4 bet. Bowery/Second Ave.
Bridge	98-100 Orchard bet. Broome/Delancey
Cherry	185 Orchard bet. Houston/Stanton
Chuck Roaste	49 Clinton bet. Rivington/Stanton
Daryl K	208 E. 6 bet. Second/Third Ave.
DDC Lab	180 Orchard bet. Stanton/Houston
D/L Cerney	13 E. 7 bet. Second/Third Ave.
Do Kham	304 E. 5 bet. First/Second Ave.
Eileen Fisher	314 E. 9 bet. First/Second Ave.
Enerla	48 E. 7 bet. First/Second Ave.
Eugenia Kim	203 E. 4 bet. Ave. A/B

NoHo / West Village

February Eleventh	315 E. 9 bet. First/Second Ave.
Fine & Klein	119 Orchard at Delancey
Foley + Corinna	108 Stanton bet. Ludlow/Essex
Foot Locker	94 Delancey bet. Ludlow/Orchard
Forman's	82 Orchard bet. Broome/Grand
Fragile	189 Orchard bet. Houston/Stanton
Gabbriel Ichak	430 E. 9 bet. First/Ave. A
Gap	133 Second Ave. at St. Marks Place
Gap (Men)	750 B'way bet. Astor Pl./8 St.
Hello Sari	261 Broome bet. Allen/Orchard
Jill Anderson	331 E. 9 bet. First/Second Ave.
Jutta Neumann	317 E. 9 bet. First/Second Ave.
Klein's of Monticello	105 Orchard at Delancey
Leather Corner	144 Orchard at Rivington
Leather Rose	412 E. 9 bet. First/Ave.A
Lina Tsai	436 E. 9 bet First/Ave. A
Lord of the Fleas	305 E. 9 bet. First/Second Ave.
MarcoArt	186 Orchard bet. Houston/Stanton
Mark Montana	434 E. 9 bet. First/Ave. A
Meghan Kinney Studio	312 E. 9 bet. First/Second Ave
Metro Bicycle	332 E. 14 bet. First/Second Ave.
New York City Custom Leather	168 Ludlow bet. Houston/Stanton
Nicole Vaughn	110 E. 7 bet. First/Ave. A
99X	84 E. 10 bet. 3/4 St.
Nova USA	100 Stanton St. at Ludlow
The Open Door Gallery	27 E. 3 bet. Second Ave./Bowery
Red Tape by Rebecca Dannenberg	333 E. 9th bet. First/Second Ave.
Resurrection Vintage	123 E. 7 bet. First/Ave. A
Selia Yang	328 E. 9 bet. First/Second Ave.
Skella	156 Orchard St. bet. Rivington/Stanton
Studio 109	115 St. Marks Place bet. Ave. A/First Ave.
TG-170	170 Ludlow bet. Houston/Stanton
Timtoum	179 Orchard bet. Houston/Stanton
Tokio 7	64 E. 7 bet. First/Second Ave.
Tokyo Joe	334 E. 11 bet. First/Second Ave.
Urban Outfitters	162 Second Ave. bet. 10/11 St.
Zao	175 Orchard bet. Houston/Stanton

NoHo / West Village *See map pages 248–249.*

Aerosoles	63 E. 8 bet. B'way/University Pl.
Aldo	700 B'way at W. 4th
Andy's Chee-pees	691 B'way bet. 3/4 St.
Antique Boutique	712-714 B'way bet. 4 St./Astor Pl.
Arche	10 Astor Place bet. Lafayette/B'way
Arleen Bowman	353 Bleecker bet. W. 10/Charles St.

Stores by Neighborhood

SoHo / NoLiTa

Athlete's Foot	60 E. 8 at B'way
Atrium	644 B'way at Bleecker
Banana Republic	205 Bleecker at Sixth Ave.
Basis Basic	710 B'way bet. Wash. Pl./4 St.
Benetton	749 B'way bet. 8 St./Astor Pl.
Blades Board and Skate	659 B'way bet. 3 St./Bleecker
Bond 07	7 Bond bet. B'way/ Lafayette
Crunch	404 Lafayette bet. Astor/E. 4 St.
Crunch	152 Christopher St. bet. Wash./Greenwich St.
Daryl K	21 Bond bet. Lafayette/Bowery
Doll House	400 Lafayette at E. 4th
Eastern Mountain Sports	611 B'way bet. Houston/Bleecker
Foot Locker	734 Broadway at 8th
French Connection	700 B'way bet. Wash. Pl./4 St.
Gap	345 Sixth Ave. at 4th
Gap Kids and Baby Gap	354 Sixth Ave. at Washington Pl.
Ghost	28 Bond bet. Lafayette/Bowery
Jungle Planet	175 W. 4 bet Sixth/Seventh Ave.
Katayone Adeli	35 Bond St. bet. Lafayette/Bowery
La Gallerie la Rue	385 Bleecker at Perry
La Petite Coquette	51 University Pl. bet 9/10 St.
Luichiny	21 W. 8 bet. Fifth/Sixth Ave.
Make 10	680 B'way bet. Bond/W. Third St.
Marc Jacobs	403 Bleecker bet. W. 11/Hudson
Milen Shoes	23 W. 8 bet. Fifth/Sixth Ave.
Original Leather	171 W. 4 bet Sixth/Seventh Ave.
Original Leather	552 LaGuardia Pl. bet. Bleecker/W. 3 St.
Patricia Field	10 E. 8 bet. Fifth/University Place
Petit Peton	27 W. 8 bet. Fifth/Sixth Ave.
Screaming Mimi's	382 Lafayette bet. Great Jones/4 St.
Skechers USA	55 W. 8 bet. Fifth/Sixth Ave.
Sleek on Bleecker	361 Bleecker bet. W. 10/Charles
Tibet Arts & Crafts	197 Bleecker bet. MacDougal/Sixth Ave.
Tupli	378 Bleecker bet. Charles/Perry
Untitled	26 W. 8 bet. Fifth/Sixth Ave.
Urban Outfitters	374 Sixth Ave. bet. Waverly/Wash. Pl.
Urban Outfitters	628 B'way bet. Houston/Bleecker
Verve	353 Bleecker bet. W. 10/Charles
Wet Seal	670 B'way at Bond St.
Wolford	52 University Pl. bet. 9/10 St.
X.O.X.O.	732 B'way at Waverly Pl.

SoHo / NoLiTa *See map pages 248–249.*

Add	461 W. B'way bet. Houston/Prince
A Détacher	262 Mott bet. Houston/Prince
Agnes B.	116 Prince bet. Wooster/Greene
Agnes B. Hommes	79 Greene at Spring
Aldo	579 B'way bet. Houston/Prince

SoHo / NoLiTa

Alexia Crawford Accessories	199 Prince bet. Sullivan/McDougal
Alice Underground	481 B'way bet. Broome/Grand
Alpana Bawa	41 Grand bet. W. B'way/Thompson
American Colors	232 Elizabeth bet. Prince/Houston
Amy Chan	247 Mulberry bet. Prince/Spring
Anna Sui	113 Greene bet. Prince/Spring
Anne Fontaine	93 Greene bet. Prince/Spring
Anthropologie	375 W. B'way bet. Broome/Spring
A.P.C.	131 Mercer bet. Prince/Spring
The Apartment	101 Crosby bet. Prince/Spring
Atsuro Tayama	120 Wooster bet. Spring/Prince
Avitto	424 W. B'way bet. Prince/Spring
A/X Armani Exchange	568 B'way at Prince
Bagutta	402 W. B'way at Spring
Banana Republic Men	528 B'way at Spring
Banana Republic Women	552 B'way bet. Prince/Spring
Barbara Bui	117 Wooster bet. Prince/Spring
Beau Brummel	421 W. B'way bet. Prince/Spring
Bebesh	425 W. B'way bet. Prince/Spring
Betsey Johnson	138 Wooster bet. Prince/Houston
Big Drop	174 Spring bet. Thompson/W. B'way
Bill Amberg	230 Elizabeth bet. Prince/Houston
Bisou-Bisou	474 W. B'way bet. Houston/Prince
Bicycle Habitat	244 Lafayette bet. Prince/Spring
Blue Bag	266 Elizabeth at Houston
Buffalo Chips Bootery	355 W. B'way bet. Broome/Grand
Calypso Enfants	284 Mulberry bet. Houston/Prince
Calypso St. Barths	280 Mott bet. Houston/Prince
Calypso St. Barths	424 Broome bet. Crosby/Lafayette
Calypso St. Barths	280 Mulberry bet. Houston/Prince
Camper	125 Prince at Wooster
Canal Jean Company	504 B'way bet. Spring/Broome
Catherine	468 Broome at Greene
Christine Ganeaux	45 Crosby bet. Spring/Broome
Christopher Totman	262 Mott bet. Houston/Prince
Chuckies	399 W. B'way bet. Broome/Spring
CK Calvin Klein Shoes and Bags	133 Prince bet. Wooster/W.B'way
Claire Blaydon	202A Mott bet. Spring/Kenmare
Club Monaco	121 Prince bet. Wooster/Greene
Club Monaco	520 B'way at Spring
Costume National	108 Wooster bet. Prince/Spring
Country Road Australia	411 W. B'way bet. Spring/Prince
C.P. Shades	154 Spring bet. Wooster/W. B'way
Crunch	623 Broadway at Houston
Cynthia Rowley	112 Wooster bet. Prince/Spring
Daang Goodman	68 Greene bet. Broome/Spring

Stores by Neighborhood

SoHo / NoLiTa

Daffy's	462 B'way at Grand
David Aaron	529 B'way bet. Spring/Prince
Deborah Moorfield	466 Broome bet. Mercer/Greene
Deco Jewels	131 Thompson bet. Prince/Houston
Detour	472 W. B'way bet. Houston/Prince
Detour	154 Prince bet. W. B'way/Thompson
Detour	425 W. B'way bet. Prince/Spring
D & G	434 W. B'way bet. Prince/Spring
DieselStyleLab	416 W. B'way bet. Prince/Spring
Do Kham	51 Prince bet. Mulberry/Lafayette
Dosa	107 Thompson bet. Spring/Prince
The Dressing Room	49 Prince bet. Lafayette/Mulberry
Eastern Mountain Sports	611 Broadway at Houston
Eddie Bauer	578 B'way bet. Houston/Prince
Eileen Fisher	395 W. B'way bet. Broome/Spring
Emporio Armani	410 W. B'way bet. Spring/Prince
Epperson Studio	25 Thompson bet. Watts/Grand
Erica Tanov	204 Elizabeth bet. Spring/Prince
Final Home	241 Lafayette bet. Prince/Spring
Find	229 Mott bet. Prince/Spring
Fortuna Valentino	422 W. B'way bet. Prince/Spring
French Connection	435 W. B'way bet. Prince/Spring
Fuchsia	126 Baxter bet. Hester/Canal
Furla	430 W. B'way bet. Spring/Prince
Goffredo Fantini	248 Elizabeth bet. Prince/Houston
Guess?	537 B'way bet. Prince/Spring
Hans Koch	174 Prince bet. Sullivan/Thompson
Harriet Love	126 Prince bet. Wooster/Greene
The Hat Shop	120 Thompson bet. Prince/Spring
Hedra Prue	281 Mott bet. Houston/Prince
Heun	543 Broadway bet. Prince/Spring
Helmut Lang	80 Greene bet. Spring/Broome
Henry Lehr	232 Elizabeth bet. Houston/Prince
Henry Lehr	268 Elizabeth bet. Houston/Prince
Hotel Venus	382 W. B'way bet. Broome/Spring
If	94 Grand bet. Mercer/Greene
Il Bisonte	72 Thompson bet. Broome/Spring
Ina	101 Thompson bet. Spring/Prince
Ina	21 Prince bet. Mott/Elizabeth
Ina	262 Mott bet. Houston/Prince
In The Black	130 Thompson bet. Houston/Prince
Institut	97 Spring bet. B'Way/Mercer
Institut	99 Spring bet. B'Way/Mercer
Iramo	89 Spring bet. Mercer/W. B'way
Jack Spade	56 Greene bet. Spring/Broome
Jamin Puech	252 Mott bet. Houston/Prince
Janet Russo	262 Mott St. bet. Houston/Prince
J. Crew	99 Prince at Mercer

SoHo / NoLiTa

Jenny B.	118 Spring bet. Mercer/Greene
Jill Stuart	100 Greene bet. Prince/Spring
John Fluevog	104 Prince bet. Greene/Mercer
Joovay	436 W. B'way at Prince
Joseph	115 Greene bet. Spring/Prince
Julian and Sara	103 Mercer bet. Prince/Spring
Juno	550 B'way bet. Prince/Spring
Kate Spade	454 Broome at Mercer
Kazuyo Nakano	223 Mott bet. Spring/Prince
Keiko	62 Greene bet. Spring/Broome
Kelly Christy	235 Elizabeth bet. Houston/Prince
Kenneth Cole	597 B'way bet. Prince/Houston
Kenzo	80 Wooster bet. Spring/Broome
Kerquelen	44 Greene bet. Grand/Broome
Kerquelen	430 W. B'way bet. Prince/Spring
Kinnu	43 Spring bet. Mott/Mulberry
Kirna Zabête	96 Greene bet. Spring/Prince
Language	238 Mulberry bet. Prince/Spring
Laundry, by Shelli Segal	97 Wooster bet. Prince/Spring
Laundry Industry	121 Spring at Greene
Le Corset	80 Thompson bet. Spring/Broome
Legacy	109 Thompson bet. Prince/Spring
LeSportSac	176 Spring bet. W. B'way/Thompson
Lilliput/SoHo Kids	265 Lafayette bet. Spring/Prince
Lilliput/SoHo Kids	240 Lafayette bet. Spring/Prince
Lisa Shaub	232 Mulberry bet. Prince/Spring
Liza Bruce	80 Thompson bet. Spring/Broome
Louie	68 Thompson bet. Spring/Broome
Louis Vuitton	116 Greene bet. Spring/Prince
Lucky Brand Dungarees	38 Greene at Grand
M-A-G	120 Wooster bet. Prince/Spring
Makie	109 Thompson bet. Prince/Spring
Malia Mills	199 Mulberry bet. Spring/Kenmare
Malo	125 Wooster bet. Prince/Spring
Marc Jacobs	163 Mercer bet. Houston/Prince
Mare	426 W. B'way bet. Prince/Spring
Margie Tsai	4 Prince bet. Elizabeth/Bowery
Marianne Novobatzky	65 Mercer bet. Spring/Broome
Mark Schwartz	45 Spring bet. Spring/Mulberry
Mary Efron	68 Thompson bet. Broome/Spring
Mavi	510 Broome bet. Thompson/W. B'way
Max Studio	415 W. B'way bet. Prince/Spring
Mayle	252 Elizabeth bet. Prince/Spring
Miu Miu	100 Prince bet. Greene/Mercer
Morgane Le Fay	67 Wooster bet. Spring/Broome
Nancy Geist	107 Spring at Mercer
Nanette Lepore	423 Broome bet. Lafayette/Crosby
New & Almost New (NAAN)	65 Mercer bet. Spring/Broome

SoHo / NoLiTa

The New York Look	468 W. B'way bet. Houston/Prince
Nicole Miller	134 Prince bet. Wooster/W. B'way
Nine West	577 B'way at Prince
The 1909 Company	63 Thompson bet. Broome/ Spring
North Beach Leather	523 B'way at Spring
Oasis	138 Spring at Wooster
Old Navy Clothing Co.	503 B'way bet. Spring/Broome
Omari	132 Prince bet. Wooster/W. B'way
O.M.G.	546 B'way bet. Spring/Prince
Original Leather	176 Spring bet. Thompson/W. B'way
Patagonia	101 Wooster bet. Prince/Spring
Pearl River	277 Canal at B'way
Peter Fox Shoes	105 Thompson bet. Spring/Prince
Peter Hermann	118 Thompson bet. Spring/Prince
Philosophy by Alberta Ferretti	452 W. B'way bet. Houston/Prince
Pierre Garroudi	139 Thompson bet. Prince/Houston
Pleats Please, Issey Miyake	128 Wooster at Prince
Plein Sud	70 Greene bet. Spring/Broome
Polo Sport	381 W. Broadway bet. Broome/Spring
Prada Sport	116 Wooster bet. Prince/Spring
Product	71 Mercer bet. Spring/Broome
Product	219 Mott bet. Prince/Spring
Quiksilver	109 Spring bet. Mercer/Greene
Rampage	127 Prince at Wooster
René Lezard	417 W. B'way bet. Spring/Prince
Replay Country Store	109 Prince at Greene
Resurrection Vintage	217 Mott bet. Prince/Spring
Reva Mivasagar	28 Wooster at Grand
Sacco	111 Thompson bet. Spring/Prince
The Sak	521 B'way bet. Spring/Broome
Sample	280 Elizabeth bet. Houston/Prince
Scarlet & Sage	7 Prince bet. Elizabeth/Bowery
Scoop	532 B'way bet. Prince/Spring
Sean	132 Thompson bet. Houston/Prince
Seize sur Vingt	243 Elizabeth bet. Houston/Prince
Sharagano	529 B'way bet. Spring/Prince
Shin Choi	119 Mercer bet. Prince/Spring
Shoe	197 Mulberry bet. Spring/Kenmare
Sigerson Morrison	28 Prince bet. Mott/Elizabeth
Silverado	542 B'way bet. Prince/Spring
Sisley	469 W. B'way bet. Prince/Houston
Shambala	92 Thompson bet. Prince/Spring
Skechers USA	530 B'way at Spring
Soco	55 Spring bet. Lafayette/Mulberry
Soho Jeans	69 W. Houston bet. Wooster/W. B'way
Stephane Kelian	158 Mercer bet. Houston/Prince
Steve Madden	540 B'way bet. Prince/Spring

Lower Manhattan / TriBeCa

Steven Alan	60 Wooster bet. Broome/Spring
Steven Alan	558 Broome bet. Sixth Ave./Varick
The Stork Club	142 Sullivan bet. Prince/Houston
Stream	69 Mercer bet. Spring/Broome
Su-zen	17 Greene bet. Grand/Canal
Sylvia Heisel	131 Thompson bet. Houston/Prince
Team Shoes	480 W. B'way bet. Houston/Prince
Ted Baker London	107 Grand bet. Mercer/B'way
Tehen	91 Greene bet. Prince/Spring
Tibet Arts & Crafts	144 Sullivan bet. Houston/Prince
Tocca	161 Mercer bet. Houston/Prince
Todd Oldham	123 Wooster bet. Spring/Prince
Tootsi Plohound	413 W. B'way bet. Spring/Prince
Tracy Feith	209 Mulberry bet. Spring/Kenmare
Transfer International	594 B'way bet. Prince/Houston
Tristan & America	560 B'way bet. Prince/Spring
Trufaux	301 W. B'way bet. Grand/Canal
TseSurface	226 Elizabeth bet. Prince/Houston
Utility Canvas	146 Sullivan bet. Houston/Prince
Varda	149 Spring bet. Wooster/W. B'way
Ventilo	69 Greene bet. Spring/Broome
Via Spiga	390 W. B'way bet. Spring/Broome
Victoria's Secret	565 B'way bet. Prince/Spring
Vilebrequin	436 W. B'way bet. Spring/Prince
Vivienne Tam	99 Greene bet. Spring/Prince
Vivienne Westwood	71 Greene bet. Spring/Broome
Wang	166 Elizabeth bet. Spring/Kenmare
Warehouse of London	581 B'way bet. Houston/Prince
Wearkstatt	33 Greene at Grand
What Comes Around Goes Around	351 W. B'way bet. Broome/Grand
Wolford	122 Greene at Prince
X.O.X.O.	426 W. B'way bet. Prince/Spring
Yaso	62 Grand bet. Wooster/W. B'way
Yohji Yamamoto	103 Grand at Mercer
Yves St. Laurent Rive Gauche Men	88 Wooster bet. Spring/Broome
Yvone Christa	107 Mercer bet. Prince/ Spring
Zabari	506 B'way bet. Spring/Broome
Zara International	580 B'way at Prince
Zero	225 Mott bet. Prince/Spring
Zion	367 W. B'way at Broome

Lower Manhattan / TriBeCa *See map pages 250–251.*

Abercrombie & Fitch	119 Water St. at S.S.S.
Aerosoles	18 John St. bet. B'way/Nassau
American Eagle Outfitters	89 South St. at S.S.S.
August Max Women	330 World Trade Ctr. bet. Church/Vesey

Stores by Neighborhood

Barami	4 World Trade Center bet. Church/Vesey
Barneys New York	2 World Fin. Ctr.
Brooks Brothers	1 Liberty Plaza at Church St.
Bu and the Duck	106 Franklin bet. W. B'way/Church
Century 21	22 Cortland St. bet. Church/B'way
Champs	89 S.S.S at Pier 17
The Children's Place	400 World Trade Center bet. Liberty/Church St.
Coach	5 World Trade Ctr. bet. Church/Vesey
Country Road Australia	199 Water at S.S.S.
Custom Shop	60 Wall St. bet. Pine/Williams
D/L Cerney	222 W. B'way bet. Franklin/White
Easy Spirit	182 B'way bet. John/Maiden Lane
Foot Locker	89 S.S.S. at Pier 17
Forman's	59 John St. at William
Gap	157 World Trade Ctr.
Gap	89 S.S.S. at Pier 17
Gap Kid and Baby Gap	89 S.S.S. at Pier 17
Gap Kid and Baby Gap	225 Liberty at the World Fin. Ctr.
Gorsart	9 Murray bet. B'way/Church
Guess?	23-25 Water at S.S.S.
Hatitude	93 Reade bet. W. B'way/Church
J. Crew	203 Front St at S.S.S.
Jimin Lee/Translatio	13 White bet. Sixth Ave./W. B'way
Johnston & Murphy	1 World Trade Ctr. bet. Liberty/Vesey
Koh's Kids	311 Greenwich St. bet. Chambers/Reade
Lady Footlocker	89 South St. at S.S.S.-Pier 17
Legs Beautiful	225 Liberty at World Fin. Ctr.
The Limited	503 World Trade Ctr. bet. Church/Vesey
Mark Christopher	80 Wall St. bet. Water/Beaver
Metro Bicycle	417 Canal at Sixth Ave.
Mika Inatome	11 Worth bet. W. B'way/Hudson
Modell's	200 B'way bet. Fulton/John
Nine West	313 World Trade Ctr.
Peanutbutter and Jane	617 Hudson bet. Jane/W. 12 St.
Pearl River	277 Canal at Broadway
Rochester Big & Tall	67 Wall St. at Pearl St.
Samuel's Hats	74 Nassau bet. John/Fulton
Seam	117 West B'way bet. Duane/Reade
Shack, Inc	137 W. B'way bet. Duane/Thomas
The Shirt Store	71 B'way bet. Rector/Exchange
Shoofly	42 Hudson bet. Duane/Thomas
Sunrise Ruby	141 Reade bet. Greenwich/Hudson
Tahari	225 Liberty at World Financial. Ctr.
Talbots	189-191 Front St. at S.S.S.
Tribeca Luggage & Leather	295 Greenwich bet. Chambers/Warren

Stores by Neighborhood

Victoria's Secret — Pier 17 at S.S.S.
Young's Hat Corner — 139 Nassau at Beekman

Brooklyn

Kleinfeld & Son — 8202 Fifth Ave.

Repairs and Services

Dry Cleaners

Mending and Alterations

Custom Design Tailors

Shoe Repairs

Leather Repair (Handbags & Luggage)

Trimmings (Ribbons, Buttons, etc.)

Thrift Shops

"Some 130 years ago, Thomas Burberry wove a new cloth called gabardine which was waterproof and nearly tearproof. The material was fashioned into a trenchcoat for soldiers in the Great War of 1914, with pockets and holders for knives and grenades. But it also became a staple for any gentleman—and icon when Bogey wore it in Casablanca."
—*Gear Magazine*

"Style is an expression of individualism mixed with charisma. Fashion is something that comes after style."
—*John Fairchild*

"Sweats are clothes." —*Rosie O'Donnell*

Repairs and Services

Dry Cleaners—Haute Couture & Bridal

Dunrite
141 West 38th Street
NYC 10018
212-221-9297
bet. B'way/7th Ave.
Mon.-Fri. 7:30-5:20

Fashion Award Cleaners
1462 Lexington Avenue
NYC 10128
212-289-5623
bet. 94/95th St.
Mon.-Fri. 7:30-6:30, Sat. 9-3

Hallak Cleaners
1232 Second Avenue
NYC 10021
212-879-4694
bet. 64/65th St.
Mon.-Fri. 7-6:30, Sat. 8-3

Jeeves of Belgravia
39 East 65th Street
NYC 10021
212-570-9130
bet. Madison/Park Ave.
Mon.-Fri. 8-6:30,
Sat. 10-2 (summer months only)

Madame Paulette
1255 Second Avenue
NYC 10021
212-838-6827
bet. 65/66th St.
Mon.-Fri. 7:30-7, Sat. 8-5

Montclair
1331 Lexington Avenue
NYC 10128
212-289-2070
bet. 88/89th St.
Mon.-Fri. 7-7, Sat. 8-5

Dry Cleaners—Leather and Suede

Leathercraft Process of America
Two locations in New York,
call for information.
212-564-8980
800-845-6155

Nilo Cleaners
1173 Lexington Avenue
NYC 10028
212-861-8071
at 80th Street
Mon.-Fri. 7-7, Sat. 8-4

Dry Cleaners—All-Purpose Cleaners

Anita Cleaners
1380 First Avenue
NYC 10021
212-717-6602
bet. 73/74th St.
Mon.-Fri. 8-7

Handy Cleaners
204 West 55th Street
NYC 10019
212-247-0922
bet. 7th Ave./B'way
Mon.-Fri. 7-7, Sat. 8-6

Meurice Garment Care
31 University Place
NYC 10003
212-475-2778
bet. 8/9th St.
Mon.-Fri. 7:30-7, Sat. 7:30-5

Meurice Garment Care & Tiecrafters
245 East 57th Street
NYC 10022
212-759-9057
bet. 2/3rd Ave.
Mon.-Fri. 8-6:30, Sat. 9-3

Midnight Express
38-38 Thirteenth Street
Long Island City
212-921-0111
800-7-MIDNITE

Will pick up and deliver for a small minimum charge.

Repairs and Services

Montclair　　212-289-2070
1331 Lexington Avenue　　bet. 88/89th St.
NYC 10128　　Mon.-Fri. 7-7, Sat. 8-5

New York's Finest French Cleaners　　212-431-4010
144 Reade Street　　bet. Hudson/Greenwich
NYC 10013　　Mon.-Fri. 7:30-6:30, Sat. 8:30-5

Tiecrafters　　212-629-5800
252 West 29th Street　　bet. 7/8th Ave.
NYC 10001　　Mon.-Fri. 8:30-5, Sat. 9-2

Young's Cleaners and Launderers　　212-473-6154
188 Third Avenue　　at 17th St.
NYC 10003　　Mon.-Fri. 7-7, Sat. 8-5

Mending and Alterations

Alfonso Sciortino Custom Alteration　　212-888-2846
57 West 57th Street, Suite 602　　at 6th Ave.
NYC 10019　　Mon.-Fri. 10-6, Sat. 10-5

Bhambi Custom Tailors　　212-935-5379
14 East 60th Street, Rm. 610　　bet. 5th/Madison Ave.
NYC 10022　　Mon.-Fri. 10-6, Sat. 10-5

Claudia Bruce (dressmaker)　　212-685-2810
140 East 28th Street　　bet. Lex./Third Ave.
NYC 10016　　Mon.-Fri. 10-5:30 by appointment only

Eddie Ugras　　212-595-1596
125 West 72nd Street　　bet. Columbus Ave./B'way
NYC 10023　　Mon.-Fri. 9:30-7, Sat. 10-6

French American Weaving Co.　　212-765-4670
119 West 57th Street, Rm. 1406　　bet. 6/7th Ave.
NYC 10019　　Mon.-Fri. 10:30-5:30, Sat. 11-2

John's European Boutique & Tailoring　　212-752-2239
118 East 59th Street, 2nd Fl.　　bet. Park/Lexington Ave.
NYC 10022　　Mon.-Fri. 9-6

Marsan Tailors (men's tailoring only)　　212-475-2727
162 Fifth Avenue　　bet. 21/22nd St.
NYC 10010　　Mon.-Fri. 9:30-6:30,
Thurs. 9:30-7:30, Sat. & Sun. 9:30-6

Nelson Ferri　　212-988-5085
766 Madison Avenue, 4th Fl.　　bet. 65/66th St.
NYC 10021　　Mon.-Fri. 9-6, Sat. 9-3

Peppino　　212-832-3844
780 Lexington Avenue　　bet. 60/61st St.
NYC 10021　　Mon.-Fri. 8:30-6:30, Sat. 9-4

Sebastian Tailors　　212-688-1244
767 Lexington Avenue　　bet. 60/61st St.
NYC 10021　　Mon.-Fri. 8:30-5:30, Sat. 9-4:30

Repairs and Services

Superior Repair Center (leather)   212-889-7211
133 Lexington Avenue   at 29th St.
NYC 10016   Mon.-Fri. 10-6, Sat. 10-3 (winter only)

Three Star (leather apparel only)   212-879-4200
790 Madison Avenue, 5th Fl.   bet. 66/67th St.
NYC 10021   Mon.-Sat. 10-6

Custom Design Tailors

Atelier Eva Devecsery   212-751-6091
201 East 61st Street   at 3rd Ave.
NYC 10021   Mon.-Fri. 9-6, Sat. 10-4 by appointment

Dynasty Custom Tailoring   212-679-1075
6 East 38th Street   bet. 5th/Madison Ave.
NYC 10016   Mon.-Fri. 9-6, Sat. 10-3

Mr. Ned   212-924-5042
137 Fifth Avenue   at 20th St.
NYC 10010   Mon.-Fri. 8-5, Sat. 8-3

Shoe Repairs

Andrade Boot and Shoe Repair   212-787-0465
379 Amsterdam Avenue   bet. 78/79th St.
NYC 10024   Mon.-Fri. 7:30-7, Sat. 9-7

Andrade Shoe Repair   212-529-3541
103 University Place   bet. 12/13th Street
NYC 10003   Mon.-Fri. 7:30-7, Sat.9-6:30

B. Nelson   212-869-3552
1221 Sixth Avenue   bet. 48/49th St.
NYC 10020 (Level C-2)   Mon.-Fri. 7:30-5

David's Shoe Repair   212-867-4338
Grand Central Corridor   at 45th and Vanderbilt
NYC 10017   Mon.-Fri. 6-6:30

Evelyn and San   212-628-7618
400 East 83rd Street   bet. York/1st Ave.
NYC 10028   Mon.-Sat. 8-6

Jim's Shoe Repair   212-355-8259
50 East 59th Street   bet. Park/Madison Ave.
NYC 10022   Mon.-Fri. 8-6, Sat. 9-4
(closed Sat. July & August)

Shoe Service Plus   212-262-4823
15 West 55th Street   bet. 5/6th Ave.
NYC 10019   Mon.-Fri. 7-7, Sat. 10-5

Top Service   212-765-3190
845 Seventh Avenue   bet. 54/55th St.
NYC 10019   Mon.-Fri. 8-6, Sat. 9-3

Repairs and Services

Leather Repair (Handbags & Luggage)

Artbag Creations   212-744-2720
735 Madison Avenue   bet. 64 /65th St.
NYC 10021   Mon.-Fri. 9:30-5:45, Sat. 10-5

John R. Gerardo   212-695-6955
30 West 31st Street   bet. B'way/5th Ave.
NYC 10001   Mon.-Fri. 9-5,
Sat. 10-2 (fall/winter only)

Superior Repair Center   212-889-7211
133 Lexington Avenue   at 29th St.
NYC 10016   Mon.-Fri. 10-6, Sat. 10-3 (winter only)

Trimmings (Ribbons, Buttons, Feathers and Odds & Ends)

A.A. Feather Company   212-695-9470
16 West 36th Street   bet. 5/6th Ave.
NYC 10018   Mon.-Thurs. 9-6, Fri. 9-3
Selection: Quality feathers like ostrich plumes and feather boas.

Feibusch - Zippers and Threads   212-226-3964
27 Allen Street   bet. Canal/Hester St.
NYC 10002   Mon.-Fri. 9-5, Sun. 9-4 (winter only)
Selection: Stocks zippers in every size, color and style with threads to match.

Buttonhole Fashions   212-354-1420
580 Eighth Avenue   bet. 38/39th St.
NYC 10018   Mon.-Fri. 8-5:30
Selection: Bound buttonholes and buttonhole eyelets.

Greenberg & Hammer   212-246-2836
24 West 57th Street   bet. 5/6th Ave.
NYC 10019   Mon.-Fri. 9-6, Sat. 10-5
Selection: Trims, notions, buttons, zippers and more.

Hyman Hendler and Sons   212-840-8393
67 West 38th Street   bet. 5/6th Ave.
NYC 10018   Mon.-Fri. 9-5, Sat. 10-2:30
(except in July and August)
Selection: The highest quality ribbons from around the world.

M&J Trimming Co.   212-391-9072
1008-1014 Sixth Avenue   bet. 37/38th St.
NYC 10018   Mon.-Fri. 9-6, Sat. 10-5
Selection: Ribbons, trimmings, buttons, rhinestones and more.

Margola   212-840-0644
48 West 37th Street   bet. 5/6th Ave.
NYC 10018   Mon.-Fri. 9-5:30, Sat. 10-4
Selection: Feather trimmings, silk flowers, ribbons, veiling and netting, beading and stones.

Repairs and Services

☆ **Mokuba**   212-869-8900
55 West 39th Street   bet. 5/6th Ave.
NYC 10018   Mon.-Fri. 9-5
Selection: Super fancy ribbons. Find them in silk, velvet, chiffon, fake fur and pleated.

☆ **Tender Buttons**   212-758-7004
143 East 62nd Street   bet. Lex./Third Ave.
NYC 10021   Mon.-Fri. 10:30-6, Sat. 10:30-5:30
Selection: An exquisite collection of buttons, from modern to antique.

Tinsel Trading   212-730-1030
47 West 38th Street   bet. 5/6th Ave.
NYC 10018   Mon.-Fri. 10-5:30
Selection: Fabrics, ribbons, soutaches, trims, cords, tassles, military braids and sword knots.

Thrift Shops

Cancer Care Thrift Shop   212-879-9868
1480 Third Avenue   bet. 83/84th St.
NYC 10028   Mon., Tues. & Fri. 11-6,
Wed. & Thurs. 11-7, Sat. 10-4:30, Sun. 12:30-5

Irvington Institute Thrift Shop   212-879-4555
1534 Second Avenue   at 80th St.
NYC 10021   Mon., Tues. & Sat. 9-5,
Wed., Thurs. & Fri. 9-8

Memorial Sloan-Kettering Thrift Shop   212-535-1250
1440 Third Avenue   bet. 81/82nd St.
NYC 10028   Mon.-Fri. 10-5:30, Sat. 11-5

Spence-Chapin Thrift Shop   212-737-8448
1473 Third Avenue   bet. 83/84th St.
NYC 10028   Mon.-Fri. 10-7, Sat. 9-5, Sun. 12-5

Health and Beauty

Barbers

Haircuts—Unisex

Haircuts—Children

Hair Salons

Hair Removal

Beauty Treatments

Manicures

Day Spas—Women

Day Spas—Men

Fitness Studios

Pilates / Mat Classes

Yoga

Massage Therapists

Tanning Salons

Bridal Consultants

Make-up Artists

Personal Shoppers

"She looked as if she had been poured into her clothes and had forgotten to say when." —*P.G. Wodehouse*

"Fashion is a form of ugliness so intolerable that we have to alter it every six months." —*Oscar Wilde*

Michael Kor's idea of the perfect accessory:
"A great body".

Health and Beauty

Barbers

UPPER EAST SIDE

Paul Mole
1031 Lexington Avenue
NYC 10021

212-535-8461
bet. 73/74th St.
Mon.-Fri. 7:30-6:30

York Barber
981 Lexington Avenue
NYC 10021

212-988-6136
bet. 70/71st St.
Mon.-Fri. 8-7, Sat. 8-6

MIDTOWN EAST

Jerry's Salon
50 Rockefeller Plaza
NYC 10020

212-246-3151
enter bet. 5/6th Ave.
Mon.-Sat. 8-6

CHELSEA

Chelsea Barbers
465 West 23rd Street
NYC 10011

212-741-2254
bet. 9/10th Ave.
Mon.-Fri. 9-7, Sat. 9-6

Haircuts—Unisex

UPPER EAST SIDE

Jean Louis David ($24-$34 cuts)
783 Lexington Avenue
NYC 10021

212-838-7372
at 61st Street
Mon.-Sat. 10-7

UPPER WEST SIDE

Jean Louis David
2111 Broadway
NYC 10023

212-873-1850
at 73rd Street
Mon.-Sat. 10-7

MIDTOWN WEST

Jean Louis David
1180 Sixth Avenue
NYC 10011

212-944-7389
at 46th Street
Mon.-Fri. 10-7

NOHO

Astor Place Hair Designers ($11 cuts)
2 Astor Place
NYC 10003

212-475-9854
bet. B'way/8th Ave.
Mon.-Sat. 8-8, Sun. 9-6

WEST VILLAGE

Ginger Rose on Bleecker ($12.95 cut)
154 Bleecker Street
NYC 10012

212-677-6511
bet. Thompson/LaGuardia
Mon.-Sat. 10-8, Sun. 12-6

Health and Beauty

LOWER MANHATTAN

Jean Louis David
30 Vesey Street
NYC 10007

212-732-4938
at Church
Mon.-Fri. 10-7

Haircuts—Children

UPPER EAST SIDE

Cozy's Cuts for Kids
1125 Madison Avenue
NYC 10028

212-744-1716
at 84/85th St.
Mon.-Sat. 10-5:30

UPPER WEST SIDE

Cozy's Cuts for Kids
448 Amsterdam Avenue
NYC 10024

212-579-2600
bet. 81/82nd St.
Mon.-Sat. 10-5:30

MIDTOWN EAST

Kids Cuts
201 East 31st Street
NYC 10016

212-684-5252
bet. 2/3rd Ave.
Tues.-Sat. 9:30-6, Sun. 1-4

Hair Salons

UPPER EAST SIDE

A.K.S.
694 Madison Avenue
NYC 10021

212-888-0707
bet. 62/63rd St.
Mon.-Sat. 9-5, Thurs. 9-7

Donsuki
19 East 62nd Street
NYC 10021

212-826-3397
bet. Madison/5th Ave.
Mon.-Fri. 9:30-5:30, Sat. 9-4

Eiji (specializes in dry cuts)
768 Madison Avenue, 2nd Fl.
NYC 10021

212-570-1151
bet. 65/66th St.
Tues-Sat. 9-6

John Frieda
30 East 76th Street
NYC 10021

212-879-1000
bet. Park/Madison Ave.
Mon.-Sat. 9-6

Julius Caruso Salon
22 East 62nd Street
NYC 10021

212-759-7574
bet. Madison/5th Ave.
Mon.-Fri. 9-6, Sat. 9-4

Minardi Salon
29 East 61st Street
NYC 10021

212-308-1711
bet. Park/Madison Ave.
Mon. 9-7, Tues., Wed.,
Thurs. 8-9, Fri. 9-7, Sat. 8-7

Peter Coppola
746 Madison Avenue
NYC 10021

212-988-9404
bet. 64/65th St.
Mon.-Sat. 9-6, Thurs. 9-7

Health and Beauty

Simon
22 East 66th Street
NYC 10021
212-5174566
bet. Madison/5th Ave.
Mon.-Sat. 9-6

Thomas Morrissey Salon
787 Madison Avenue
NYC 10021
212-772-1111
bet. 66/67th St.
Mon.-Sat. 9-5, Thurs. 9-7:30

MIDTOWN EAST

Bumble & Bumble
146 East 56th Street
NYC 10022
212-521-6500
bet. Lexington/3rd Ave.
Tues.-Sat. 7:30-8:30

Frederic Fekkai
15 East 57th Street,
Level T1
NYC 10022
212-753-9500
bet. Madison/5th
in the Chanel Bldg.
Mon., Tues. & Sat. 9-6, Wed.-Fri. 9-7

Garren Salon
712 Fifth Avenue
NYC 10019
212-841-9400
at Henri Bendel bet. 55/56th St.
Mon.-Sat. 10-6

Jacques Dessange
505 Park Avenue
NYC 10022
212-308-1400
bet. 59/60th St.
Tues.-Fri. 9-7, Sat. 9-5

John Barrett Salon
754 Fifth Avenue, 9th Fl.
NYC 10019
212-872-2700
at Bergdorf Goodman
Mon.-Sat. 8-6, Thurs. 8-8

John Sahag
425 Madison Avenue, 2nd Fl.
NYC 10017
212-750-7772
at 49th St.
Tues.-Sat. 9-6

Kenneth Salon
301 Park Avenue
NYC 10022
212-752-1800
at The Waldorf Astoria Hotel
Mon.-Sat. 9-6, Wed. 9-8

Pierre Michel
131 East 57th Street
NYC 10022
212-593-1460
bet. Lex./Park Ave.
Mon.-Sat. 10-6

Louis Licari Color Group
693 Fifth Avenue
NYC 10021
212-517-8084
at Takashimaya bet. 53/54th St.
Mon.-Sat. 8-5

Oribe
691 Fifth Avenue
NYC 10022
212-319-3910
at Elizabeth Arden bet. 54/55th St.
Mon.-Sat. 9-6

Oscar Blandi
768 Fifth Avenue
NYC 10019
212-593-7930
at The Plaza Hotel at 58th St.
Mon.-Sat. 8-6, Thurs. 8-7

Stella Salon
41 East 57th Street
NYC 10022
212-753-6078
bet. Park/Madison Ave.
Tues.-Sat. 9-5

Health and Beauty

SOHO

Oscar Bond
42 Wooster
NYC 10013
212-334-3777
bet. Broome/Grand
Tues. & Wed. 10-8,
Thurs. & Fri. 11-9, Sat. 10-6, Sun. 11-6

Devachan Hair Salon & Day Spa
558 Broadway
NYC 10012
212-274-8686
bet. Spring/Prince
Tues.-Fri. 11-7, Sat. 10-5

Dop Dop Salon
170 Mercer Street
NYC 10012
212-965-9540
bet. Houston/Prince
Mon.-Wed., Fri., Sat., 11-6, Thurs. 12-7

Prive @ The Soho Grand
310 West Broadway
NYC 10013
212-274-8888
bet. Grand/Canal
Tues.-Fri. 10-8, Sat. 11-7, Sun. 11-6

John Masters Organic Haircare
79 Sullivan Street
NYC 10012
212-343-9590
bet. Spring/Broome
Mon.-Fri. 11-6:30, Sat. 9-8

Space
155 Sixth Avenue
NYC 10013
212-647-8588
at Spring
Tues.-Fri. 11-7, Sat. 10-6

CHELSEA

Suite 303 @ The Chelsea Hotel
222 West 23rd Street
NYC 10011
212-633-1011
bet. 7/8th Ave.
Tues.-Fri. 12-6:45, Sat. 12-4:45

WEST/VILLAGE

Red Salon
323 West 11th Street
NYC 10014
212-924-1444
bet. Greenwich/Washington
Mon.-Sat. 12-8

Robert Kree Salon
375 Bleecker Street
NYC 10014
212-989-9547
bet. Charles/Perry
Tues.-Fri. 11-8, Sat. 10-7, Sun. 12-7

Hair Removal

UPPER EAST SIDE

Bernice Electrolysis
29 East 61st Street, 2nd Fl.
NYC 10021
212-355-7055
bet. Park/Madison Ave.
Mon., Tues., Fri. & Sat. 8-6,
Wed. & Thurs. 8-8

Completely Bare
764 Madison Avenue
NYC 10021
212-717-9300
bet. 65/66th St.
Mon.-Thurs. 10-8, Fri. & Sat. 9-5

Isabella Electrolysis
794 Lexington Avenue
NYC 10021
212-832-0431
bet. 61/62nd St.
Mon.-Sat. 10-7

Health and Beauty

Miriam Vasicka   212-734-1017
897 Park Avenue   at 79th St.
NYC 10021   daily 8-6 by appointment

Steven Victor, M.D.   212-249-3050
30 East 76th Street   bet. Park/Madison Ave.
NYC 10021   daily by appointment

UPPER WEST SIDE

Vanishing Point   212-362-1327
102 West 73rd Street   bet. Columbus/Amsterdam Ave.
NYC 10023   Mon. & Thurs. 10-9,
Tues., Wed., Fri., Sat & Sun. 10-7

MIDTOWN EAST

Smooth   212-759-6997
133 East 58th Street, Suite 507   bet. Park/Lexington Ave.
NYC 10022   Mon.-Fri. 10-7

FLATIRON

Vanishing Point   212-255-3474
4 West 16th Street   bet. 5/6th Ave.
NYC 10011   Mon. & Thurs. 10-9, Tues.-Sun. 10-7

Beauty Treatments

UPPER EAST SIDE

Bernice   212-355-7055
29 East 61st Street, Suite 210   bet. Park/Madison Ave.
NYC 10021   Mon., Tues., Fri. & Sat. 8-6,
Wed. & Thurs. 8-8

Eastside Massage Therapy Center   212-249-2927
351 East 78th Street   bet. 1st/2nd Ave.
NYC 10021   Mon.-Fri. 9-8:30, Sat. 9-7, Sun. 9-6

Sirene   212-737-3545
1044 Madison Avenue   bet. 79/80th St.
NYC 10021   Mon.-Sat. 10-7, Sun. 10:30-6

Yasmine Djerradine   212-588-1771
30 East 60th Street   bet. Park/Madison Ave.
NYC 10022   Mon.-Sat. 8:30-7

UPPER WEST SIDE

Gemayel Salon   212-787-5555
2030 Broadway   at 70th St.
NYC 10023   Mon.-Fri. 9-8, Sat. 9-6

MIDTOWN EAST

Diane Young   212-753-1200
38 East 57th Street, 8th Fl.   bet. Park/Madison Ave.
NYC 10022   Mon.-Thurs. 10-8, Fri. 10-6, Sat. 9-5

Health and Beauty

Elizabeth Arden
691 Fifth Avenue
NYC 10022
212-546-0200
at 54th St.
Mon.-Sat. 8-6:30, Wed. 8-7:30, Sun. 9-5

Janet Sartin
500 Park Avenue
NYC 10022
212-751-5858
bet. 58/59th St.
Mon.-Fri. 10-7, Sat. 10-6, Sun. 11-6

Lia Schorr Skin Care
686 Lexington Avenue, 4th Fl.
NYC 10022
212-486-9670
bet. 56/57th St.
Mon.-Fri. 9-8, Sat. & Sun. 9-5

Mario Badescu
320 East 52nd Street
NYC 10022
212-758-1065
bet. 1/2nd Ave.
Mon., Tues. & Fri. 8:30-6,
Wed. & Thurs. 8:30-8:30, Sat. 9-5

SOHO/FLATIRON

Ling Skin Care
12 East 16th Street
NYC 10003
212-989-8833
bet. 5th Ave. & Union Square
Mon.-Fri. 10-7, Sat. 9:30-5

Oasis Day Spa
108 East 16th Street
NYC 10003
212-254-7722
bet. Irving Pl./Union Sq.
Mon.-Fri. 10-10, Sat. & Sun. 9-9

Soho Sanctuary
119 Mercer Street
NYC 10012
212-334-5550
bet. Prince/Spring
Tues.-Fri. 10-9, Sat. 10-6, Sun. 12-6

Manicures

UPPER EAST SIDE

Ellegee Nail Salon
22 East 66th Street
NYC 10021
212-472-5063
bet. Madison/5th Ave.
Mon.-Fri. 9-7, Sat. 8:30-5:30

Nails by Nina
129 East 80th Street
NYC 10021
212-288-8130
bet. Lexington/Park Ave.
Mon.-Fri. 10-6

Sirene Beauty Spa
1044 Madison Avenue
NYC 10021
212-737-3545
bet. 79/80th St.
Mon.-Sat. 10-7, Sun. 10:30-5:30

UPPER WEST SIDE

167 Nail Plaza
167 Amsterdam Avenue
NYC 10023
212-496-7155
bet. 67/68th St.
Mon.-Fri. 9:30-8,
Sat. 9-7:30, Sun. 10:30-7

Paul LaBrecque
160 Columbus Avenue
NYC 10023
212-595-0099
bet. 67/68th St.
Mon.-Fri. 8-11, Sat. 9-8, Sun. 10-8

Health and Beauty

MIDTOWN EAST/MIDTOWN WEST

Four Seasons   212-350-6420
57 East 57th Street   bet. Park/Madison Ave.
NYC 10022   Mon.-Sun. 10-6

Warren-Tricomi   212-262-8899
16 West 57th Street   bet. 5/6th Ave.
NYC 10019   Mon.-Sat. 10-7

Day Spas—Women

UPPER EAST SIDE

Ajune: Ctr. for Beauty Synergy   212-628-0044
1294 Third Avenue   at 74/75th St.
NYC 10021   Mon., Tues. & Fri. 9-6,
Wed. & Thurs. 9-8, Sat. 9-5

Anhouska Institute   212-355-6404
241 East 60th Street   bet. 2/3rd Ave.
NYC 10022   Mon. 10-6, Tues. & Thurs. 10-8,
Wed. & Fri. 10-7, Sat. 9-6

Helen Lee Day Spa   212-888-1233
205 East 60th Street   bet. 2/3rd Ave.
NYC 10022   Mon.-Sat. 9-6, Wed. & Thurs. 10-8

Karen Wu Beauty & Wellness Spa   212-737-3545
1044 Madison Avenue   bet. 79/80th St.
NYC 10021   Mon.-Sun. 10-7

Karen Wu Beauty & Wellness Spa   212-585-2044
1377 Third Avenue   bet. 78/79th St.
NYC 10021   Mon.-Sun. 10-8

The Townhouse Day Spa   212-439-6664
East 76th Street   bet. Fifth/Mad. Ave
NYC 10021   Mon.-Fri. 9-5

MIDTOWN EAST/FIFTH AVENUE

Allure Day Spa   212-644-5500
139 East 55th Street   bet. 3rd/Lexington Ave.
NYC 10022   Mon.-Fri. 11-8, 10-6

The Avon Center   212-755-2866
725 Fifth Avenue, 14th Fl. at Trump Tower bet. 56/57th St
NYC 10022   Mon.-Sat. 9-6, Wed. & Thurs. 9-8

Away   212-407-2970
541 Lexington Avenue, 4th Fl.   bet. 49/50th St.
NYC 10022   at the W Hotel
Mon.-Fri. 6 a.m.-10, Sat. & Sun. 8:30-7

Bliss Spa   212-219-8970
19 East 57th Street, 3rd Fl.   bet. Madison/Fifth Ave.
NYC 10022   Mon.-Fri. 9:30-8:30, Sat. 9:30-6:30

Health and Beauty

Gazelle **212-751-5144**
509 Madison Avenue bet. 52/53rd St.
NYC 10022 Mon.-Sun. 9-6, Thurs. & Fri. 9-7

Georgette Klinger **212-838-3200**
501 Madison Avenue bet. 52/53rd St.
NYC 10022 Mon.-Thurs. 9-7, Fri.-Sun. 9-5

The Greenhouse Day Spa **212-644-4449**
127 East 57th Street bet. Lexington/Park Ave.
NYC 10022 Mon.-Sat. 9-6

The Peninsula Spa **212-903-3910**
700 Fifth Avenue at 55th St.
NYC 10022 Mon.-Fri. 8:30-9, Sat. & Sun. 9-8:30

Repechage Spa de Beaute **212-751-2500**
115 East 57th Street bet. Park/Lexington Ave.
NYC 10022 Mon. & Thurs. 10-8,
Tues., Wed. & Fri. 10-6:30, Sat. 10-6

The Stress Less Step **212-826-6222**
115 East 57th Street, 5th Fl. bet. Park/Lexington Ave.
NYC 10022 Mon.-Fri. 8-11 p.m., Sat. & Sun. 8-10 p.m.

Susan Ciminelli Day Spa **212-872-2650**
754 Fifth Avenue at Bergdorf Goodman
NYC 10019 Mon.-Sat. 10-7

MIDTOWN WEST/UPPER WEST SIDE

Dorit Baxter Day Spa **212-371-4542**
47 West 57th Street, 3rd Fl. bet. 5/6th Ave.
NYC 10019 Mon.-Sat. 9-8

Gemayel Salon & Spa **212-787-5555**
2030 Broadway at 70th St.
NYC 10023 Mon.-Fri. 9-8, Sat. 9-6

SOHO

Bliss Spa **212-219-8970**
568 Broadway at Prince
NYC 10012 Mon.-Fri. 9:30-8:30, Sat. 9:30-6:30

Haven **212-343-3515**
150 Mercer Street bet. Prince/Houston
NYC 10012 Mon.-Fri. 11-7, Sat. 10-6

The HR Beauty Gallery **212-343-9963**
135 Spring Street bet. Greene/Wooster
NYC 10012 Tues. 10-7, Wed. 11-9,
Thurs. & Fri. 11-8, Sat. 10-6, Sun. 12-6

Shiseido Studio **212-625-8821**
155 Spring Street bet. Wooster/W. B'way
NYC 10012 Sun. & Mon. 12-6, Tues. 11-6, Wed.-Sat. 11-7

FLATIRON

Oasis Day Spa **212-254-7722**
108 East 16th Street bet. Irving Pl./Union Square East
NYC 10003 Mon.-Fri. 10-10, Sat. & Sun. 9-9

Health and Beauty

Day Spas—Men

UPPER EAST SIDE

Equinox Spa   212-750-4671
140 East 63rd Street   at Lexington Ave.
NYC 10021   Mon.-Thurs. 9-10,
Fri. 9-9:30, Sat & Sun. 9-8:30

Equinox Spa   212-396-9611
205 East 85th Street   bet. 2/3rd Ave.
NYC 10028   Mon.-Thurs. 9-10, Fri. 9-9,
Sat. & Sun. 9-8

Kozue Aesthetic Spa   212-734-8600
795 Madison Avenue, 2nd Fl.   bet. 67/68th St.
NYC 10021   Mon.-Sun. 10-6

MIDTOWN EAST

Bliss Spa   212-219-8970
19 East 57th Street, 3rd Fl.   bet. Madison/Fifth Ave.
NYC 10022   Mon.-Fri. 9:30-8:30, Sat. 9:30-6:30

The Stress Less Step   212-826-6222
115 East 57th Street, 5th Fl.   bet. Park/Lexington Ave.
NYC 10022   Mon.-Fri. 8-11, Sat. & Sun. 9-8:30

SOHO/NOLITA

Aveda Institute   212-807-1492
233 Spring Street   bet. 6th Ave./Varick
NYC 10013   Mon.-Sun. 10-6

Bliss Spa   212-219-8970
568 Broadway   at Prince
NYC 10012   Mon.-Fri. 9:30-8:30, Sat. 9:30-6:30

Prema NoLiTa (holistic skincare)   212-226-3972
252 Elizabeth Street   bet. Houston/Prince
NYC 10012   Tues.-Sun. 11-7

FLATIRON

Carapan Spa   212-633-6220
5 West 16th Street   bet. 5/6th Ave.
NYC 10001   Mon.-Sun. 10-9:45

Fitness Studios

UPPER EAST SIDE

Classic Bodies   212-737-8440
189 East 79th Street   at Lexington Ave.
NYC 10021   call for class schedule

David Barton Gym   212-517-7577
30 East 85th Street   bet. Madison/5th Ave.
NYC 10028   Mon.-Fri. 5:30 a.m.-11, Sat. & Sun. 8-9

Health and Beauty

The Equinox
205 East 85th Street
NYC 10028
212-439-8500
bet. 2/3rd Ave.
Mon.-Thurs. 5:30-10:30,
Fri. 5:30-10, Sat. & Sun. 8:30-9

The Equinox
140 East 63rd Street
NYC 10021
212-750-4900
at Lexington Ave.
Mon.-Thurs. 5:30-11,
Fri. 5:30-10, Sat. & Sun. 8-9

Lotte Berk Method
23 East 67th Street
NYC 10021
212-288-6613
bet. 5th/Madison Ave.
Mon.-Fri. 7:15-8,
Sat. 8:30-2, Sun. 9:30-2:15

Studio Uma
20 East 68th Street
NYC 10021
212-249-7979
bet. Madison/Fifth Ave.
Mon.-Fri. 7-10, Sat. 7-9, Sun. 9-6

Synergy Fitness Center
1438 Third Avenue
NYC 10028
212-879-6013
bet. 81/82nd St.
Mon.-Fri. 6-11, Sat. & Sun. 9-8

UPPER WEST SIDE

Crunch
162 West 83rd Street
NYC 10024
212-875-1902
bet. Amsterdam/Columbus Ave.
Mon.-Thurs. 6-11, Fri. 6-10,
Sat. & Sun. 8-9

The Equinox
344 Amsterdam Avenue
NYC 10024
212-721-4200
at 76th St.
Mon.-Thurs. 5:30-11,
Fri. 5:30-10, Sat. & Sun. 8-9

The Equinox
2465 Broadway
NYC 10025
212-799-1818
bet. 91/92nd St.
Mon.-Thurs. 5:30-11,
Fri. 5:30-10, Sat. & Sun. 8-9

Reebok
160 Columbus Avenue
NYC 10023
212-362-6800
at 67th St.
Mon.-Thurs. 5-11,
Fri. 5-10, Sat & Sun. 7-9

MIDTOWN EAST

Crunch
1109 Second Avenue
NYC 10022
212-758-3434
bet. 58/59th St.
Mon.-Fri. 8:30-9, Sat. 8:30-8:30

The Equinox
250 East 54th Street
NYC 10022
212-277-5400
at 2nd Ave.
Mon.-Thurs. 5:30-11,
Fri. 5:30-10, Sat. & Sun. 8-9

**The Sports Club/LA
in New York (membership)**
45 Rockefeller Plaza
NYC 10111
212-218-8600
at 51st Street
Mon.-Thurs. 5-11,
Fri. 5-10, Sat & Sun. 8-6

Health and Beauty

Synergy Fitness Center   212-545-9590
4 Park Avenue   bet. 33/34th St.
NYC 10016   Mon.-Fri. 6-11, Sat. & Sun. 9-7

MIDTOWN WEST

Crunch   212-594-8050
560 West 43rd Street   at 11th Ave.
NYC 10036   Mon.-Fri. 6-10, Sat. & Sun. 9-7

Crunch   212-869-7788
144 West 38th Street   bet. B'way & 7th Ave.
NYC 10018   Mon.-Fri. 5:30-10, Sat. & Sun. 8-5

Radu   212-581-1995
24 West 57th Street, 2nd Fl.   bet. 5/6th Ave.
NYC 10019   Mon., Wed. & Fri. 7-7,
Tues. & Thurs. 8-7, Sat. & Sun. 10-12

SOHO/NOHO

Crunch   212-420-0507
623 Broadway   bet. Houston/Bleecker
NYC 10012   Mon.-Fri. 6-12, Sat. 8-8, Sun. 9-8

Crunch   212-614-0120
404 Lafayette   bet. Astor/E. 4th St
NYC 10003   Mon.-Fri. open 24 hrs, Sat. to 9, Sun. 8-9

WEST VILLAGE/TRIBECA

Crunch   212-475-2018
54 East 13th Street   bet. B'way/University Pl.
NYC 10003   Mon.-Fri. 6-10, Sat & Sun. 8-8

Crunch   212-366-3725
152 Christopher Street   bet. Wash. St./Greenwich St.
NYC 10014   Mon.-Fri. 6-11, Sat. & Sun. 8-9

CHELSEA/FLATIRON

David Barton Gym   212-727-0004
552 Sixth Avenue   bet. 15/16th St.
NYC 10011   Mon.-Fri. 6-12, Sat. 9-9, Sun. 10-11

The Equinox   212-780-9300
897 Broadway   bet. 19/20th St.
NYC 10003   Mon.-Thurs. 5:30-11,
Fri. 5:30-10, Sat & Sun. 8-9

The Sports Ctr. at Chelsea Piers   212-339-6000
Pier 60, West Side Hwy.   at W. 23rd St.
NYC 10011   Mon.-Fri. 6-11, Sat. & Sun. 8-9

Pilates/Mat Classes

FLATIRON

Power Pilates   212-627-5852
49 West 23rd Street   bet. 5.6th Ave.
NYC 10011   Mon.-Fri. 7-8, Sat. & Sun. 9-2

Health and Beauty

TRIBECA/NOHO

The Kane School of Core Integration 212-463-8308
7 East 17th Street bet. 5th/B'way
NYC 10003 Mon.-Fri. 9-5 or by appointment

re: AB 212-420-9111
33 Bleecker Street at Mott
NYC 10012 Mon.-Fri. 7-8, Sat. 9-2, Sun. 10-4

Tribeca Bodyworks 212-625-0777
177 Duane Street bet. Greenwich/Hudson
NYC 10013 Mon.-Thurs. 7:30-9,
Fri. 7:30-8, Sat. & Sun. 9-3

Yoga

UPPER WEST SIDE

Integral Yoga Institute 212-721-4000
200 West 72nd Street, Room 41 at Broadway
NYC 10023 call for class times

SOHO

Soho Sanctuary 212-334-5550
119 Mercer Street bet. Prince/Spring
NYC 10012 Mon.-Thurs. 10-7:15,
Fri. 10-6, Sat. 10-2:30, Sun. 10-5:15

NOHO/WEST VILLAGE

Integral Yoga Institute 212-929-0586
227 West 13th Street bet. 7/8th Ave.
NYC 10011 Mon.-Fri. 10-8:30, Sat. 9-5, Sun. 10-2

Jivamukti Yoga Center 212-353-0214
404 Lafayette Street bet. W. 4th St./Astor Place
NYC 10003 Mon.-Sun. 7-8:30

CHELSEA/FLATIRON

Om Yoga Center 212-229-0267
135 West 14th Street bet. 6/7th Ave.
NYC 10011 Mon.-Fri. 7-9, Sat. 9-6, Sun. 9-7

Massage Therapists *(office & home visits)*

Back-To-Work 212-696-9069
$60 to $75 per hour

Knead-a-Break Enterprises 212-460-1879
$70 per hour

New York Massage Company 212-427-8175
$60 per hour

Health and Beauty

Tanning Salons

UPPER EAST SIDE

Portofino Sun Center　　　　212-988-6300
1300 Third Avenue　　　　　　　　　at 75th St.
NYC 10021　　Mon.-Fri. 9-9:15, Sat. 9-8, Sun. 9-6

UPPER WEST SIDE

Portofino Sun Center　　　　212-769-0200
104 West 73rd Street　　　　　at Columbus Ave.
NYC 10023　　Mon.-Fri. 9-10, Sat. 9-9, Sun. 10-7

MIDTOWN EAST

Portofino Sun Center　　　　212-355-2772
38 East 58th Street　　　　bet. Park/Madison Ave.
NYC 10022　　　　Mon.-Sat. 9-10, Sun. 10-7

SOHO

Portofino Sun Center　　　　212-473-7600
462 West Broadway　　　　　bet. Houston/Prince
NYC 10012　　　　　Mon.-Sat. 9-9, Sun. 11-7

WEST VILLAGE

Portofino Sun Center　　　　212-627-4775
64 Greenwich Avenue　　　　　　　at 7th Ave.
NYC 10011　　Mon.-Fri. 9-10, Sat. 9-9, Sun. 10-7

Bridal Consultants

Ober, Onet & Associates　　　212-876-6775
205 East 95th Street　　　　　　bet. 2/3rd Ave.
NYC 10128　　　　　　　　Contact: Polly Onet

Marcy Blum Associates　　　　212-688-3057
251 East 51st Street　　　　　　bet. 2/3rd Ave.
NYC 10022　　　　　　　Contact: Marcy Blum

Saved by the Bell　　　　　　212-874-5457
11 Riverside Drive　　　　　　　bet. 73/74th St.
NYC 10023　　　　　　　　Contact: Susan Bell

Make-up Artists

Kathy Pomerantz　　　　　　　212-772-3865
518 East 80th Street, 1B

Kimara Ahmeert　　　　　　　　212-452-4252
1113 Madison Avenue

Rochelle Weithorn　　　　　　212-472-8668
431 East 73rd Street

Health and Beauty

Personal Shoppers

Barneys New York 212-826-8900
660 Madison Avenue bet. 60/61st St.
NYC 10021 Mon.-Sat. 10-6:30

Bergdorf Goodman 212-872-8772
754 Fifth Avenue bet. 57/58th St.
NYC 10019 Mon.-Fri. 9:30-5:30
Contact: "Solutions" by Betty Halbreich

Bloomingdale's 212-705-2000
1000 Third Avenue at 59/60th St.
NYC 10022 Mon.-Fri. 10-8:30, Sat. 10-7, Sun. 11-7

Henri Bendel 212-373-6353
712 Fifth Avenue bet. 55/56th St.
NYC 10019 Mon.-Sat. 10-7
Contact: Michael Palladino

Lord & Taylor 212-391-3344
424 Fifth Avenue bet. 38/39th St.
NYC 10018 Mon. & Tues. & Sat. 10-7,
Wed. & Thurs. 9-8:30, Fri. 10-8:30, Sun. 11-7

Paul Stuart 212-682-0320
Madison Avenue at 45th Street
NYC 10017 Mon.-Fri. 8-6:30, Thurs. 8-7,
Sat. 9-6, Sun. 12-5

Saks Fifth Avenue 212-940-4145
611 Fifth Avenue bet. 49/50th St.
NYC 10022 Mon.-Sat. 10-7, Thurs. 10-8, Sun. 12-6
Contact: Nanette Difalco

Macy's 212-494-4181
Broadway at Herald Square
NYC 10001 Mon.- Sat. 10-7:30, Sun. 11-6
Contact: Linda Lee

Glossary of Terms

What was created in the 1800's for King Edward VII of England to wear on his yacht, and first appeared Stateside in 1896 when one enterprising dandy wore it to an exclusive country club? *Answer: White tie and tails*

Marci Klein, Calvin's daughter, once complained, "Every time I'm about to go to bed with a guy, I have to look at my dad's name all over his underwear."

Levi Strauss left New York in 1849 for the California gold rush and by the time he got there the only thing he had to sell was canvas. So he started making pants out of it for goldminers who needed pants with pockets strong enough to lug around heavy gold nuggets. When he ran out of canvas, he switched to a French fabric called denim.

Glossary of Terms

Avant-garde: Forward thinking or advanced. When referring to art or costume, sometimes implies erotic or startling. French derivative "advance guard."

Couture: French word used throughout fashion industry to describe the original styles, the ultimate in fine sewing and tailoring, made of expensive fabrics, by designers. The designs are shown in collections twice a year—spring/summer and fall/winter.

Custom-made: Describing garments made by tailor or couture house for an individual customer following couturier's original design. Done by either fitting a model form adjusted to the customer's measurements or by several personal fittings.

Ensemble: The entire costume, including accessories, worn at one time. More than one item of clothing designed and coordinated to be worn together.

Fashion trend: Direction in which styles, colors, and fabrics are moving. Influenced by political events, films, personalities, dramas, social, and sports events.

Faux: False or counterfeit, imitation: used in connection with gems, pearls and leathers.

Haberdashery: A store that sells men's apparel and furnishings.

Haute couture: Top designers of custom-made clothes. French derivative "highest-quality dressmaking." Term originally applied to designers in France.

Knock-off: Trade term for the copying of an item of apparel, e.g., a dress or a coat, in a lower price line. Compare with piracy.

Made-to-measure: Dress or suit made according to individual's measurement. No fittings required.

Pret-a-porter: French term for ready-to-wear clothes. French derivative "ready to be carried."

Ready-to-wear: Apparel that is mass produced in standard sizes. Records of ready-to-wear industry tabulated in U.S. Census of 1860 included hoop skirts, cloaks, and mantillas; from 1890 on, shirtwaists and wrappers were added; and, after 1930, dresses.

Tailor-made: Garment made specifically for one individual by a tailor—customer's measurements are taken and several fittings are necessary.

Website Shopping Directory

When asked which New Yorker he would most like to create an ensemble for and what would it be? Kor's replied, "99-year-old Brooke Astor—gray flannel trouser and a gray cashmere turtleneck."

"A woman's first duty in life is to her dressmaker. What the second duty is no one has yet discovered."
—*Oscar Wilde*

"Blue Laws" first appeared in New Haven, Connecticut, in 1781. These ordinances, which forbade shops to open on Sundays, were printed on blue paper.

Website Shopping Directory

Accessories

www.bestpashmina.com - Devoted exclusively to selling pashmina shawls, scarves, blankets, and ponchos guaranteed to arrive within 48 hours.

www.thecashmerecompany.com - Shop the world's largest direct seller of cashmere and pashmina. It's the same quality found in exclusive shops around the world, but sells for 30% to 50% less. Pashmina shawls start at $129 and cashmere sweaters at $99.

www.indulge.com - Devoted to selling a range of products and services. Shop for pashminas, cashmere hats, handbags, hair accessories, jewelry, and beauty products.

www.luxlook.com - A luxury goods site offering 2,000 women's and men's designer accessories. The selection includes handbags, scarves, belts, ties, eyewear, jewelry and watches with brand names like Etro, Bulgari, Valentino, Loro Piana, Ferre, and Versace.

Activewear/Sports

☆ www.lucy.com - A shopping site specializing in women's activewear and sports apparel. Shop major brand labels like Champion and Columbia Sportswear.

www.puma.com - Dedicated to a smattering of Puma products. Shop for running wear, athletic wear and footwear. Also read about Puma-sponsored athletes or even e-mail tennis star Serena Williams or boxer Oscar de la Hoya.

www.fogdog.com - A sport's retailing site that allows consumers to browse by store destinations like Hockey Shop, Golf Shop, Soccer Shop, Snowboarding Shop and Outdoor Shop. Ask their knowledgeable online sales staff to help you find the right product for your needs. A large selection of Nike products.

Baby & Maternity

☆ www.babystyle.com - An online baby and maternity site devoted to one-stop shopping for expectant moms and their bambinis. Mothers can shop for maternity basics, baby gear, nursery items, playtime ideas, gifts and more. In addition, get the latest word from first-time mom and super model Cindy Crawford by clicking onto the Cindy's Corner icon.

www.imaternity.com - "The maternity everything store" for expectant mothers on the run. Shop for clothing for all times of day, including career wear, casual basics, dresses, denim, sleepwear & lingerie and nursewear.

www.pumpkinmaternity.com - Young, fun maternity clothes, using natural fibers enhanced with enough stretch

Website Shopping Directory

to go the distance. Find looks like long Lycra skirts, cuff shirts, castaway shorts, a "Mothers-in-Motion" athletic wear line, and Jagger vintage jeans.

Beauty

☆ www.eve.com - The "beauty authority" on the internet with the "hottest" and "best" brands on the market. Choose from fragrances, cosmetics and skincare to bath & body, hair and accessories. You'll also get the latest tips and trends in make-up and skincare. Brand names include Calvin Klein, Cellex-C, Urban Decay, Erno Laszlo, Orlane, Elizabeth Arden, Philosophy, and Club Monaco.

www.beautyjungle.com - Shop five beauty boutiques offering specialty, foreign and American brands for men and women. Labels include Cellex-C, Baignoire, Bloom, Calypso, Joey New York, L'Oreal, Cover Girl, Max Factor, and Oil of Olay.

www.gloss.com - Shop the latest in beauty and fashion trends for make-up, fragrances, beauty treatments, accessories and handbags. Cosmetic brand names include Clinique, Estee Lauder, and Bobbi Brown Essentials. Find designer fragrances by Anna Sui, Yohji Yamamoto, and Calvin Klein.

Designer/Discount

www.designeroutlet.com - Discount designer fashions for men, women, and children. Shop for designer overstocks by DKNY, Diesel, Hugo Boss, Cynthia Rowley, Susan Lazaar, Easel, Ralph Lauren, Free People and French Connection. Jewelry, handbags and accessories also available.

www.bluefly.com - The Loehman's of the internet, featuring men's, women's and children's clothing up to 75% off. The ultimate online shopping site for end-of-season apparel and accessories by designers like Ralph Lauren, Helmut Lang, Prada, Clavin Klein, Gucci and Dolce & Gabbana. It's like having an outlet store in your very own home.

www.pieceunique.com - This is the first online site to feature new and pre-owned designer duds and accessories. A virtual consignment shop with the ultimate in luxury labels like Prada, Valentino, Armani, Yohji Yamamoto, Louis Vuitton, and Hermes.

Juniors

www.accessstyle.com - Shop girls' clothing by body type, price point or fashion category. Best feature is "Prom Shop", an extensive section to get you ready for the prom. Choose your prom dress or design your very own.

Website Shopping Directory

www.blueasphalt.com - Part magazine and part shopping catalog for juniors in search of the latest trends and styles. Shop for Blue Asphalt apparel, accessories and footwear.

☆ **www.delia's.com** - A core site for girls in search of hip and trendy fashions at affordable prices. Shop for dresses (casual or fancy), skirts, tops, swimwear, pants, outerwear, accessories, shoes and more. Threads guaranteed to please teen fashionistas.

www.rampage.com - A sportswear clothing company that caters to juniors seeking trendy fashions. Shop for denim, sportswear, dresses, outerwear, intimates, footwear, handbags, and accessories.

Legwear/Hosiery

www.alexblake.com - A hosiery site featuring a large selection of designer and top legwear brands like Hue, Oroblu, DKNY, Evan Picone, Cosabella, Round the Clock and Hippies. Also available in plus sizes.

www.gazelle.com - Devoted exclusively to your legs. Shop for leading brands of designer hosiery, casual socks, seductive evening sheers, as well as luxury legcare products that will make your legs look and feel great.

Lifestyle/Trends

☆ **www.girlshop.com** - For girls who want to shop for the "hottest" downtown fashion designers. Click onto a designer's individual boutique, including Built by Wendy, Amy Chan, Plum, Trufaux, and Easel. They even offer a messenger delivery service to your home.

☆ **www.fashionmall.com** - "Fashion's most powerful click." Shop four locations: Madison Avenue, Soho, Galleria and Main Street. A wide spectrum of products, from cutting-edge clothing and luxury labels to beauty and make-up. Stores include Old Navy, Brooks Brothers, Coach, Banana Republic, T. Anthony, and Dolce & Gabbana. Fun extras like Style Experts allow you to e-mail designers such as Todd Oldham or Kate Spade for style advice.

www.Ilook.com - A shopping and style guide for fashion and home furnishings. Users may shop by price, look or style, or get linked to a specific brand sites.

www.purpleskirt.com - Known for her stand-up comedy routines, Tracey Ullman shifts gears and rolls out her new online site. Shop her click-and-buy boutique for clothes, gifts and accessories by hip labels like Trina Turk, Chaiken, William B, Katayone Adeli, and Velvet. Accessories include purses, hair apparel, shoes and jewelry. Also share fashion tips, as well as get advice from celebrity stylists and costume designers.

Website Shopping Directory

☆ www.style365.com - An online site that features every department under the sun from top fashion labels. Find designer, sportswear, activewear, lingerie, handbags, shoes, and eyewear by coveted brands like Dolce & Gabbana, Louis Vuitton, Helmut Lang, Wolford, Eres, La Perla, Lacoste, Tanne Krolle, and Bottega Veneta.

☆ www.net-a-porter.com - A London-based site designed to provide you with the best high fashion from around the world. Shop the latest in clothing, accessories, and jewelry from pages like Designer Focus, Fashion Fix, Editorial Favorites, and Fashion Features. Designer labels include Anya Hindmarch, Clements Ribeiro, Jimmy Choo, Mathew Williamson, Patch NYC, Boyd, Vanessa Paradise, and Paul & Joe.

Lingerie/Sleepwear

☆ www.carolehochman.com - Devoted to sleepwear and loungewear. Designer Hochman's goal: to provide women with comfortable and fashionable sleepwear. Styles include caftans, short chemises, long sleep gowns, pajama sets and tunic tops.

www.figleaves.com - An online store featuring innerwear apparel that includes underwear, bras, panties, hosiery, socks, sleepwear and loungewear. Brand names include Calvin Klein Underwear, Donna Karan Intimates, Maidenform, Barely There and Wonderbra.

www.heatherbloom.com - A tastefully designed site for high-end collection of lingerie and sleepwear. Labels include Hanro, On Gossamer, and Cherry Pie.

www.herroom.com - Enjoy shopping for lingerie at this new site equipped with cyber-fitting rooms. Find European and American brand names like Simone Perelle, Rigby & Pellar, Schiesser, Maidenform, Hanro, Wonderbra and Barely There.

Luxury

☆ www.bestselections.com - Luxury merchandise that can be navigated by item, collection, store or city. From pony skin sling-backs and Moo Roo's custom handbags to luxurious cashmere from Palm Beach's Trillion, it's all accessible here. Other shops include Alan Flusser Custom Shop, Au Chat Botte, David Cenci, Scoop, and Golf & Ski. In addition, you can shop for children, antiques, jewelry, food, and the home.

www.eluxury.com - Luxury across the board, from designer clothing to travel, home and gourmet. Click on the designer shop icon and find collections by Louis Vuitton, Michael Kors, Dior, Givenchy, Celine, Thomas Pink, Wolford, and Malo.

Website Shopping Directory

www.fashion500.com - A luxury website that will challenge upscale designer shops like Bergdorf Goodman and Neiman Marcus. Shop high-profile apparel and accessories. You can also work with one of their 30 personal shoppers.

www.luxuryfinder.com - Quality, high-end merchandise is their niche. Shop for handbags by Lulu Guiness, children's clothing by Monica Noel, Lejaby lingerie, Lambertson Truex handbags, Lacoste shirts and dresses, Ghurka travel accessories, Alexandre de Paris hair accessories, T. Anthony leathergoods, pashmina shawls, jewelry, linens, jets and rare books.

Mens Shirts

www.thomaspink.co.uk - Instead of purchasing your Pink shirt duty-free at airports, order it online and save yourself the trip. Choose from shirts of all kind, cufflinks and more.

☆ **www.harvieandhudson.com** - Since 1948 H & H has dressed gents with their Kent-collared shirts. Choose from end-on-end cotton poplins, solids and checks, request a sleeve length and cuff style. Ties and cufflinks also available.

www.hilditch.co.uk - The *London Times* claims these are the best shirts in the world. Log onto their website and decide for yourself. Shop for bespoke or off-the-rack shirt styles in dandified patterns and hues.

Mens Large Sizes

www.bigmen.com - Dedicated to big and tall clothing for men. Shop for suits, sportcoats, slacks, jeans, swimwear, hats, socks and shoes. Waist sizes run from size 32 to 88, neck sizes up to 28 and shoe sizes from 6 to 20 inch widths.

Petites

www.itsybits.com - For petite fashionistas seeking clothing and accessories. Shop for dresses, suits, activewear, tops, bottoms, underbits, accessories, and beauty. Labels include J. Crew, Esprit, 3 Dot, City Lights, and Bisou Bisou.

Plus Size

☆ **www.alight.com** - Plus-sized clothing for women seeking updated fashions, as well as a "Hip and Happening" section for the junior market featuring sportswear items (sari-inspired dresses, embroidered jeans), and T-shirts from labels like Bongo, and LA Movers.

www.dianachibas.com - Plus-sized models Diana Chibas and Suzanne Donovan have developed their own line of sexy lingerie for larger-sized women. Styles include saucy chemises, romantic sleepwear and other shapely intimates.

Website Shopping Directory

www.realsize.com - Find plus-size career wear, casual wear, eveningwear, swimwear, and lingerie from the Delta Burke collection.

Mens Ties

☆ www.luxuryties.com - Choose from 16 Saville Row ties and see how they look against the ten shirt styles offered on the site, or scan your own shirt and then match the ties to it online.

www.tiemasters.com - Italian made silk scarves at 20% to 50% off the retail price. Labels include Fendi, Versace, Dolce & Gabbana, and Moschino.

☆ www.raffaelloties.com - A fabulous selection of Italian designer ties, scarves and leather briefcases. Shop top-of-the-line labels like Armani, Gucci, Zegna, Valentino, and Mila Schon. Save up to 50%.

www.thetieguys.com - One of the largest distributors of neckwear in the USA, The Tie Guys feature a wide selection of neckwear styles that include wovens, silks, jacquards, as well as custom logo neckwear, and novelty ties.

Vintage

www.vintagesilhouettes.com - For the discriminating collector seeking authentic clothing from the 1830's to 1965. Shop for vintage clothing, hats, jewelry, and accessories that recognize the style of these periods.

☆ www.vintagecouture.com - The créme de la créme of vintage sites for collectors and consumers (and sellers, too). Shop a regularly updated list of treasures like a 70's Chanel suit, a 50's Dior dress, and a 60's Yves Saint Laurent mohair coat.

Note from the Authors

As we are all aware, the retail landscape of New York City is constantly changing. What may have once been considered a down-and-out area is likely to be the "in place" to shop; a good example is downtown NoLiTa. Every neighborhood, from Wall Street to the Upper West Side, with its every nook and cranny, has a place in the shopper's heart. When reviewing these shops, the authors have endeavored to be as accurate as possible, but as we all know, things change with time. Therefore, please don't hold us responsible for each and every detail as the store, its merchandise, its ownership, its address and hours can change at the drop of a hat (no pun intended). In fact, Where to Wear will be updated annually to keep you informed of all the latest changes in New York City retailing.

The information compiled for this guide is based on the authors' individual research, as well as the opinions of what they believe are the fashion views of reliable New York shoppers. The authors have neither financial nor personal interests in the stores listed in this guide, nor were any fees or services rendered for the store's inclusion. While every attempt has been made to include the newest shops of 2000, deadlines must be met. However, for convenience, we have included a small section entitled "Notable 2000/2001 Openings" which lists the stores scheduled to open in the Fall/Winter 2000-2001, see page 6.

Your comments and suggestions are important to us. Please send them to:

Where to Wear
666 Fifth Avenue
PMB 377
New York, NY 10103

TEL 212-969-0138
FAX 212-315-1534
TOLL-FREE 1-877-714-SHOP (7467)
E-MAIL wheretowear@aol.com

—D.C. and J.F.M.

Where to Wear
Shopper's Questionnaire

Where to Wear wants to hear from you.

NAME: _____

ADDRESS: _____

_____ ZIP _____

E-MAIL: _____

I'd like to comment on:

SHOP NAME: _____

LOCATION: _____

_____

_____

Merchandise for (check all that apply):
- ❏ Women ❏ Men ❏ Children ❏ Unisex

Recommended for (check all that apply):
- ❏ Career / Business ❏ Classic ❏ Casual
- ❏ Contemporary ❏ Juniors ❏ Designer
- ❏ Vintage & Retro ❏ Maternity ❏ Bridal
- ❏ Young & Trendy ❏ Petites ❏ Plus Size

- ❏ Ballet, Dance ❏ Athletic, Sports, Workout
- ❏ Accessories ❏ Evening, Special Occasion
- ❏ Cashmere ❏ Formal Wear & Tuxedos
- ❏ Furrier ❏ Jeans ❏ Outerwear

- ❏ Custom Tailoring ❏ Hosiery ❏ Swimwear
- ❏ Lingerie & Sleepwear ❏ Shirts ❏ Shoes
- ❏ Handbags, Briefcases & Leathergoods ❏ Hats
- ❏ Discount ❏ Thrift Shop / Consignment

COMMENTS: _____

_____

_____

_____

_____

_____

_____

_____

_____

I'd like to nominate the following:

SHOP NAME: _____

LOCATION: _____

❏ Best Picks ❏ Shhh! (Best-Kept Secrets)
❏ Designers: Rising Stars ❏ Where Designers Shop
❏ Affordable Chic ❏ Penny Wise
❏ Best Sales ❏ Staff with Attitude
❏ Unique Interiors
❏ Where Hollywood Shops (celebrity sightings): _____

_____

_____

❏ Source of "Must-Haves" (specify): _____

_____

_____

❏ Best Website: _____

_____

_____

❏ Other (specify): _____

_____

_____

COMMENTS: _____

_____

_____

Mail or fax completed form (or copy) to:

Where to Wear
666 Fifth Avenue
PMB 377
New York, NY 10103

TEL 212-969-0138
FAX 212-315-1534
TOLL-FREE 1-877-714-SHOP (7467)
E-MAIL wheretowear@aol.com